MAYO CLINIC
FITNESS *for* EVERYBODY

Diane Dahm, M.D.

Jay Smith, M.D.

Editors in Chief

Mayo Clinic
Rochester, Minnesota

Mayo Clinic Fitness for EveryBody provides reliable, practical, comprehensive, easy-to-understand information on issues relating to fitness and exercise. Much of its information comes from physicians, research scientists and other health care professionals at Mayo Clinic. This book is intended to supplement the advice of your personal physician, whom you should consult about your individual fitness plan and any medical condition that you may have. *Mayo Clinic Fitness for EveryBody* does not endorse any company or product. MAYO, MAYO CLINIC, MAYO CLINIC HEALTH INFORMATION and the Mayo triple-shield logo are marks of Mayo Foundation for Medical Education and Research.

Published by Mayo Clinic Health Information, Rochester, Minn. Distributed to the book trade by Kensington Publishing Corp., New York, N.Y.

For bulk sales to employers, member groups and health-related companies, contact Mayo Clinic Health Management Resources, 200 First St. S.W., Rochester, MN 55905, or send email to SpecialSalesMayoBooks@Mayo.edu.

Stock photography from Artville, Brand X, Corbis Images, Digital Stock, Digital Vision Ltd., PhotoDisc and Stockbyte. The individuals pictured in these photos are models, and the photos are for illustrative purposes only. There is no correlation between the individuals portrayed and the condition or subject being discussed. Equipment photos on pages 108, 109 and 122 from Stamina Products. All photos in the "Exercise guide," pages 135-187, and on pages 119 and 262 from Mayo Clinic.

Library of Congress Control Number: 2004116612

ISBN-13:   978-1-893005-37-2
ISBN-10:   1-893005-37-2

Printed in the United States of America

First Edition

2 3 4 5 6 7 8 9 10

Preface

It's safe to say that almost everyone would like to be considered "fit." However, when it comes to designing and carrying out a plan to achieve physical fitness, many people feel a little overwhelmed. It may be lack of time, energy, resources or motivation that prevents us from starting an exercise program. Or perhaps an illness or injury has led to a decline in physical activity. Whatever the reason, more than 60 percent of American adults are not active on a regular basis. This large group of people is missing an opportunity to decrease stress, to prevent disease and illness, and to age more gracefully.

Mayo Clinic Fitness for EveryBody is designed to help you achieve the goal of becoming physically fit, regardless of your age, size, physical ability or overall health. You'll find information in this book on the various components of fitness and the specific health benefits of each component, as well as detailed and practical information on designing a personal fitness program that can be successful, enjoyable and cost-effective. In the illustrated "Exercise guide" that begins on page 134, we personally demonstrate more than 150 exercises, and offer suggestions for making them more, or less, challenging according to your level of fitness. We offer practical tips on how to train for many common sporting activities, and how to reduce your risk of injury while training and playing. In addition, we discuss ways to optimize nutrition during exercise.

Myths and outrageous claims abound in the world of fitness advertising, and we have taken great care to ensure that the information in this book is accurate and scientifically based. Our reviewers include specialists in the fields of sports medicine, internal medicine, cardiology, orthopedic surgery, physical medicine and rehabilitation, nutrition and personal training.

Using the strategies outlined in this book, along with the guidance of your personal physician, you can experience the tremendous benefits of an active lifestyle. We truly believe that fitness is for everybody.

Diane Dahm, M.D.
Jay Smith, M.D.
Editors in Chief

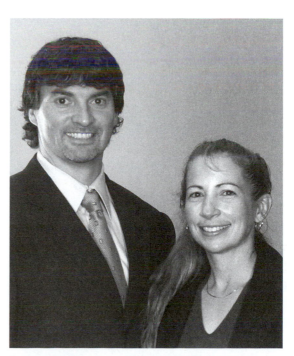

Jay Smith, M.D., and Diane Dahm, M.D., are a husband-wife team, and staff physicians in the Sports Medicine Center at Mayo Clinic.

Editorial staff

Table of contents

CHAPTER 1

Why

Imagine that a new wonder drug has been created. It will help prevent illness and disease — including cancer. It will help you lose excess weight — and keep it off. It will slow the aging process, making you look and feel younger than your years. It will give you energy and increase your self-esteem. It will reduce stress, fight depression and anxiety, and put you in a better mood. It will make you stronger and healthier. It will improve your posture, your flexibility, your balance and your endurance. It will even help you sleep better.

Now imagine that this drug doesn't cost a penny and that you can take it several times a day or just once a day and still see results. In fact, you'll start seeing results within two weeks of your first dose.

Sounds pretty appealing, doesn't it? Would you take it?

This miracle drug is available right now — and you can start taking it today. It's called exercise.

Regular, old-fashioned, sweat-inducing exercise is probably the single most

stay fit?

important thing you can do to age successfully. Even in moderate amounts, exercise can help you enjoy life and avoid diseases that many people mistakenly believe automatically come with age. It truly is a wonder drug.

Unfortunately, most people don't exercise. According to a 1996 report from the U.S. Surgeon General titled *Physical Activity and Health,* more than 60 percent of American adults aren't active on a regular basis. Worse yet, 25 percent of adults aren't active at all. And, sadly, they're leading by example. Nearly half the young people in the United States ages 12 to 21 aren't getting the exercise they need on a regular basis.

Simply put, Americans are out of shape. They don't give their bodies the exercise they need to function efficiently. And they're paying the price. Their arteries are clogging, their blood pressure is rising, they're overweight, and their muscles are weakening with every inactive day that goes by.

Americans are also more vulnerable to disease and illness because of inactivity.

Nearly 1 million people in the United States die of cardiovascular diseases each year. Twenty-seven percent of adult Americans are obese. Worldwide, 200 million people have the bone-thinning disease osteoporosis. And that's just the beginning of a very long list.

REVERSING THE TREND

By introducing a moderate amount of physical activity into your daily life, you can significantly improve your overall health, well-being and quality of life. These benefits can be achieved by virtually everyone, regardless of age, sex, race or physical ability.

Whatever exercise you choose — and your activity of choice may vary from day to day — the key is to aim for 30 to 60 minutes of moderate-intensity physical activity on most days of the week. How you get it is up to you.

Don't like vigorous exercise? That's OK. Discouraged by trying to adhere to a strict exercise program? No problem. Physical activity takes many forms, a number of which you may already enjoy, such as walking, gardening, dancing, swimming, playing basketball, biking, skating, shoveling snow, raking leaves and washing your car. Almost anything that gets your heart rate up qualifies.

Here's some more good news. The more you exercise, the more you benefit. Even a modest increase in daily activity can help improve your health and quality of life. If you're already getting 30 minutes of physical activity a day, adding just one more mile to your evening walk or taking the stairs instead of the elevator at work can make your heart, muscles and lungs even healthier.

Almost anyone can exercise. Few people are too old, too young, too sick, too poor or too busy to be active. Exercise is an equal-opportunity activity. Older adults can use strength training to reduce the risk of falling and breaking bones. People with chronic conditions can improve their stamina, mental outlook and ability to perform daily tasks with exercise. People who are too tired to exercise find they have increased energy after just a few regular sessions of physical activity. Truth be told, very few people have a valid excuse for not engaging in some form of exercise.

Becoming physically fit doesn't require strenuous, high-intensity workouts, boring or monotonous routines or an expensive health club membership. You simply need some comfortable shoes (unless you're a swimmer), a regular program of exercise and a healthy diet.

You may even save money by exercising. A study by the Centers for Disease Control and Prevention found that, on average, physically active people had lower annual direct medical costs than did inactive people. It also found that physically active people had fewer hospital stays and doctor visits and used less medication than did inactive people. And in an era of increasing health care costs and insurance co-pays, these facts alone are significant.

It's never too late to establish a lifetime commitment to an exercise program. Whether you're 25 or 85, regular, repetitive physical activity can provide the benefits you need to help you look better, feel better and enjoy better health. Make physical activity a part of your lifestyle today. The time to start is now!

'Use it or lose it.' It doesn't get any simpler than this. If you don't stay active by getting some form of exercise nearly every day, you'll pay the price with your health. You'll have a higher risk of dying prematurely and succumbing to any number of diseases — including cancer — and, eventually, you'll lose the ability to do the everyday things you enjoy.

You may believe that if you aren't active, you'll simply maintain your current health and wellness levels. That's not true. If you don't exercise, you'll lose muscle mass and flexibility, bone density, lung capacity, joint mobility — and many other factors of health — every day. So it's a "Use it or lose it" proposition.

With regular exercise, you can reduce, prevent or slow many of the adverse effects of aging. You might not know that many of your basic bodily functions start to decline at a rate of about 2 percent a year after age 30. This is an undeniable fact of the aging process. But with exercise you can slow this decline to a rate of about half a percent a year.

What does this mean for you? Consider this example. People who get no physical activity will lose 70 percent of their functional ability by the time they reach age 90. But people who engage in regular physical activity will lose only 30 percent of their functional ability by that age. Which end of the spectrum do you want to be on? When you commit to being physically active as you age, you'll feel younger, look younger and have the energy to do the things you really want to do.

Even a moderate amount of physical activity has benefits. You don't need to run a marathon, climb Mount Kilimanjaro or become an aerobics instructor to benefit from physical activity. Regular, moderate activity on most days of the week will help you become fit and enjoy the benefits of good health.

What's moderate activity? You may be surprised to learn that activities that you already enjoy qualify. When getting a moderate amount of activity, you should be able to feel yourself working but still be able to hold a conversation.

The benefits of moderate activity affect all aspects of your life. When you become fit, you have more energy, lower your risk

Physical activity vs. exercise

The terms *physical activity* and *exercise* are used throughout this book. And although they're closely related — and often overlap — there's a difference.

Physical activity refers to any body movement that burns calories, such as mowing the lawn, walking up stairs, making the bed or walking the dog. *Exercise* is a more structured form of physical activity. It involves a series of repetitive movements designed to strengthen or develop some part of your body and improve your cardiovascular fitness. Exercise includes walking, swimming, bicycling and many other activities. Therefore, exercise is a form of physical activity, but not all physical activity fits the definition of exercise. Either way, the good news is that many health benefits may be gained through regular physical activity, even if it's not in the form of structured exercise.

of disease, enhance your mood, manage stress better, sleep more soundly — and reduce your risk of dying prematurely by almost half.

Enjoy the absence of illness. One of the greatest myths about health is that illness is an inevitable part of aging. This isn't true. Although illness and disease do occur more often as people get older, this is as much a result of inactivity as it is age.

This is very good news. It means that with exercise you can counter many of the negative effects of aging and inactivity, such as osteoporosis, heart disease and arthritis. Regular exercise decreases the chance of illness or death from all causes and even helps reduce anxiety and depression.

With a lower incidence of the illnesses that may accompany aging, you can be more active and enjoy a longer, more fulfilling life.

MAINTAINING HEALTH AND QUALITY OF LIFE

People of all ages, races and cultural backgrounds gain substantial health benefits from regular physical activity. When you commit yourself to a regular program of exercise, you're giving yourself the gift of fitness, health and well-being. You'll feel better, look better, be stronger and more able and live longer. Your life will change.

Regular exercise has beneficial effects on most, if not all, of your organ systems. As a result, it helps to prevent a broad range of health problems and diseases.

No matter what your specific health and fitness goals are, you'll likely feel and see a difference in both your mental and physical health within one month of beginning an exercise program.

Fighting disease and illness

When it comes to preventing and postponing the onset of disease and illness, there truly isn't a better tool than exercise. Regular physical activity reduces the risk of developing or dying of some of the leading causes of illness in the United States. By starting a regular program today, you'll help your body prevent disease and illness, and you may find it easier to manage and control a disease or illness that you're already facing, such as those listed below.

Cardiovascular disease

The term *cardiovascular disease* refers to many types of heart and blood vessel diseases. Hardening of the arteries, heart attack, stroke, heart failure and coronary artery disease all fall under this umbrella. Each year in America, about 960,000 people die of cardiovascular diseases. That's more than 40 percent of all the deaths in the United States, making heart disease the nation's No. 1 killer of both women and men.

Cardiovascular disease develops when the arteries that supply the heart with blood slowly become clogged from a buildup of cells, fat and cholesterol. When the blood flow gets blocked, a heart attack or stroke can occur.

Regular physical activity reduces the risk of dying of cardiovascular disease. When you exercise regularly, you reduce the amount of harmful low-density lipoprotein (LDL) cholesterol in your blood. This is the bad cholesterol that clogs arteries, cuts off blood flow and helps cause heart attack and stroke. At the same time, regular physical activity increases the concentration of high-density lipoprotein (HDL) cholesterol, the "good" cholesterol that helps prevent clogging of blood vessels. Walking as little as eight to 10 miles a week may increase this good form of cholesterol.

Exercise also strengthens your heart so that it can pump your blood more efficiently and bring oxygen and nutrients to the rest of your body. It increases the flexibility of blood vessel walls and reverses hardening of the arteries. Exercise also helps prevent and control other risk factors for cardiovascular disease, including high blood pressure, diabetes and obesity.

High blood pressure

Fifty million Americans have high blood pressure (hypertension). Blood pressure is the force of blood pushing against the walls of your blood vessels. It's measured in millimeters of mercury (mm Hg) and is written as a pair of numbers. The first (top) number is the pressure exerted when the heart contracts (systole). That's your systolic pressure. The second (bottom) number is the pressure when the heart rests between beats (diastole). That's your diastolic pressure.

You have high blood pressure if either your systolic pressure is 140 mm Hg or higher or your diastolic pressure is 90 mm Hg or higher. People with hypertension have a significantly higher risk of cardiovascular disease, congestive heart failure, hardened arteries, stroke, kidney disease and coronary artery disease.

Regular exercise reduces the risk of developing high blood pressure, even if you're already at increased risk of it. Most studies have found that blood pressure is

Classifying blood pressure

(Blood pressure measurements in millimeters of mercury — mm Hg)

Condition	Systolic (Top number)		Diastolic (Bottom number)	What to do
Normal	119 or lower	and	79 or lower	Maintain a healthy lifestyle
Prehypertension	120-139	or	80-89	Adopt a healthy lifestyle
Hypertension *Stage 1*	140-159	or	90-99	Lifestyle changes plus a medication
Stage 2	160 or higher	or	100 or higher	Lifestyle changes plus more than one medication

Note: *Normal blood pressures above apply to all people 18 and older. Blood pressure conditions are usually diagnosed based on the average of two or more readings taken at two different visits to your doctor, in addition to the original screening visit. However, if you have a systolic pressure of 210 mm Hg or higher or a diastolic pressure of 120 mm Hg or higher, a diagnosis may be based on a single measurement.*

Source: National Institutes of Health, 2003

reduced relatively early — three weeks to three months — after the start of an exercise program.

Physical activity — both low- and moderate-intensity exercise — also helps lower the blood pressure in people who already have hypertension. Exercise has also been shown to reduce mortality in individuals initiating an exercise program even if they remain hypertensive.

Although the generally recommended amount of exercise — 30 to 60 minutes most days of the week — is sufficient to

make these positive changes, there's one important caveat. When you stop your exercise program, blood pressure typically returns to its prior, higher level.

Obesity

Obesity has become a significant health problem in the United States. Nearly 50 million adults ages 20 to 74 — or 27 percent of the adult population — are obese. Obesity is most commonly measured by body mass index (BMI). See the table on page 9 to determine your BMI.

In addition to the daily toll on your body and self-esteem, obesity carries with it serious health risks. People who are obese have an increased risk of premature death, type 2 diabetes (formerly called adult-onset or noninsulin dependent diabetes), cardiovascular disease, stroke, hypertension, gallbladder disease, a deterioration of the cartilage and bone in joints (osteoarthritis), sleep apnea, asthma, certain cancers, high cholesterol, menstrual irregularities and stress incontinence. Obesity also increases surgical risk, risk of pregnancy complications, psychological disorders such as depression, and psychological difficulties as a result of being socially stigmatized.

Physical activity combats these health risks. Coupled with a healthy diet, exercise can help obese people lose weight and achieve a healthy body composition, alleviating the problems associated with being seriously overweight. And yet people who are overweight can reap some of the benefits of exercise even without

Almost everyone can exercise

Even if you're obese, disabled or a wheelchair user, you can still find ways to exercise.

Medical research shows that physical activity is both safe and beneficial for people with arthritis, osteoporosis and other chronic conditions of the bones and joints. In fact, lack of physical activity can make your condition worse — or at least make it more difficult to live with.

One study even showed that frail, wheelchair-using nursing home residents in their 80s and 90s improved their strength and overall functional ability after joining a weightlifting program.

So if you find exercise to be difficult, get creative. If you have arthritis, for instance, consider water exercise. If you're especially busy, find exercise in common household chores and lifestyle activities, such as walking the dog, washing the car or raking the yard. Talk with a doctor about what will work best for you. (See Chapter 8 for details on exercising with a medical condition.)

Body mass index (BMI)

BMI	Healthy		Overweight					Obese				
	19	24	25	26	27	28	29	30	35	40	45	50
Height							Weight in pounds					
4'10"	91	115	119	124	129	134	138	143	167	191	215	239
4'11"	94	119	124	128	133	138	143	148	173	198	222	247
5'0"	97	123	128	133	138	143	148	153	179	204	230	255
5'1"	100	127	132	137	143	148	153	158	185	211	238	264
5'2"	104	131	136	142	147	153	158	164	191	218	246	273
5'3"	107	135	141	146	152	158	163	169	197	225	254	282
5'4"	110	140	145	151	157	163	169	174	204	232	262	291
5'5"	114	144	150	156	162	168	174	180	210	240	270	300
5'6"	118	148	155	161	167	173	179	186	216	247	278	309
5'7"	121	153	159	166	172	178	185	191	223	255	287	319
5'8"	125	158	164	171	177	184	190	197	230	262	295	328
5'9"	128	162	169	176	182	189	196	203	236	270	304	338
5'10"	132	167	174	181	188	195	202	209	243	278	313	348
5'11"	136	172	179	186	193	200	208	215	250	286	322	358
6'0"	140	177	184	191	199	206	213	221	258	294	331	368
6'1"	144	182	189	197	204	212	219	227	265	302	340	378
6'2"	148	186	194	202	210	218	225	233	272	311	350	389
6'3"	152	192	200	208	216	224	232	240	279	319	359	399
6'4"	156	197	205	213	221	230	238	246	287	328	369	410

Modified from National Institutes of Health's Clinical Guidelines on the Identification, Evaluation, and Treatment of Overweight and Obesity in Adults, 1998

Calculating your weight risk

The body mass index (BMI) is the most commonly used tool to determine whether a person is overweight or obese. Here's how it works. BMI measures your weight in relation to your height. The formula is your weight in pounds divided by the square of your height in inches, multiplied by 703, like this: (pounds ÷ inches^2) x 703 = BMI.

For example, a 175-pound person who is 5 feet 5 inches (65 inches squared equals 4,225) tall would have a BMI of 29.1.

According to clinical guidelines published by the National Institutes of Health in 1998, you're overweight if your BMI is between 25 and 29.9. You're obese if your BMI is 30 or greater.

Your age and your weight

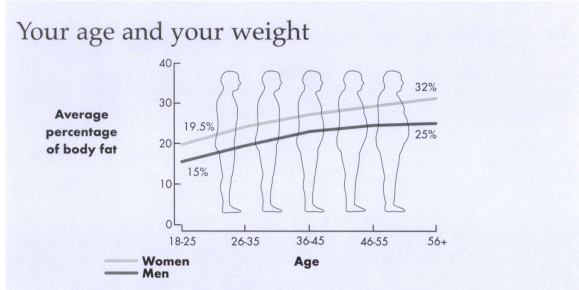

Getting older usually means getting fatter. With age, the amount of muscle tends to decline and fat accounts for a greater percentage of body weight.

losing weight. In one study, overweight women increased their daily activity and significantly improved their health by lowering their blood pressure — without dieting or weight loss.

Diabetes

Diabetes, a disease in which the body doesn't produce or properly use insulin, is one of the leading causes of disability and death in the United States. According to the American Diabetes Association, 18.2 million people in the United States, or 6.3 percent of the population, have diabetes.

There are two forms of diabetes — type 1 and type 2. Type 1 diabetes (formerly called juvenile or insulin-dependent diabetes) results from the body's failure to produce insulin, a hormone that regulates the use of blood sugar by converting sugar, starches and other foods into energy.

Type 2 diabetes occurs when the body doesn't use insulin properly, allowing the concentration of sugar in the blood to increase. A significant relationship exists between type 2 diabetes, obesity and a lack of physical activity. Approximately 90 percent to 95 percent of Americans with diabetes have type 2 diabetes, and one in four older adults is at risk of developing it.

Regular physical activity and a healthy diet reduce the risk of developing type 2 diabetes and can help control all forms of diabetes in those who already have it. This is because mild to moderate exercise helps insulin work better, lowering blood sugar levels. Regular exercise prevents glucose from accumulating in the blood by helping muscles convert glucose in the bloodstream into energy. And by burning calories, exercise helps achieve and maintain a healthy weight, an important factor in the risk and management of type 2 diabetes.

As with other benefits from physical activity, if you don't use it, you'll lose it. Exercise is a long-term aid to preventing and managing diabetes only when you do it on a regular basis.

Osteoporosis

Osteoporosis, a condition marked by decreased bone density and deterioration of bone, affects more than 25 million Americans. Bones affected by osteoporosis become weak, porous and fragile.

Because osteoporosis leads to fragile bones, it's a major contributor to bone fractures — a significant health risk for older adults. By the time Americans reach age 90, about one-third of the women and about one-sixth of the men will have suffered a hip fracture. This means that in the United States, about 250,000 people are hospitalized each year with hip fractures due to osteoporosis. An even more sobering fact is that between 15 percent and 20 percent of those with hip fractures die within the following year.

Physical activity is likely the single most important influence on maintaining bone density and makeup. It plays several roles in preventing and treating osteoporosis. Perhaps most important is that exercise strengthens your bones. Bones, like muscles, grow stronger when they're physically stressed through exercise. Weight-bearing exercises, such as walking and jogging, and strength training exercises, such as lifting weights or working with resistance bands, stimulate bone growth, increase bone density and protect against the decline of bone mass, making your bones healthier.

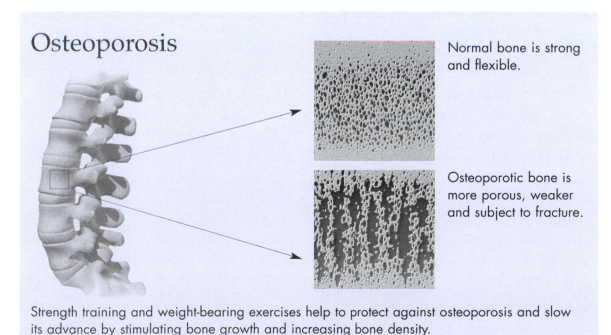

Osteoporosis

Normal bone is strong and flexible.

Osteoporotic bone is more porous, weaker and subject to fracture.

Strength training and weight-bearing exercises help to protect against osteoporosis and slow its advance by stimulating bone growth and increasing bone density.

You don't need a gym membership or home exercise equipment to do osteoporosis-fighting exercises. Even simple activities, such as repeatedly lifting a soup can, may be helpful.

Regular exercise will also help you maintain good balance and coordination so that you're less likely to fall and suffer a disabling fracture. Studies show a lower risk of hip fracture among active adults — an important fact, since hip fractures are associated with more deaths, permanent disability and medical care costs than are all other osteoporosis-related fractures combined.

It's never too early to prevent osteoporosis. Through regular physical activity, even children and adolescents can build greater bone mass, which helps maintain strong bones during adulthood. Bone mass continues to increase slightly when you're in your 20s, and your skeleton usually reaches its maximum mass at about age 30. This is known as peak bone mass — the highest amount of bone mass that you're able to attain as a result of normal growth.

Arthritis

Although many people believe that arthritis prevents them from exercising at all, just the opposite can be true. In fact, it's important that people with arthritis get regular exercise.

Arthritis, which comprises more than 100 different diseases and conditions, affects nearly 70 million Americans.

Osteoarthritis

Normal spine

Disk

Nerve

Vertebra

Osteoarthritis

Narrowed disk

Bone spur

In a normal spine, your vertebrae are cushioned by elastic structures called disks, which help to keep the spine flexible. When you have osteoarthritis in the spine, the disks narrow, leading to bony lumps along the sides of the vertebrae. Pain and stiffness may occur where bone surfaces rub together.

It's most prevalent in people over age 55, but it affects younger adults, too.

Osteoarthritis, the most common form of arthritis, is characterized by deterioration of cartilage around the joints. People with osteoarthritis experience pain, aching, stiffness and swelling in or around their joints. As a result, osteoarthritis can make it difficult to do everyday activities, such as typing on a computer keyboard or writing a grocery list.

Rheumatoid arthritis is another common form of arthritis. It primarily affects the lining of the joints (synovium), which become chronically inflamed, causing stiffness, swelling and pain.

Regular exercise can help people with osteoarthritis and rheumatoid arthritis in a couple of ways. After doing appropriate, regular physical activity, people with both types of arthritis have had a significant reduction in joint swelling. Regular physical activity has also been found to raise the pain threshold and improve the energy level of people with osteoarthritis.

It's important to note that moderate physical activity isn't associated with joint damage or the development of osteoarthritis. On the contrary, a lack of physical activity can aggravate osteoarthritis. This is because weak muscles around joints can lead to further joint distress.

Although moderate-intensity exercises such as swimming or pool walking are good ways to start, there are many types of exercise that can help strengthen your joints and the surrounding muscles, relieve joint stiffness and reduce pain.

If you have arthritis, be sure to talk with your doctor before beginning an exercise program.

Cancer

Regular exercise may help lower the incidence of some cancers, in particular, cancers of the colon, prostate, uterine lining (endometrium) and breast.

About 107,000 people are newly diagnosed with colon cancer each year. One way in which the disease can develop is when food remains in the colon for extended periods of time, causing irritations that can lead to cancer. Exercise combats colon cancer by helping digested food move through the colon more quickly.

In the United States, breast cancer is the leading cancer among women. Exercise lowers the risks of breast cancer by reducing body fat, which produces the female hormone estrogen. Estrogen, in turn, has been shown to support the growth of some female cancers, including breast and endometrial cancers.

ACTIVE AGING

Older adults can reap significant health benefits with a moderate amount of physical activity. Daily — or almost daily — activities such as walking or swimming can make a big difference in fitness levels.

It's never too late to start. Whether you're 39 or 93, there are literally dozens of reasons why regular exercise is a powerful contributor to healthy aging.

In addition to the great number of diseases that exercise can help prevent or postpone, regular physical activity offsets the loss of muscle mass and strength typically associated with normal aging. It improves your posture, flexibility and balance — all areas that begin to fail as you age.

Regular physical activity also contributes to longevity. One recent study showed that white women age 65 and older who increased their physical activity to the equivalent of walking one mile a day lowered their risk of death during the six-year follow-up period by between 40 percent and 50 percent. In another study, men who improved from unfit to fit reduced their mortality risk by 44 percent during a five-year follow-up period.

Exercise leads to a healthier, happier, more independent lifestyle — significantly enhancing your quality of life. It boosts your confidence and self-esteem and helps you to remain active longer.

Consider the following aging-related benefits derived from regular exercise.

Maintains muscle tone and elasticity

Regular exercise — particularly strength training — slows the loss of muscle mass, helps mobility and balance, and strengthens your muscles as you age. But did you know that it also offers cosmetic rewards?

As you age, a loss of muscle strength is normal. A person's total muscle mass decreases by nearly 50 percent between the ages of 20 and 90. As this happens, muscles naturally lose their tone and texture (elasticity). As your muscles become

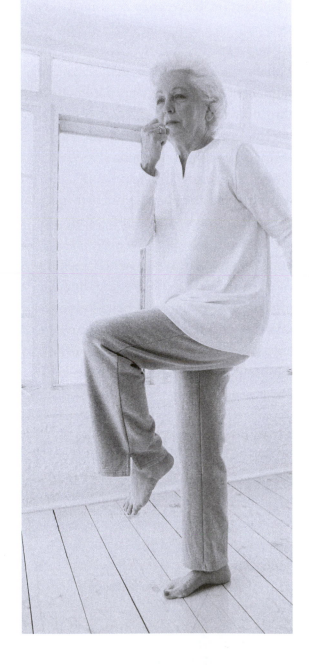

Balance as you age

As you get older, maintaining your balance is an important part of avoiding falls. You can work on your balance throughout the day. Practice standing on one leg while waiting in line or doing housework, for instance, or rise up on your toes while washing the dishes or ironing.

stiff and sag from the constant pull of gravity, your body begins to show the signs of aging.

By engaging in a regular strength training program, you can fight this trend. You can maintain your muscle mass and tone and counteract the effects of gravity. You'll achieve what hundreds of beauty products promise. You'll look younger longer.

Generates energy to do things

Many older adults complain that they don't have the energy to do the things they once did. They assume that their chronic fatigue and lack of energy is a result of old age, when in truth, it's largely the result of inactivity.

Popular endurance exercises, such as walking, swimming, jogging, biking and rowing, can be done by people at any age to improve stamina and energy. After just a few weeks in a walking program, for instance, even previously inactive older adults found they had more energy to do things such as gardening, traveling and spending time with grandchildren.

Types of fitness

True physical fitness is a combination of different components, including aerobic fitness, muscular fitness, flexibility and body composition. Take these into account in your exercise program, and you'll be on your way to living a long, healthy life:

- **Aerobic fitness.** The body's ability to take in and use oxygen to produce energy
- **Muscular fitness.** The strength and endurance of your muscles
- **Flexibility.** The ability to bend joints and stretch muscles through their full range of motion
- **Body composition.** The amount of fat you have in comparison with muscle, bone and other tissue

Helps maintain a positive outlook on life

When you look good, feel good and enjoy an active lifestyle, it's easy to adopt the attitude of an optimist. People of all ages who exercise regularly report having an improved outlook on life, an enhanced self-image and an overall sense of well-being.

The social aspects of physical activity may be especially valuable to older adults.

Overall physical activity level

Age	Never active	Low	Medium	Medium-high	High
18-24 years	4.4%	14.2%	29.9%	27.5%	24.1%
25-44 years	5.3%	15.0%	34.0%	25.2%	20.5%
45-64 years	10.1%	17.4%	33.0%	22.5%	17.1%
65 years and older	22.5%	15.8%	27.9%	18.4%	15.3%

A 2000 report conducted by the Centers for Disease Control and Prevention's National Center for Health Statistics shows the percentage of individuals in various age ranges and the amount of physical activity in which they engage.

Instead of succumbing to inactivity — which leads to poor health — active older adults have the opportunity to engage in group activities such as dancing, golf and exercise classes. Such activities not only create a social network but also help make life interesting and fun.

LOSING AND MANAGING WEIGHT

Maintaining a healthy weight is critical to your health. If you're overweight or obese, you have an increased risk of a number of health problems, including heart disease, diabetes, arthritis and back pain.

When it comes to losing weight and keeping it off, no cabbage, grapefruit, or wonder-pill diet will ever deliver the results of good nutrition coupled with a regular exercise program. The bottom line is clear. Physical activity is a necessary component in any weight-loss or weight management program.

A weight-loss tool

Regular physical activity, when combined with proper nutrition, does what hundreds of fad diets promise. It helps you lose weight and keep it off. Simply put, exercise burns calories. And when you burn more calories than you take in, you can reduce your body fat.

Here's how it works. Your body requires a certain amount of energy to maintain the functions you need to sustain life. When you exercise, your

> # Did you know?
> - When it comes to physical activity, it's either "Use it or lose it." Once you stop exercising, the benefits begin to diminish within two weeks — and will completely disappear in two to eight months.
> - Getting 30 to 60 minutes of physical activity most days of the week is recommended to improve health and fitness.
> - Most Americans overestimate how much activity they get each day and underestimate how many calories they take in.

body works harder and needs more fuel (calories) to function. Even after you stop exercising, your body continues to burn calories at a modestly increased rate for a few hours. The more intensely you exercise, the more calories you burn.

There's more good news. As long as you maintain your exercise program while watching your diet, you can achieve long-term weight loss while preserving lean muscle mass. As you become more physically fit and increase your endurance and the intensity of your exercise program, you can lose even more body fat, helping you to reach your healthy-weight goal.

According to the American College of Sports Medicine (ACSM), people trying to lose weight should aim for 2 1/2 hours of moderate-intensity exercise a week. Moderate-intensity exercise includes activities such as brisk walking, biking and swimming. To determine whether you're working at the right intensity, see page 70 in Chapter 4. If you're seriously overweight or obese and can't reach the 2 1/2-hour goal right away, that's OK. Work toward it. And don't be satisfied once you've reached it! It's been shown that increasing your weekly activity by just 1 to 3 1/2 hours of exercise each week aids in achieving long-term weight loss.

Don't underestimate the role of diet in this formula. Proper nutrition, including eating plenty of fresh fruits and vegetables, is vital to any weight-loss program. Talk with your health care provider about the number of calories that you need each day.

A final note: Don't think an exercise program is unnecessary if you're taking weight-loss medications. Good nutrition and regular physical activity are the keys to achieving long-term weight loss.

A weight-maintenance tool

Physical activity helps you to not only lose weight but also keep it off. That's why once you've reached your goal weight, it's important to stick to your exercise program. There are a couple of reasons for this. Individuals who are at a healthy weight require just as much physical activity as do overweight people. By itself, being thin doesn't create a healthy heart. Regular physical activity can.

Both modest and large weight gains are associated with an increased risk of disease. Maintaining your exercise program will help you burn calories, maintain a desirable body weight and a healthy percentage of body fat — in turn, boosting your confidence and self-esteem.

Remember, even if you don't lose weight, regular exercise can yield other health benefits, such as a reduced cholesterol level and lower blood pressure.

ENHANCING PSYCHOLOGICAL WELL-BEING

You know that exercise can make you stronger and healthier and help you to live longer. But did you know that it's also good for your mental health?

The same regular exercise routine that wards off disease and builds muscle can also improve your psychological well-being. There's considerable evidence that regular physical activity can help reduce stress, manage mild or moderate depression and anxiety — and possibly other psychiatric disorders — improve your mood, fight fatigue, help you sleep and boost your self-esteem.

Reduces stress

Stress comes in many forms. You may feel overwhelmed by a busy schedule, anxious about an upcoming vacation or worried about significant changes at home or work. Whatever the source of your stress, one thing is certain. Chronic stress can take its toll on your health.

You may feel your stress in tension headaches, in persistent feelings of panic or in a vague sense of unease. Stress may also affect your immune system — decreasing your ability to fight off illness. In one study, older adults with chronic stress had higher than normal elevations of interleukin-6, an immune system protein in the blood. The result? An acceleration of age-related conditions such as heart disease, diabetes, arthritis, osteoporosis, frailty and certain cancers.

Regular physical activity can reduce and manage the stress in your life — and thus reduce these negative effects of stress on your body. Here's how:

- Exercise is relaxing and soothing — used by many as a form of meditation. Even as you exert your body during physical activity, your mind maintains a sense of calm and control. You feel a sense of command over your body and your life and a heightened sense of well-being. It's no wonder that many people who exercise regularly have normal blood pressure even when under stress.

- Physical activity also serves as a positive coping strategy — a sort of timeout from the problems and stressors of everyday life. While exercising you tend to concentrate on the task at hand — and not the tensions of your day.

- According to the Society of Behavioral Medicine, people who participate in high levels of physical activity may actually reduce the amount of stress they experience — using the exercise as a stress buffer.

The bottom line is this: People who exercise are better able to cope with stress and, according to research, are less likely to be depressed and anxious.

Helps combat depression

People who are inactive are twice as likely to have symptoms of depression as are people who are active. Depression is a serious condition marked by sadness, low self-esteem, pessimism, hopelessness and despair. Although depression is classified as a mental illness, physical fitness can play a very real part in the treatment of mild or moderate depression.

Exercise fights depression by activating neurotransmitters — chemicals used by your nerve cells to communicate with one another — that are associated with depression. Those neurotransmitters are serotonin and norepinephrine. When you experience depression, the level of serotonin, norepinephrine or both may be out of balance. Exercise may help synchronize those brain chemicals.

Exercise also stimulates the production of endorphins — other neurotransmitters that produce feelings of well-being. This phenomenon is commonly referred to as runner's high. Many people will feel this uplifting rush just 12 minutes into a workout.

One study found that depressed people experienced significantly less depression after exercising for 20 minutes to an hour three times a week for five weeks. Another study suggested that exercise may stimulate the growth of new brain cells that enhance memory and learning — two functions hampered by depression. It has even been suggested that regular physical activity may reduce or prevent the risk of developing depression, although further research on this topic is needed.

Work exercise into your life

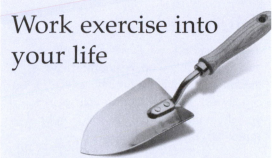

Most of us have many opportunities for regular physical activity, but relatively few of us take advantage of them. Indeed, only about 22 percent of American adults engage in regular, sustained physical activity during their leisure time. Although it's recommended that you adopt a regular exercise program, you can also make small lifestyle changes that add regular physical activity to your daily routine so that you begin to experience some of the health benefits of increased activity. Consider these activities for giving each day a boost:

- Walk or bike on short errands instead of driving your car.
- Do some gardening. Planting seeds, pulling weeds and tending the soil work your joints, muscles and heart.
- Park at a distance from your destination and walk the rest of the way.
- Walk the stairs instead of taking the elevator. If you work or live on a high floor, take the elevator only partway up.
- Walk your dog. If you don't have one, offer to walk the dog of a neighbor or friend.
- Do your own yardwork. Mow your lawn, rake your leaves and shovel your walk.
- When it's practical, hold walking meetings at work instead of sitting at a table.
- While golfing, walk instead of riding in a cart.
- Go dancing.
- Play charades with your family instead of having a TV night.

If you suffer from clinical depression, don't try to cure yourself with exercise. Talk with your doctor, who can recommend a treatment plan.

Helps combat anxiety

People who suffer from anxiety often feel tense, uncertain, helpless, nervous and apprehensive of something they can't define. Anxiety is more than worry — it's an ongoing tension that can negatively affect your self-esteem.

Activities such as walking have been shown to reduce chronic anxiety for the same reasons that exercise helps manage mild or moderate depression. The activity serves as a diversion, giving an anxious mind a break — and a chance to refocus.

Studies of athletes, firefighters and police officers have shown that exercise and improved physical fitness may reduce anxiety. One study found that a single session of exercise — in this case, walking — was as effective as a prescribed tranquilizer in reducing tension, and the benefit of the exercise lasted longer.

Improves mood and self-esteem

Exercise creates a powerful snowball effect on your mood and self-esteem. When you make the decision to start an exercise program, you're taking control of your life. You'll improve your strength, endurance and appearance. You may even lose weight. As a result, you'll feel better about yourself. This new confidence will carry over into your everyday life — improving your outlook. You'll have a new bounce in your step and a feeling that you can accomplish anything you commit to doing.

Reduces fatigue

If you frequently lack energy, you know that fatigue is no fun. No one likes to feel tired — especially when that feeling prevents you from doing the activities you want to do, such as playing with your children or grandchildren or enjoying a favorite hobby.

That afternoon slump or evening exhaustion you feel may not be the result of too little sleep. It may be the result of inactivity.

Instead of trying to cure your fatigue with daily catnaps, try spending time exercising. When you're fit, your heart, blood vessels, lungs and muscles have the energy to carry out their daily tasks, and to meet unexpected physical challenges.

Regular aerobic exercise increases your ability to take in and use oxygen. When your body efficiently transports oxygen, you can make better use of it to produce energy. Your body's ability to do this is called aerobic capacity. When your aerobic capacity is high, your heart, lungs and blood vessels are able to transport and deliver greater amounts of oxygen to your body tissues. When this happens, you don't fatigue as quickly, and your body is able to produce more energy for the activities you want and need to do, whether it's going for a long hike in your favorite park or doing lawn and garden work.

Did you know?

If you're unable to talk while exercising, you're probably working too hard. Although you should be breathing hard or be slightly out of breath during your workout, you should also be able to speak in brief sentences. If you can't, slow down.

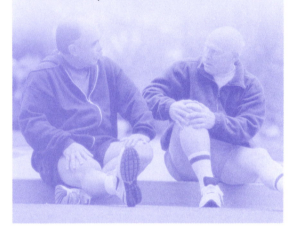

Enhances sleep

A good night's sleep helps maintain your physical and mental health. Exercise can help you get much-needed rest. Studies show that moderate exercise at least three hours before bedtime can help you relax and sleep better at night.

WHAT'S AHEAD?

Whether you're looking to slow the aging process, prevent disease, reduce stress or lose weight, physical activity is an integral part of achieving these goals. In the chapters ahead, you'll learn how to make exercise a part of your daily life. You'll find tips on staying motivated, on choosing exercise equipment that best suits your needs, and how to stay fit even if you have a medical condition that may limit physical activity. There's also a chapter on nutrition to help you select foods that complement your fitness plan. And there's information about choosing a sport that's best for you. Read on and good luck as you move toward a healthier, more fit lifestyle.

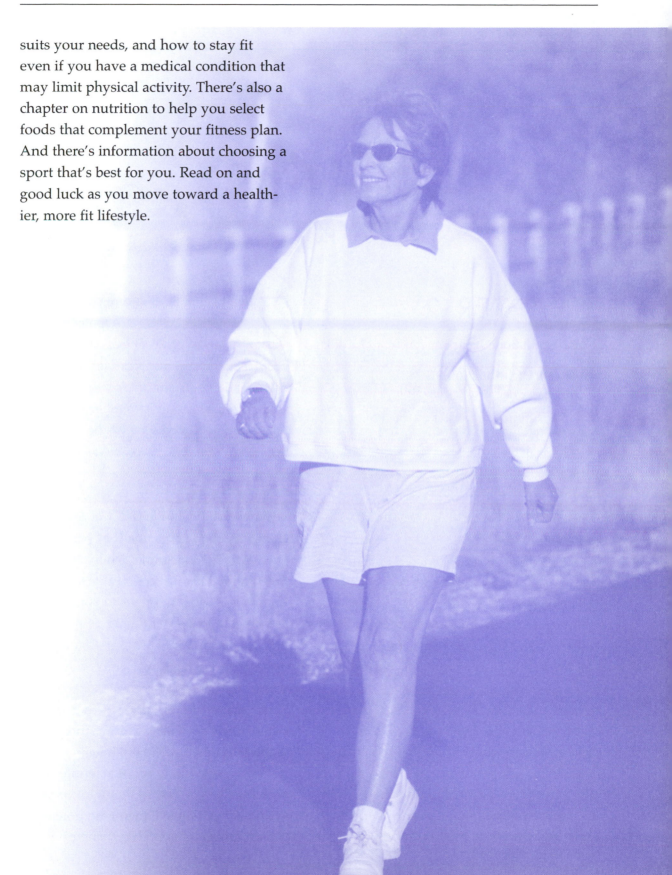

Anatomy & aging

CHAPTER 2

The human body is a remarkable set of systems capable of an amazing variety of physical feats. Whether your fitness achievements are record-setting, personal best goals or just mowing the lawn, your body's intricate system of muscles, bones and nerves gets the job done. As finely tuned as your body may be, though, with time you'll naturally lose some of your edge. But how much may be up to you.

Change is inevitable. Most of the changes in body function that you experience with age are subtle, while others can significantly affect your lifestyle. To understand what happens to your body as you get older — and the role physical activity plays in this process — you first need to understand how your body works. In this chapter, you'll learn how your muscles, bones and nerves work together to help you perform. And you'll learn about the body's three main energy systems and what types of activities they fuel. Finally, you'll find that while body systems inevitably change with time, you can do things to slow that change.

MUSCLE AND BONE BASICS

Bones, muscles, tendons, ligaments and joints form the musculoskeletal system that allows your body to move. This system enables you to do everyday activities — from walking to the mailbox to riding a bike to simply pouring a glass of water.

Each part of the musculoskeletal system is interconnected and is essential for movement. Your bones form the frame of your body — giving it shape, protecting your vital organs and providing a foundation to which muscles and tendons are attached. Combined with your joints, bones help make movement possible. Muscles, tendons and ligaments, the elastic tissues that connect bones and joints, also are crucial for movement.

Bones. Your body has 206 bones — ranging from the large bones in your legs to the small bones in your wrist. Bones consist of a harder, outer portion (compact bone) and a softer, inner portion (cancellous bone).

Inside your bones is marrow, where most of your blood cells are made. Bones also contain large amounts of minerals, including phosphorus and sodium. Calcium, the mineral that makes your bones hard and able to support weight, is also stored in your bones. Your bones release calcium as your body needs it. Your diet directly affects how much calcium is stored in your bones, which is just one reason it's essential to consume a healthy, vitamin- and mineral-rich diet.

Muscles. When it comes to numbers, your muscles have your bones beat by a mile. Your body has more than 660 muscles. Simply put, muscles are in the business of contracting to create movement. To do that, each muscle contains thousands of cells that make up muscle fibers. The length of each of these fibers varies depending on what it's used for. Eye muscles, for instance, require small fibers that may be only a few millimeters (about a tenth of an inch) in length. Larger muscles, however, such as those in your leg, may have fibers reaching nearly 30 centimeters (about 12 inches) in length.

Cardiac muscle
(Muscle of the heart)

Skeletal muscle
(Voluntary muscle
attached to bones)

Smooth muscle
(Involuntary muscle, such
as that lining the stomach
and other organs)

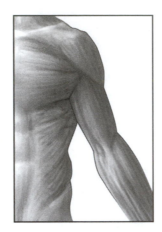

There are three kinds of muscles that create different types of movement:

- Skeletal muscles (voluntary muscles) are made up of fibers that can become shorter and tighter (contract) quickly and powerfully, although they tire relatively easily and have to rest between heavy activity. They're found in many forms throughout the body and vary in size and shape depending on where they're located. The size and shape of a muscle plays a role in how much force it can generate, how quickly it can contract and how much endurance it has. For more information, see "Skeletal muscle fibers" on page 25.

- Smooth muscles (involuntary muscles) also are made up of fibers and are smooth in appearance. These muscles, found in the walls of your stomach and intestines, are controlled by your central nervous system. You can't consciously control them.

- Cardiac muscle is found only in your heart. The walls of your heart and its chambers (ventricles and atria) are made almost entirely of muscle fibers. Like smooth muscle, cardiac muscle is also involuntary. When cardiac muscle contracts, it forces blood out of the heart, producing your heartbeat. Cardiac muscle is quick and powerful and doesn't fatigue as skeletal muscles do.

Tendons. Muscles are connected to bones by tough, cord-like tissues called tendons. Tendons allow your muscles to pull on your bones, causing movement. You can easily identify some of the tendons on your body. The cord-like area on the back of your ankle that leads to your calf is called the Achilles tendon. The narrow bands on the tops of your hands are tendons, too. When you move your foot or your fingers, you can watch and feel these tendons lengthen and shorten.

Skeletal muscle fibers

You have two distinct types of skeletal muscle fibers. These fibers use the energy systems discussed beginning on page 27 to power their activities. The fibers have innate "preferences" for how they produce energy and movement. Type I (slow-twitch) muscle fibers generate energy and movement primarily through aerobic pathways. These fibers are slower to fatigue compared with type II (fast-twitch) fibers. For this reason, slow-twitch fibers sustain continuous activities and are associated with long-duration, aerobic activities.

Type II muscle fiber has a high capacity for generating energy and movement without oxygen (anaerobically). These fibers are used during activities that involve frequent changes of pace or stop-and-go activities, such as basketball and tennis. They're also important for efforts that require rapid, powerful movements or increased force, such as running or vigorous cycling up a hill.

Type II muscle fibers contract faster and more forcefully than do type I fibers and use their energy relatively fast. Unlike type I muscle fibers, type II fibers don't have much aerobic energy machinery and aren't activated for most low-intensity activities. Many physical activities require fairly slow, sustained muscle actions interspersed with bursts of powerful effort, like those used in soccer. In these activities, both muscle fiber types are activated.

All muscles contain both types of fibers, but the ratio of one type to the other varies in each person. This ratio is determined genetically, which can account in part for a person's natural ability in a given sport.

The different muscle fiber types become larger in response to the specific type of physical activity you do. For example, people who are trained in an aerobic activity, such as distance running, have larger slow-twitch fibers than fast-twitch fibers in the same muscle. On the other hand, people trained in anaerobic power activities have larger fast-twitch fibers. With appropriate training, both type I and II muscle fibers can be made more efficient. In addition, some type II fibers can take on type I properties.

Your tendons connect both ends of a muscle to the outside covering of the bone (periosteum). The link between your tendons and bones is so strong that only very severe stress or injury can tear or pull the tendons away from the bone.

Ligaments. Tendons connect muscle and bone, and ligaments connect bone to bone. These long, flat, strap-like fibers wrap around your joints, fastening bone to other bone. Like tendons, ligaments are quite strong.

Joints. Joints are the junctions of bones that allow them to move as muscles pull them. Some open and close like a hinge (fingers and elbows), and others allow bones to move backward, forward and sideways, and to rotate, as in the shoulders.

Most of the joints used for movement are lined with a tissue called synovium, which generates synovial fluid. This fluid serves as a lubricant that allows your joints to move freely and easily. Examples of synovial joints are your hips, knees and shoulders.

Your body has other types of joints, as well. Partially movable joints (cartilaginous joints) move just a little. Part of your spine is made up of these partially movable joints. Each vertebrae in your spine is linked to the vertebrae above and below it by these joints. They're made of cartilage, which increases flexibility.

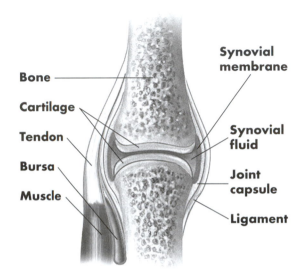

Bone

Cartilage

Tendon

Bursa

Muscle

Synovial membrane

Synovial fluid

Joint capsule

Ligament

GOING THROUGH THE MOTIONS

Before you make a movement, your brain sends a message to your muscles. Your muscles, in turn, work with your tendons and ligaments to coordinate and execute the movement, and finally, send a message back to your brain to confirm that the movement has been made.

Flexors and extensors

Muscles, with the help of tendons and ligaments, move bones by contracting and then relaxing. Muscles can pull bones, but they can't push them back to their original position. So they work in pairs of flexors and extensors — one always doing the opposite of the other.

On one side of the formula is the flexor, which contracts to bend a limb at a joint and bring it closer to the body. On the other side is the extensor, which contracts to extend or straighten the limb at the same joint. When the flexor contracts, the extensor relaxes, and vice versa.

Take, for example, your biceps and triceps — the muscles in your upper arm. The biceps muscle, in the front of the arm, is a flexor. The triceps muscle, at the back of the arm, is an extensor. In every movement, they do the opposite of each other. So when you contract your biceps, and thus relax your triceps, your elbow bends. When you contract your triceps, and relax your biceps, your elbow straightens.

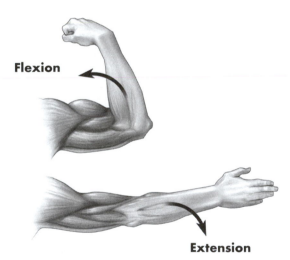

Flexion

Extension

Did you know?

Muscle tissue burns more energy than does fat tissue. Because men naturally have more muscle than women do, they burn between 10 percent and 20 percent more calories than women do, even at rest.

Movement

Muscles don't contract on their own. Every movement you make — from the smallest tap of a finger to the longest strides of an all-out run — is part of a specialized chain of events. In order to carry out action, your muscles rely on your brain for direction and the food you eat for energy.

Think of your body as a fine-tuned machine in which all the parts must work together — much like a car. Your brain is the electrical system that dictates how your frame and engine parts (your bones, muscles and joints) move. In order to power the car and get where you need to go, you need the right fuel (proper nutrition). And, like your car, your body needs regular tuneups (exercise) in order to stay strong and resilient.

ENERGY SYSTEMS AND THE FUEL FOR MOVEMENT

If you've ever run out of gas, you know all too well that for a car to move, the engine has to have fuel. It's no different with your muscles. For them, the fuel is a chemical compound called adenosine triphosphate (ATP). When ATP is "burned" in muscle cells, it provides the energy for muscle fibers to contract. The complex process of producing and using this energy source is called metabolism.

Nutrients in the foods you eat provide the raw materials for metabolism. Carbohydrates are broken down into glucose, which circulates in your blood.

Glucose can be used to produce ATP in your cells. If not needed immediately, glucose is stored in the form of glycogen in your muscles or liver. In some cases, it may be converted into fat for long-term storage. Although fats and proteins from foods can be immediately processed to make ATP, fats are normally stored as a long-term energy reserve, and proteins are normally used to build muscle and enzymes that support the body's structure and function.

Your body manages this fuel supply process through three major energy systems. Although your body draws on all three in almost every physical activity, which one is predominantly used at any given time depends on the duration and intensity of the activity. The three systems can be classified as:

- **Immediate energy.** In this system, ATP and phosphocreatine (PC), a compound that can assist in ATP production, are stored in muscle tissue for quick access.
- **Short-term energy.** This system produces ATP from stored glycogen.
- **Long-term (endurance) energy.** ATP from this system is produced by the metabolism of stored fats, proteins and carbohydrates.

Immediate energy — ATP and PC

When you lift a weight, the ATP needed to make your muscles contract and accomplish the lift was already in your muscle tissue. PC was there, too, ready to help replenish the phosphorus in ATP. This is your immediate energy system at work.

Aerobic and anaerobic

Aerobic means "with oxygen." *Anaerobic* means "without oxygen." In reference to physical activity, the terms relate to which of the body's three energy systems — immediate, short-term or long-term — is the primary supplier of fuel during a given activity.

Your body's immediate energy system doesn't use oxygen to break down adenosine triphosphate (ATP) or replenish ATP with phosphocreatine (PC), so it's anaerobic. Your long-term (endurance) energy system does use oxygen in the chemical process that produces ATP and therefore is aerobic. The short-term energy system can break down glycogen either in the presence or absence of oxygen. With oxygen, the process occurs more slowly and is aerobic.

For most activities, your body blends the use of these three systems depending on the intensity and duration of whatever you're doing. For example, a soccer player may be relying primarily on his or her aerobic energy system while jogging, but the dependence shifts to the immediate system for quick bursts or to the short-term system for relatively intense runs of a minute or so.

For some activities, though, one system predominates. Distance running is primarily aerobic and therefore long-term energy system dominant — except for the sprint at the end — while golf (with use of a cart) draws primarily on the anaerobic immediate energy system to power the swing.

Aerobic activities tend to be "steady state" or "pay as you go," meaning that you're able to breathe in enough oxygen to keep up with the rate that oxygen is being used in the production of ATP. If your intensity level rises to the point where your breathing can no longer keep up, energy production shifts to anaerobic, and fatigue sets in more quickly. People who have developed strong and efficient cardiovascular and respiratory systems, such as distance runners or cross-country skiers, are able to maintain a fairly intense level of activity for a long duration because of their ability to take in and use oxygen. They have a high aerobic capacity.

Aerobic vs. anaerobic activities

	Mode	Intensity	Duration
Aerobic activities	Continuous, long-duration activities	Less intense (60% to 85% of maximum heart rate)	A few minutes to several hours
Anaerobic activities	Explosive or intense, short-duration activities	More intense (75% to 100% of maximum effort)	A few seconds to two minutes

Adapted from Daniel Arnheim and William Prentice, Principles of Athletic Training, 10th Edition, McGraw-Hill, 2000

The immediate energy system provides ATP for short-duration activities, just a few seconds long. Your muscles can store only a small amount of ATP, so the higher the intensity of the activity, the faster you burn through the ATP and the shorter the time you can continue at that intensity. The immediate energy system can sustain all-out muscle effort for only about five to 15 seconds. After that, your body needs to supply fuel from one of the other two energy systems, or both.

All activities use the immediate energy system, but some rely on it more than others. For example, swinging a golf club, throwing a baseball, serving a tennis ball, lifting a weight or sprinting for a short distance all use the immediate energy system for a quick burst of energy. (See "Aerobic vs. anaerobic activities, page 28.)

Short-term energy — Glycogen

After a few seconds of intensive exercise, the small supply of ATP and PC in your working muscle cells is used up, and your body quickly shifts to glucose circulating in your blood and to stored glycogen in the muscles as its primary sources of energy. The short-term energy system breaks these down to produce fresh supplies of ATP and PC (a process called glycolysis). If this process needs to happen fast, then oxygen isn't used and anaerobic glycolosis occurs. Consequently, this energy system is also referred to as the lactic acid system.

Activities that rely primarily on the short-term energy system last from about 10 seconds to two minutes. Examples include playing hockey (where players skate intensively for short shifts and then rest on the bench), downhill skiing and strength training with lighter weights and more repetitions.

The immediate and short-term energy sources together provide enough fuel to power exercise for only a few minutes. Muscular activities that last longer need the much greater energy provided by the aerobic system, which uses oxygen to break down fats and other nutrients.

Lactic acid

Lactic acid (lactate) is created as a result of the process in which glucose is broken down to obtain energy for working muscles. As lactic acid is produced in the muscles, it spreads into the blood and is carried around the body. Lactic acid begins to accumulate in your muscles once you start exercising at an intensity above about 85 percent to 90 percent of your maximum heart rate. (To calculate your maximum heart rate, see page 42.) If this continues, your muscles will fatigue very quickly, typically in less than a minute.

As oxygen is delivered to your muscles, the lactic acid is converted back to usable energy (ATP). Aerobic training stimulates the growth of small blood vessels (capillaries) in your muscles, allowing for more efficient oxygen delivery and removal of lactic acid. Anaerobic training increases tolerance to lactic acid. Lactic acid is in part responsible for the burn you feel in your muscles when you're exercising hard and for the muscle soreness you might experience in the 48 hours following a hard workout.

Long-term energy — Fat and the aerobic system

For lower intensity, longer duration exercise, most of the energy comes from aerobic metabolism. This energy system uses oxygen — shuttled to your muscles by your respiratory and cardiovascular systems — to form ATP from glycogen stored in muscles and the liver, and from fats and proteins. Your cardiorespiratory system also helps clear lactic acid from the blood.

As glycogen supplies are reduced over time during activity, your body relies more heavily on fats stored in fat tissue to meet its energy need. Although energy from fat isn't available as quickly as from glycogen, the supply is much larger and therefore available for a longer period of time. In fact, the longer your physical activity lasts, the more fat that's used, especially toward the end of an endurance event such as a long run. By comparison, the anaerobic systems produce more power more quickly, but the energy is shorter lived.

The aerobic system is more important during low-intensity, long-duration (endurance) activities, such as distance running, distance cycling and cross-country skiing.

PHYSIOLOGY OF AGING

You know that your body changes as you age. Your skin wrinkles, and your hair grays. And while some of these changes are only cosmetic, other age-related changes that can significantly affect your life are occurring beneath your skin — in your bones, muscles and organs.

As a rule, you're in the best physical shape of your life in your 20s. As you enter your early 30s, though, subtle physiologic decline typically begins.

You may begin to lose muscle mass, strength, lung capacity and flexibility.

The good news is that these declines aren't inevitable. They can be prevented, or at least delayed. In fact, most of the changes blamed on aging are actually the result of inactivity and other lifestyle choices. If you make healthy choices and establish positive habits, you can maintain your health — and independence — as you age.

The single most important way to prevent, minimize and cope with physical changes related to aging is regular exercise. This can't be stressed enough. If you don't get regular exercise on an almost daily basis, your fitness level will decline. It *will not* just stay the same. It *will* decline. If you maintain an active lifestyle, you may find one day that you're a 50-something grandparent with the athletic endurance of a 40-year-old.

The bottom line is that being physically fit can help forestall the physiologic declines associated with aging, keep you stronger and give you better balance, flexibility and coordination. Ultimately, the result is continuing independence, health, happiness and quality of life as you age.

Aging muscle. Your muscles lose strength and flexibility as you age. This is because as you get older, muscles shrink and lose mass. Although the decline begins as early as your late 20s, major declines don't take place until after age 40. By the time you are 80, you may have half the muscle mass you had in your prime. Although this is a natural process, an inactive lifestyle certainly accelerates it.

Even if you lead an active life, your muscles will have lost some of the strength they had in your younger years by the time you're 60. You may find that you've lost some of your flexibility and your reflexes have slowed. You may also find it more difficult to accomplish tasks such as opening a jar. In older adults, this strength loss can make it harder to get around and can increase the risk of accidents, such as falls.

Regular physical activity — especially strength training — is a powerful way to slow the normal loss of muscle mass and strength. In one study, a group of 70-year-old men who had done strength training exercises since age 50 had the same muscle cross-section measurements and strength as a group of 28-year-olds.

Even in your 90s, vigorous exercise programs will improve muscle strength and help to minimize and even reverse physical frailty.

Aging ligaments and tendons. As you age, the amount of water in your tendons and ligaments decreases. This causes them to lose elasticity, becoming increasingly stiff and weak, which may lead to decreased joint motion. However, the rate

Lifelong exercise

Were you on the college swim team? A 20-something triathlete? Great! But that's not necessarily going to ensure your good health later in life. Athletic participation as a young adult doesn't equal good health and longevity in later years. What does result in lifelong health and longevity? Maintaining physical activity and fitness throughout life.

Older means weaker?

It wasn't that long ago that scientists believed that a substantial loss of strength was an inevitable part of aging. After all, some decrease in muscle mass is a normal part of getting older. But it's now clear that if you're dedicated to maintaining your strength, you can make great strides in doing so as you get older.

Studies have shown that strength can be maintained and perhaps increased at any age — even in your 80s and beyond. The key is to dedicate yourself to a regular and progressive program of strength exercises.

In one study, people in their late 80s and early 90s performed regular strength training exercises over a 12-week period. The results showed an increase in the strength of the participants' upper thigh (quadriceps) muscles by an average of 175 percent. They also improved their balance, found climbing stairs to be easier and could rise out of a chair without pushing off with their hands.

at which this occurs depends greatly on your lifestyle. In one study, for example, participants ranging in age from 65 to 88 completed 12 weeks of exercise and dance classes. They showed significant improvements in ankle, knee, wrist, shoulder and neck motion when compared with the participants who didn't exercise. This is an example of the use-it-or-lose-it phenomenon.

Aging joints. Joints, too, become less mobile as you age — primarily because of the changes that take place in your tendons and ligaments. Arthritis is the bigger problem that affects joints. After decades of use, the cartilage that cushions your joints can begin to deteriorate, causing them to become stiff, inflamed and sore. The cartilage can eventually wear away, allowing the bones of the joint to painfully grate against each other.

More than 80 percent of older adults have some degree of osteoarthritis, also called degenerative arthritis. Osteoarthritis can cause considerable pain and stiffness. Previous trauma, such as a broken knuckle or hip, can speed the process of osteoarthritis.

Arthritis is chronic and can worsen over time, slowing you down considerably — especially if you were inactive before problems developed. To compound the problem, people often react to arthritis by not moving their painful joints. This, in turn, can cause them to use the surrounding muscles less frequently, resulting in reduced muscle mass and a loss of strength.

Fitness and longevity

In an expansive 20-year study of the lifestyles and exercise habits of 17,000 male Harvard University alumni, researchers established the importance of regular exercise. The study showed that moderate-intensity exercise — equivalent to jogging about three miles a day — not only promoted good health but added years to the lives of the participants. Here are some of the results.

- Men who exercised at the equivalent of a light sport activity had a higher life expectancy than did sedentary men.
- Regular exercise countered the life-shortening effects of cigarette smoking and excess body weight.
- Those with high blood pressure who exercised regularly had half the death rate of those who didn't exercise.
- Men who walked nine or more miles each week showed a 21 percent lower mortality rate than did men who walked three miles or less each week.
- Regular exercise countered genetic tendencies toward early death. Individuals with one or both parents who died before age 65 reduced death risk by 25 percent with a lifestyle of regular exercise.
- Men with the most active lifestyles — those who completed vigorous regular exercise — had the greatest life expectancies. This was due largely to fewer deaths from cardiovascular disease.

Regular activity actually helps arthritic joints. In fact, regular exercise — especially the low-impact kind — can help strengthen your joints and the surrounding muscles, relieve joint stiffness and reduce arthritis pain.

Did you know?

Losing excess weight helps reduce stress and strain on your muscles and joints.

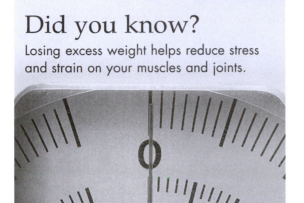

Aging bones. Your bones reach their maximum mass between the ages of 25 and 35. In the years that follow, your bones decline slightly in size and density. Another consequence is that your bones become increasingly weak and brittle.

About 25 million Americans have osteoporosis, which is caused by the gradual loss of mineral content from bones, making them thinner, weaker and more prone to fracture. In fact, bone mass can decrease by 30 percent to 50 percent in people older than age 60.

Although both men and women can get osteoporosis, it's a disease that primarily affects postmenopausal women. In fact, women are twice as likely as men to experience osteoporosis-related injuries. Still, one-third of men have some osteoporosis by the time they're age 75.

Osteoporosis leads to more than 1 million fractures each year in the United States — usually in the spine, hip or wrist. It's responsible for almost all hip fractures in older men and women. In the spine, osteoporosis sometimes causes the bones to simply deteriorate and collapse, resulting in a so-called dowager's hump, that sometimes stooped-over appearance of an older person's back.

Some bone-related injuries, especially hip fractures, can profoundly affect your quality of life. Although surgery to repair fractures is usually effective, the recovery period may be lengthy, and complications, including death, can occur.

Because osteoporosis is due, in part, to lack of exercise and calcium intake, life-long physical activity is key to building strong bones and avoiding this disease. Regular exercise in childhood and young adulthood, coupled with adequate calcium and vitamin D intake, can increase the density of your bones and help prevent or delay osteoporosis.

Even if you weren't a dedicated exerciser in your 20s, yours isn't necessarily a lost cause. You can, at any age, still help to reverse the damage of osteoporosis with regular weight-bearing and strength training exercises. For more on keeping fit with osteoporosis, see Chapter 8.

Your bones

Your body's 206 bones do much more than give your body its shape. Consider this list of your bones' essential functions:

- Protect vital organs, including your brain
- Store crucial minerals, such as calcium
- Produce blood cells
- Serve as attachment sites for muscles and tendons

Aging and your cardiovascular system. Like your bones, your heart and blood vessels change with age. Your heart muscle becomes less elastic and less efficient at pumping blood. You may also lose some of the so-called pacemaker cells, which control your heart's activities. Blood vessels and arteries also lose elasticity and are more likely to become clogged and damaged, although the latter is due in large part to diet.

The changes in your cardiovascular system occur gradually, and the heart usually remains strong enough to meet normal demands. However, it may have less reserve capacity for overcoming injury or handling the sudden demands of stress or illness as you age.

Regular aerobic exercise — such as brisk walking, swimming or biking — is an essential part of maintaining cardio-vascular health as you age. It can help increase your heart's capacity to pump and keep your blood pressure in check. It reduces the risk of cardiovascular disease and can help prevent stroke.

The body's aerobic capacity — the ability of the heart, lungs and blood vessels to deliver enough oxygen to muscles during physical activity — declines a small percentage each year in adult men and women. The rate of decline is largely up to you. If you're overweight or inactive, you'll experience a higher rate of decline. If you maintain a regular exercise program, you may experience less decline in your aerobic capacity.

Aging and your lungs. When you inhale, air enters your mouth and nose and travels down your windpipe (trachea). The trachea branches into two main air passageways, which then branch into

Effects of aging ... and exercise

Condition or system	Aging effect	Exercise effect
Heart	Decline	Improvement
Blood pressure	Increase	Decrease
Diabetes	Increased risk	Decreased risk
Falls	Increased risk	Decreased risk
Bone density	Decline	Slowed or no decline
Muscle mass	Decline	Maintained or improved
Arthritis	Increased pain	Decreased pain
Cognitive performance	Decline	Improvement
Body fat	Increase	Decrease
Response time	Slowed	Maintained
Joint mobility	Decline	Improved
Aerobic capacity	Decrease	Maintained or increased
Stroke and heart attack	Increased risk	Decreased risk

Keeping your balance

Falls are a common problem in older adults. More than just an inconvenience, falls are a major cause of broken hips and wrists and other injuries that often lead to long-term disability. In fact, 90 percent of hip fractures in older adults are the result of falls.

Doing balance exercises regularly can help older adults avoid falls — and walk with more confidence. Many balance exercises, such as briefly standing on one leg, can be done during your normal daily activities. Others, such as tai chi and yoga, also will help build your flexibility. Be sure to get proper training to do balance exercises correctly.

progressively smaller passageways and tubes called bronchioles. The smallest bronchioles end in tiny air sacs. Blood vessels called pulmonary capillaries carry blood to these air sacs, where they release carbon dioxide and absorb oxygen.

Healthy adult lungs contain about 300 million of these air sacs. As you age the number of these air sacs decreases,

resulting in a decline of lung function. This decline is especially noticeable if you don't exercise, and can contribute to that out-of-breath feeling after completing even low-intensity activity. If you lead an active life as you age, you may not even notice the gradual change in lung function. Regular aerobic exercise has been shown to slow the decline in lung function associated with aging.

Aging and your brain and nervous system. As you age, the speed with which your brain processes information slows down. It has been suggested that a physically active lifestyle slows this age-related decline in mental performance. Older adults who stay active for at least 20 years, for instance, show the same — or greater — reaction speeds as inactive people in their 20s.

Aging and your bowels. Constipation, the passage of hard stools or less than three bowel movements a week, is a common condition for older adults. This may be due to a number of factors, including certain medications, inactivity,

Physical activity and cardiovascular disease

When it comes to risk factors for cardiovascular disease, an inactive lifestyle ranks high. One study found inactivity to be a more important gauge of death than any other significant cardiovascular disease risk factor. The least fit men and women in the study were nearly twice as likely to die of cardiovascular disease as were their fit counterparts. Poor physical fitness was a greater cardiovascular risk factor than were high blood pressure, high cholesterol, obesity *and* family history.

Increased physical fitness was also shown to counter the negative effects of other coronary artery disease risk factors. Moderately fit smokers with high cholesterol, for instance, lived longer than did healthy but sedentary nonsmokers.

illness, dehydration and poor diet. Increasing your physical activity and eating a balanced diet can help lessen the risk of constipation.

Aging and your urinary tract. Many postmenopausal women experience what's called stress incontinence. This may happen for a variety of reasons. The muscles around the opening of the bladder can lose strength. In addition, as estrogen levels decline, the tissues lining the tube through which urine passes (urethra) become thinner. And pelvic muscles often become weaker, reducing bladder support. Pelvic floor exercises (Kegel exercises) can help relieve mild-to-moderate stress incontinence in both women and men (see page 269 for details).

Aging and sleep. Rest is an important component of any exercise program. In fact, your body needs regular exercise, proper nutrition and sufficient rest in order to achieve its best health. Unfortunately, many people find that getting enough sleep is more difficult the older they get.

The amount of sleep you need remains fairly constant throughout your life. If your body requires about six hours a night now, for instance, it's likely that you'll need about six hours of sleep each night 10 years from now. Despite this fact, aging can cause you to sleep less soundly. The inability to fall asleep (insomnia) becomes more prevalent with age.

Sleep often becomes less restful between the ages of 50 and 60. Not only do you typically spend less time in deep sleep, but also you get tired earlier in the evening and wake up earlier in the morning. There are a number of possible rea-

Why do we age?

The exact causes of aging aren't fully understood, but most scientists think that it's due to a combination of factors. Two categories of aging theories exist:

- Programmed theories argue that biological factors, or programs, in your body cause aging to occur on a set timeline. One theory suggests that aging is caused by the programmed decline of your immune system, resulting in disease, and therefore aging and death.
- Damage or error theories suggest that aging is a result of environmental factors

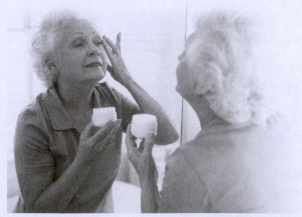

that gradually damage your body and interfere with its normal function. One such theory suggests that the cells and tissues in your body simply give in to wear and tear over time.

Before you begin

You can exercise at any age — even if you've never previously exercised. However, before you jump into an exercise program, it's wise to pay a visit to your doctor. He or she may perform a physical exam and can recommend an exercise program. This is a good time to ask whether any medications you're taking may affect your exercise plan. Seeing your doctor is especially important if:

- You've been inactive for some time
- You have a family history of heart disease
- You have heart or lung disease
- You have high blood pressure, diabetes, arthritis or asthma
- You smoke
- You're unsure about your health

sons for this. Changes in your activity level and health can disrupt your sleep schedule. Chronic pain, depression, anxiety and stress also are common culprits. Medications, including some antidepressants, high blood pressure medications and steroid medicines, also can interfere with sleep. Daily physical activity can help you sleep better at night. Aim to finish a workout at least two hours before bedtime.

Aging and recovery. If you're in good physical condition before an injury, an illness, surgery or even overexertion, you'll likely recover more quickly. This is especially important as you age, tire more quickly and generally take longer to recover.

Regular exercise can reduce the amount of disability and pain that can occur after an older adult falls. And as was previously mentioned, regular strength training exercises can lessen joint pain and improve physical performance in people with osteoarthritis.

THE PAYOFF

Longevity is affected by some things that you just can't control, such as a family history of various illnesses. But of the things you can control that have proved to both extend life and improve the quality of life, fitness ranks high on the list.

Regardless of your age, the time you invest now in getting and staying fit is likely to pay off in the years to come.

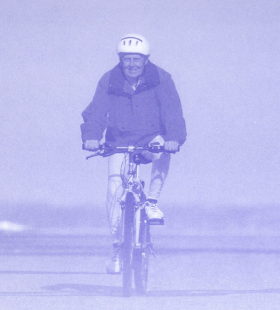

CHAPTER 3

Fitness —

Hundreds of exercises are available to help you reach your fitness goals. Some are exercises designed to strengthen your heart and some are designed to strengthen your biceps. Some exercises build your endurance and some enhance your flexibility. Other exercises can help you stay balanced, and still others help build bone mass. Each may have a place in your exercise program depending on your situation and goals.

Different exercises affect your body in different ways. For example, lifting hand weights may help you build major muscles in your arms (triceps and biceps), but it won't improve your cardiovascular endurance or your flexibility. And walking is great for maintaining balance, building aerobic capacity and strengthening your leg muscles, but it won't necessarily increase your flexibility or strengthen your arms.

For optimal fitness, include these five types of exercise in your program:
- Aerobic
- Strength (resistance)

What's **best** for me

- Core stability
- Flexibility
- Balance

If you're doing the math right now and fear you'll be exercising three hours a day to fit everything in, you'll be happy to hear that many activities include more than one exercise type, and there's no need to do each exercise every day. You can rotate exercises through the week and, often, do two or three types of exercise with one activity.

Some balance exercises, for instance, also help strengthen your core muscles. And many aerobic exercises, such as walking or bicycling, also help build strength in your lower body muscles and help maintain balance. Balance exercises, in fact, can effectively be combined with strength training exercises.

Incorporating these exercises into your lifestyle delivers many benefits (review Chapter 1 if you're still a nonbeliever). But perhaps the greatest reward is that you'll become fit, and that's a powerful thing.

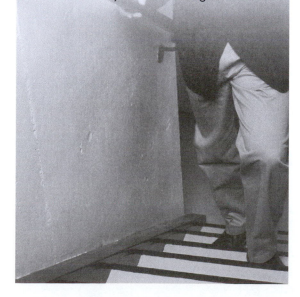

Am I fit?

How do you know if you're reaching your fitness goals? Consider these indicators. You're fit when:

- You have enough energy to enjoy the leisure activities you want to do, from water skiing to walking the dog.
- You have no problem carrying out the daily tasks of your life.
- You can hold a brief conversation while doing light-to-moderate-intensity exercise.
- You can walk a mile without feeling winded or fatigued.
- You can easily climb three flights of stairs.

An overview of each of the recommended types of exercise — aerobic, strength (resistance), core stability, flexibility and balance — is found at the beginning of the "Exercise guide" on page 134. Each section of the guide includes photos of various exercises along with detailed instructions on how to perform them.

AEROBIC EXERCISE

Aerobic exercise — activities during which oxygen plays an important role in the release of energy in your muscles — includes some of the most popular, accessible and fun exercises you'll do.

It includes low-to-moderate-intensity walking, dancing, biking and swimming. For more on how the aerobic system works, see Chapter 2.

No matter what your age, aerobic exercise will help you in your daily activities. It will help your heart, blood vessels, lungs and muscles complete routine tasks and rise to unexpected challenges. It will increase your stamina and endurance so that you can do the things you want to

Choosing the right exercise for you

You want to become more fit, and you know that the best exercise program combines the five types of exercise: aerobic, strength, balance, flexibility and core stability. But which exercises are best for you? Well, that depends. Ask yourself these questions before choosing activities for your exercise program:

- What are my goals? Which exercises will help me meet them?
- What kinds of activities do I enjoy doing?
- What are my limitations? Which exercises can't I do?
- Do I prefer to exercise alone or with others?
- When will I exercise?
- Do I own the equipment necessary to do the activities I enjoy, or will I have to buy equipment or join a health club?

Exercise for healthy joints

If you're worried about joint health or have joint problems that restrict your movement, take into account the degree of strain that each of the following activities puts on your joints:

Easy on your joints
Swimming
Water aerobics
Cross-country skiing
In-line skating
Cycling
Rowing
Elliptical machines

Moderate on your joints
Stair climbing machines
Walking
Hiking
Low-impact aerobics

Hard on your joints
Skipping rope
Running
Aerobics that involve jumping and hard running, such as soccer and basketball

do, whether it's playing hide-and-seek with your grandchildren or training for your first marathon.

Any activity you do — from taking a walk to doing the dishes — requires oxygen. Regular aerobic exercise increases your body's ability to use oxygen. How well you use it is called your aerobic capacity. When your aerobic capacity is high, your heart, lungs and blood vessels efficiently transport and deliver large amounts of oxygen throughout your body. As a result, you can produce more energy and you won't fatigue as quickly.

If you don't get enough aerobic exercise, you may use your entire aerobic capacity while walking up a flight of stairs. You'll get to the top and feel out of breath and in need of a break. On the other hand, if you're fit, you can climb the flight of stairs and then hop on a stationary bike for a 30-minute workout. That's because your aerobic capacity is higher.

Aerobic exercise does far more than increase your endurance. It can increase your life span and improve the overall

Aerobic basics

- A beginning goal is to exercise at least three days a week and work up to at least five days a week.
- Before doing any aerobic activity, warm up for at least five minutes.
- Work toward a goal of exercising for 30 to 60 minutes each day, either continuously or in divided sessions throughout the day.
- Spend at least five minutes cooling down at the end of your workout.
- Do some activity every day, even on busy days. If you can't fit in your regularly scheduled exercise, replace it with another activity.
- Take steps to increase your physical activity each day, even if it's not a scheduled exercise day. Jog in place while waiting for the bus or take the stairs instead of the elevator at work.

Aerobic workouts should include three parts

- **Warm-up.** Before each session, spend five to 10 minutes preparing for exercise. This general warm-up should let you break a sweat but not be too strenuous. If you have a tight or previously injured muscle, also do some stretching of that muscle. Otherwise, save stretching until after your workout. (See "Stretching, flexibility and when to stretch" on page 78.)
- **Conditioning.** Doing at least 30 minutes of aerobic exercise develops your aerobic capacity by increasing your heart rate, depth of breathing and muscle endurance. You'll also burn calories. How many calories you burn depends on how fast and how long you exercise and how much you weigh. The more you weigh, the more calories you'll burn.
- **Cool-down.** After each session, spend about five to 10 minutes cooling down. Stretch your calf muscles, upper thighs, hamstrings, lower back and chest. This after-workout stretch is important because it allows your heart rate and muscles to return to normal. It also helps develop and maintain muscle and joint flexibility.

function of your entire body — helping you feel happier and healthier. And that's just for starters. Consider these benefits of regular aerobic exercise:

- Burns calories. Aerobic exercise burns calories. To burn fat calories, choose an activity that's of low-to-moderate intensity and takes longer, such as brisk walking, swimming or square dancing. Exercise duration, and not necessarily intensity, is the key to weight loss. Combined with a healthy diet and appropriate strength training, aerobic exercise will help you lose weight and maintain your healthy weight.
- Reduces disease. Aerobic exercise reduces the risk of such conditions as heart disease, high blood pressure, stroke, diabetes and some forms of cancer. In fact, a regular walking program can reduce the risk of having a heart attack by up to 50 percent.
- Challenges your heart and stimulates it to grow stronger and become more efficient. Having a strong heart helps you live a longer, healthier life.
- Improves mental health. Regular aerobic exercises release endorphins, your body's natural painkillers. Endorphins help reduce stress and anxiety, increase your self-esteem, boost your mood and help fight depression.

How much aerobic activity is enough?

To achieve the heart-healthy benefits of physical activity, try to exercise at an intensity that feels somewhat hard or hard. How do you know if you're working at a somewhat hard level? Watch for these signs:

- Your breathing has increased.
- You're developing a light sweat.
- You're feeling some strain in your muscles.
- You sense you're working at over 50 percent of your maximum capacity.
- You can speak in brief sentences but can't sing a song.
- You're reaching your target heart rate. To calculate your exercise heart rate, use the following formula:
1. Estimate your maximum heart rate: 220 - your age = maximum heart rate.
2. Determine your lower limit exercise heart rate by multiplying your maximum heart rate by 0.6: maximum heart rate x 0.6 = lower limit exercise heart rate.
3. Determine your upper limit exercise heart rate by multiplying your maximum heart rate by 0.85: maximum heart rate x 0.85 = upper limit exercise heart rate.
4. Your exercise heart rate range is between your lower (60 percent of maximum heart rate) and upper (85 percent of maximum heart rate) limits.

For example, if you're 40 years old, your maximum heart rate would be about 180 beats a minute (220 - 40). Your lower limit exercise heart rate would be around 108 beats a minute (180 x 0.6), and your upper limit exercise heart rate would be about 153 beats a minute (180 x 0.85).

So how do you use this information? While exercising, find your pulse. To do this, place two fingers on the inside edge of your wrist and press gently. Count your pulse for 10 seconds and multiply that number by 6 to determine your heart rate in beats a minute. If it's within the range you calculated above, you're working at about the right level.

- Increases stamina. Although you may become tired during and right after exercise, in the long run, regular workouts increase your stamina and reduce fatigue. They'll also give you more energy throughout the day.
- Helps you sleep better at night.
- Improves muscle health. Aerobic exercise stimulates the growth of tiny blood vessels (capillaries) in your muscles. This not only helps your body deliver oxygen to your muscles more efficiently but also removes metabolic waste products, such as lactic acid. This can lessen your pain if you have chronic muscle pain, fibromyalgia or chronic lower back pain.
- Helps control your appetite.
- Reduces arthritis pain by mobilizing your joints.

Regardless of the exercise you choose, you'll know you're working at the right intensity — and in a good aerobic range — when you're breaking a sweat and breathing faster but are still able to exercise comfortably for 30 to 40 minutes. As a general rule of thumb, you should be able to speak briefly — but not sing — during aerobic exercise.

Examples

The key to a successful and sustained aerobic exercise program is to find activities that you enjoy and can do regularly. You needn't limit yourself to a single activity, such as swimming, for a successful exercise program. Add variety and increase your motivation by trying different types of activity. The most important thing is that you do some form of aerobic activity most days of the week, whether it's dancing, biking or taking a water aerobics class.

To get the most benefit from aerobic activity, keep your heart rate safely elevated for a sustained length of time. And you don't necessarily need to choose strenuous activities in order to improve your endurance. The idea is to start slowly with exercises you enjoy, then work up to a more intense pace as necessary.

Each type of exercise has advantages and disadvantages. For example, walking is an extremely popular aerobic activity that's relatively easy on the joints. But walking burns fewer calories than do some other exercises, such as running, which is more intense. Unfortunately, for some people running may lead to knee or foot pain. Swimming is a low-impact exercise that's easy on both your joints and your muscles because your body weight is supported by water. The downside? It may not be as convenient as walking, and because swimming is not a weight-bearing exercise, it doesn't help prevent osteoporosis. It also isn't a great exercise for weight loss. In studies of land exercises versus swimming exercises at similar intensities, swimmers lost less weight.

Your best bet is to incorporate different kinds of aerobic activities and get the benefits of each. Here's more on a few of the most popular forms of aerobic exercise.

Walking. A brisk walk 30 to 60 minutes most days of the week can help deliver many of the benefits of aerobic exercise.

Even walking slowly can lower your risk of heart disease, although faster, farther and more frequent walking offers even greater health benefits.

When you gradually increase the amount of exercise you do, your body responds by improving its capacity for exercise and your fitness level improves. In just eight to 12 weeks, you may begin to feel noticeable improvements.

To condition your heart and lungs safely, include the following aspects in your program:

■ **Intensity.** Walking doesn't have to be strenuous to be beneficial. But what's a desirable range of exercise intensity for you? Here are two simple tools to find out:

1. Talk test. While you walk, you should be able to talk with a companion but not sing a song. If you can sing, your workout is too easy. If you can't talk, it's too hard. Slow your pace.

2. Perceived exertion. This refers to the total amount of physical effort you experience. Work at a level that feels somewhat hard to you. (See the Borg ratings of perceived exertion scale on page 71.)

Get the most out of your walking program

■ **Make an appointment with your doctor.** If you're over age 40 or have a chronic health problem, talk to your doctor about setting up a safe walking program.

■ **Start slowly.** If you try to do too much too fast, you'll likely wind up with pain and burnout. Instead, walk at a lower intensity for your first two to three weeks. Then gradually increase the intensity and length of your walks. *Lower intensity* means that you're working at about 60 percent of maximum heart rate or 11 to 12 on the Borg ratings of perceived exertion scale. See page 71 for details.

■ **Establish a regular program.** If you simply decide to walk more, you'll likely find that your good intentions go by the wayside when your schedule gets busy. But if you make a commitment to a regular schedule of exercise, you're more likely to continue it. Plan, for instance, to walk Monday, Wednesday and Friday mornings from 6:30 to 7:00 a.m. Write it on your calendar and follow through.

■ **Set goals.** Decide what you want to gain from your aerobic exercise program, then write it down. Make sure your goals are realistic and specific and include short-term as well as long-term goals. Instead of writing, "I want to lose weight," try writing, "I want to lose 5 pounds by the end of this month, and 20 pounds by the end of this year."

■ **Buy the right equipment.** Good shoes are essential for your walking program. Although you don't need to spend a lot of money on shoes designed specifically for walking, do choose shoes that give your feet adequate protection and stability. And after about a year of regular wear — about 500 miles — you'll be ready for a new pair. To see if your shoes are breaking down, line them up side by side. Does either shoe tilt to the right or left? Have the soles started to separate from the uppers? If you answer yes to either of these questions, it's time to buy new shoes. For details on selecting shoes, see Chapter 5.

- **Frequency and duration.** Walk a minimum of three times a week for at least 30 minutes or more for general cardiovascular and health benefits. A good goal is to build up to walking three to four hours a week. If you've never exercised regularly or you haven't exercised for a long time, start at a level that's comfortable for you. It may be no more than five minutes at first. (See "A 12-week walking schedule" on page 46.)
- **Stretch.** Spend a few minutes stretching your muscles before and after your walk. Stretch your back, shoulders and arms in addition to your legs. If your time is limited, save stretching for after your walk.

Running. Like walking, running also is an excellent form of aerobic exercise. And like walking, running doesn't have to be strenuous to have a positive effect. Even when done at low intensity, running is a good way to increase cardiovascular fitness.

Planning is an important part of any running program. Start by deciding on your goal. Do you simply want to increase cardiovascular fitness, or do

- **Dress appropriately.** Loosefitting, comfortable clothes are best for walking. Layers are recommended for most days because you can peel them off as your body temperature rises. Bright colors trimmed with reflective fabric or tape also are good choices. Wear sunscreen, sunglasses and a hat to protect your skin.
- **Don't neglect the stretch.** Make sure to stretch, especially after walking.
- **Stay hydrated.** Drink plenty of water before and after your workout. Carry a water bottle with you if you walk for more than 20 minutes or if the weather is hot.
- **Take safety precautions.** Walk with a partner and only in safe, well-lit areas. Spend time checking out your routes. Avoid a course above your ability level, such as one with steep terrain or uneven surfaces. Avoid trails or paths with cracked or uneven ground or narrow passages. Stay away from busy streets, especially at night, opting instead for sidewalks or walking paths.

- **Pay attention to your body's signals.** Although it's natural to feel some muscle soreness when you first start out or increase the intensity of your program, shortness of breath, a feeling that you can't catch your breath or joint soreness indicates that it's time to slow down. Walking should feel comfortable, not painful. If you have chest pain, chest pressure, heart irregularity or severe shortness of breath during or right after exercise, seek emergency medical attention immediately.
- **Have fun.**
  If your walking program begins to feel like an obligation, take a day off. Then replace your scheduled walk with another activity that you enjoy, such as biking or dancing. You'll still get exercise and be able to return to your walking program refreshed.

you want to run a marathon? Running for 30 minutes three times a week can help achieve cardiovascular fitness, but it won't prepare you to complete a marathon. There are many running programs available in books, in magazines and on the Web. Look for one that increases frequency and intensity gradually over several weeks and that's designed to help you meet your goal.

- **Intensity.** Use the talk test and the Borg ratings of perceived exertion scale as measures of intensity when running. In addition, try to keep your heart rate between 60 percent and 85 percent of your maximum heart rate for optimal aerobic training effect.

- **Frequency and duration.** How often you run will depend on your goal. If you're just starting out, take it easy and build frequency and duration gradually. You may find it works best to run for a few minutes and then walk for a few minutes. Eventually, you'll be running more and walking less.

- **Stretch.** Stretch your legs, back, shoulders and arms. In addition, try to ease into your run by walking first. If your

A 12-week walking schedule

Consider this sample program, in which you slowly progress in the frequency and duration of your walking workout.

Week	Time (minutes)	Days a week	Total hours a week
1	20*	3	1
2	20	3	1
3-4	25	3	1.25
5-6**	30	3-4	1.5-2
7-8	35	4-5	2.5-3
9-10	40	4-5	3-3.5
11-12	40	5-6	3.5-4

*Older adults and people whose fitness is very limited may start out with just five to 10 minutes.
**If the days on which you can exercise are limited, you may choose to continue to walk three or four days a week but gradually extend each walk to 45 or 60 minutes. On the other hand, if you have relatively little time on most days, you may benefit from more frequent but shorter sessions.

This program can be adapted to many ability levels. A beginner might get a sufficient workout from a 10-minute walk around the neighborhood, and a more experienced walker can focus on increasing his or her speed, stride lengths or route, to make the workout more intense. Walking in a hilly area, for instance, may be a good choice for someone looking to boost endurance and build additional muscle tone in his or her legs. Note that walking with hand or ankle weights isn't recommended because adding these weights increases the stress and strain on your body.

time is limited, save stretching for after your run.

Hiking. Essentially off-road walking, hiking is a popular way to get aerobic exercise while enjoying the beauty of the outdoors. Many state and local parks have hiking trails. You may even find some paths marked with distances so that you can more easily track your progress.

Hiking can be as intense a workout as you want it to be. A beginner can stick to short, level trails, and an advanced hiker can attempt a trek through miles of hilly terrain. Hiking helps to increase your endurance as well as your muscle strength and, depending on your route, it works some different muscles than does simply walking.

If you decide to try hiking, consider these safety tips:
- Hike with a friend or your dog.
- Never go hiking after dark.
- Wear comfortable shoes.
- Dress in layers.

How many calories does it use up?

Exercise that's equivalent to burning about 1,000 calories a week significantly lowers your overall risk of a heart attack. This chart shows the estimated calories used while performing various activities for one hour. The figures represent a moderate-intensity level for many activities. The more you weigh, the more calories you use. Note that the figures are estimates — actual calories used vary from person to person.

Activity (1-hour duration)	Calories used 140- to 150- lb. person	Calories used 170- to 180- lb. person	Activity (1-hour duration)	Calories used 140- to 150- lb. person	Calories used 170- to 180- lb. person
Aerobic dancing	416-442	501-533	Racquetball	448-476	539-574
Backpacking	448-476	539-574	Rope jumping	640-680	770-820
Badminton	288-306	347-369	Running, 8 mph	864-918	1,040-1,107
Bicycling (outdoor)	512-544	616-656	Skating (ice or roller)	448-476	539-574
Bicycling (stationary)	448-476	539-574	Skiing (cross-country)	512-544	616-656
Bowling	192-204	231-246	Skiing (downhill)	384-408	462-492
Canoeing	224-238	270-287	Stair climbing	576-612	693-738
Dancing	288-306	347-369	Swimming	384-408	462-492
Gardening	256-272	308-328	Tennis	448-476	539-574
Golfing (carrying bag)	288-306	347-369	Volleyball	192-204	231-246
Hiking	384-408	462-492	Walking, 2 mph	160-170	193-205
Jogging, 5 mph	512-544	616-656	Walking, 3.5 mph	243-258	293-312

For other body weights, you can calculate approximate calories used by selecting the number of calories used from the column for a 170- to 180-pound person. Multiply it by your weight and divide by 175. For example, if you weigh 220 pounds, jogging uses $\frac{656 \times 220}{175} = 825$ calories an hour.

- Carry water in a backpack or waist pack. If you'll be out for more than an hour, carry a snack as well.
- Wear insect repellent and sunscreen. Take extra with you if you'll be out for some time.
- Drink at least 4 ounces of water every 20 minutes in any weather.
- Bring a fully charged cell phone and double-check that you have coverage in the area.
- Know the weather report.
- Tell someone where you're going and when you'll be back.
- Carry flares or some other type of emergency signal.
- Carry a Mylar blanket and a lighter, just in case.

Water exercise. If you want a low-impact activity that exercises your entire body, swimming may be for you. Because swimming is a low-impact activity, it's often recommended for people with muscle and joint problems. If lap swimming isn't your style, consider water aerobics or just walking in the pool. Walking in water about chest-high greatly reduces the impact load on your joints. Water exercise is great for working all of your muscles, and it's easy on your joints. The water's buoyancy prevents falls and helps support you if you have balance problems. The buoyancy may aid circulation in people with lower body blood flow problems or in those who are susceptible to swelling. Both swimming and water aerobics are great for people with arthritis or balance problems. Most local YMCAs, health

Exercise for weight loss

If you want to lose weight, aerobic exercise can play a key role in your weight loss program. Aim first for at least 2 ½ hours of moderate-intensity exercise each week. Once you've achieved that milestone, work toward about 3 ½ hours of moderate-intensity exercise each week. Walking, biking and aerobic dancing are popular and effective exercises for losing weight. A healthy, low-fat diet also plays an important role in weight loss.

Strength training can be a key component of weight loss. During times of increased aerobic activity, particularly when accompanied by reduced calorie intake, your body may break down muscle for energy. Strength training may minimize or prevent this. Additionally, muscle is metabolically active, which means that it burns calories all the time. One way to improve your resting metabolic rate — the amount of calories you need just to stay alive — is to increase your muscle mass through strength training.

Did you know?

- With regular, long-term exercise, you may reach a level of fitness comparable with that of an inactive person 10 to 20 years younger.
- The more vigorously you exercise, the greater the benefits. Add intensity gradually to avoid injury.
- The "no pain, no gain" mentality is outdated. Exercise should feel good. In fact, none of the exercises you do should cause pain.

Interval training

You can shake up your workout and be rewarded with some powerful benefits by interval training. Interval training consists of alternating short bursts of intense activity with less intense activity.

For example, if walking is your exercise of choice, you can add interval training by walking for a few minutes, then running or jogging for a few minutes throughout your workout. If you're less fit, you can alternate walking at a leisurely pace for a few minutes with walking fast for a few minutes. The intensity and length of each interval are up to you and depend on how you feel and what your goals are.

Interval training not only helps you increase the intensity of your workout in a way that doesn't burn you out, but also increases the number of calories you're burning. Perhaps the biggest benefit is the change in routine that adds variety to your exercise program.

clubs with pools and aquatic centers offer a range of water exercise options, from swimming to fitness classes. Many classes are conducted with music and fun routines, which can add variety to your workout.

Although water may be great for toning your muscles and building your aerobic capacity, it may not be the best method to facilitate weight loss. So if weight loss is one of your goals, consider supplementing your water workout with other forms of exercise, such as walking.

Bicycling. Low-to-moderate-intensity bicycling revs up your cardiovascular fitness while strengthening your leg muscles. Biking offers a great deal of freedom, it offers a welcome change of scenery from one session to the next, and it's a good low-impact activity.

If you're worried about traffic or don't care to chance the elements, a stationary bike is a good choice. Stationary bikes can be upright or reclining (recumbent). Though recumbent bikes may be more comfortable for people with back or neck pain and are a good choice for people with balance problems, one type of stationary bike isn't inherently better than another. You can also ride your regular bike indoors when you fit it with rollers. All stationary bikes can be fitted with toe clips that hold your feet in place while pedaling. Toe clips may be of particular help if one leg is weaker than the other or doesn't function properly, as is sometimes the case during recovery from a stroke. Biking may also be a low-impact alternative for people with arthritis who find walking any distance to be painful. See "Biking" beginning on page 282 for a full discussion of exercising with a bike.

Aerobic dancing. This popular exercise is often offered through community education programs, senior centers and gyms. If you'd prefer to work out in the privacy of your home, you'll find a variety of videotapes and DVDs offering aerobic dance instruction.

Low-impact aerobic dance exercises the whole body while you move to music. Classes are usually offered for a variety of levels, although at any time you can alter your movements to whatever intensity you choose. Of course, the intensity will determine the benefits you derive.

Aerobic stepping. Like aerobic dancing, stepping is a popular exercise for people of all abilities. Instruction can be found in community centers and gyms as well as on videotapes and DVDs.

Using a short, stable platform-type bench, exercisers step up and down to music during each session. Low-impact stepping can be a fun, motivating way to exercise — increasing your endurance and lower body muscle strength. Vigorous stepping, on the other hand, provides many of the cardiovascular benefits of running while placing somewhat less stress on the joints.

If you'd like to try aerobic stepping, consider these tips:

- Make sure the steps are at the proper height for your ability level. If you're a beginner, start with a platform height of 4 to 6 inches. Check to make sure that you're not bending your knees more than 90 degrees.
- Keep your neck straight and relaxed.
- Don't lock your knees.
- Practice good posture. Keep your shoulders back and your pelvis tucked under. Exercising in front of a mirror can help you check your posture.
- Don't arch your back.
- Place your entire foot on the platform with every step.
- Don't stomp. Pounding can stress the knees and ankles.
- Don't use hand weights, which can put too much stress on your joints.

If you have trouble keeping up in a stepping class, stop doing the arm motions until you've become acclimated.

STRENGTH TRAINING

When it comes to overall fitness, investing in a set of weights or other strength training equipment may pay dividends just as great as those gained with a pair of walking shoes. The more fit your muscles are, the easier your daily tasks become, whether they include lifting children, shoveling snow or pushing a vacuum cleaner.

Strength training safety

To begin a safe and effective strength training program, follow these guidelines:

- Always use proper form.
- Avoid lower body exercises with weight if you have had a hip or knee repair or replacement. Use the weight of your leg as resistance and discuss how to safely increase resistance with your doctor.
- When using free weights, aim for smooth, steady motions. Don't jerk weights into position.
- Stop if you feel pain. Though mild muscle soreness is normal after doing resistance exercises, sharp pain, sore joints and pulled muscles are signs of injury. Joint swelling, too, is a sign that you've overdone it.
- Don't lock your joints. Keep some bend in your knee and elbow joints while performing the exercises.

Strength training involves the use of free weights, your own body weight, resistance bands or a weight (resistance) machine to increase muscle strength and endurance. Adults of all ages can benefit from strength training. If you're inactive, you can lose up to 10 percent of your lean muscle mass each decade after age 30. If you do strength training, however, you can preserve and enhance your muscle mass.

Strength training can help you in a number of ways. Here's how:

- Strength training increases the strength of your muscles, tendons and ligaments and can decrease your risk of injury.

- Doing strength exercises increases the density of your bones, reducing the risk of osteoporosis. If you already have osteoporosis, strength training can lessen its impact.

- Because strength training contributes to better balance, coordination and agility, it may help prevent falls in older adults.

- Strength training increases your lean muscle mass. This helps to raise your metabolic rate, making it easier to maintain a healthy body weight.

- Those with chronic lower back pain often experience less pain after launching a program to strengthen their lumbar region and abdominal area. For many, this significantly increases their ability to perform daily tasks.

- Strength training helps you perform your daily routine. As you grow stronger, such tasks as doing housework, carrying groceries and mowing the lawn take less effort.

- Regular strength training can improve your mental health and reduce the risk of depression.

- Those who commit to a regular strength training program have less insomnia.

What is it?

What's strength? The ability of your muscles to exert a force. When a force is exerted for more than 30 to 60 seconds, it's considered strength endurance.

What's flexibility? The ability to bend joints and stretch muscles through a full range of motion.

What's your core? Your body's foundation or trunk, linking your upper body and lower body. It includes the rib cage, lower back and abdominal areas. Core stability training includes components of flexibility, strength and balance exercises.

Did you know?

- *Strength training* and *resistance training* mean the same thing.
- Even a previously unfit person can increase his or her strength 50 percent or more in six months with regular strength training.
- During strength training, the order in which you work muscles is important. The recommended sequence is large before small, multiple-joint before single-joint and higher before lower intensity exercises.
- Keeping a daily exercise log of your activity and progress is a great way to stay motivated.

- Strength training can improve your glucose tolerance and insulin sensitivity, lowering the risk of diabetes.
- Strength training has been shown to have a modest effect on decreasing the pressure when your heart is relaxed (diastolic blood pressure).

Examples

You needn't spend 90 minutes a day lifting weights to benefit from strength training. In fact, it's better that you not lift weights every day. Strength training sessions lasting 20 to 30 minutes and done just two to three times a week are sufficient for most people and can result in significant, noticeable improvements in just a few weeks.

Strength training is typically done in four ways — with free weights, body weight, machines and resistance bands or tubing. A fifth method that's also discussed here is called plyometrics. You can choose one method or combine them for greater variety. Before trying any of the following strength training exercises, it can be helpful to spend some time with a professional trainer who can help you design a resistance program and advise you on safety issues.

- **Free weights.** The term *free weights* refers to items such as barbells and dumbbells. These are the basic tools of strength training. Although homemade weights, such as plastic soft drink bottles filled with water or sand may work for you, store-bought weights are best.

  When using weights, make all movements slowly and deliberately. If you experience pain in any of your joints when using weights, reduce the amount of weight or switch to a different exercise. When appropriate, such as when lifting heavy weights, use a spotter, someone who can take the weight from you if you lose control. Examples of strength training with free weights are found beginning on page 150.

Strength training exercises to avoid

Strength training is a powerful way to increase your fitness and strength, but only if it's done correctly. Here's a list of exercises you may want to avoid, and why.

Exercise	Problem
Deep knee bends (beyond 90 degrees)	Strain knees
Jumping jacks	Strain inside of knee joint
Full sit-ups	Not effective for abdominals, strain lower back
Straight-leg sit-ups	May strain lower back
Double-leg lifts	May strain lower back
Donkey kicks	Hyperextend back
Bicycle kicks	Strain neck and back
Squat thrusts	Strain back and knees

■ **Resistance machines and home gyms.** These typically work different parts of your body with controlled weights and resistance. Some have stacked weights, others have bendable plastic pieces, and still others have hydraulic components. Each of these devices works by providing resistance to motion in one way or another. Most gyms will have a selection of resistance machines to work muscles in each of your major muscle groups. Resistance machines often must be adjusted to your height in order to ensure proper form during exercises. Overall, they're considered safe and easy to use. See Chapter 5 for details on choosing equipment that's right for you.

■ **Resistance bands or tubes.** These are elastic-like cords, tubes or flat bands that offer weight-like resistance when you pull on them. They come in different tensions to fit a range of abilities and are usually color-coded by the manufacturer. Resistance bands are very portable and an inexpensive alternative to a home gym and can add variety to your workout. Remember that it's sometimes hard to determine the difference in resistance levels between bands just by using them, so make sure you understand the color coding.

■ **Plyometrics.** Plyometrics training is a specialized form of strength training that capitalizes on the ability of muscles to generate more force after they've been stretched slightly. This slight stretching is sometimes referred to as stretch-shortening. The stretching part of the plyometric movement (loading) can be equated to the stretching of a rubber band, and the shortening part (unloading) to the letting go of the rubber band. Plyometric movements are common in sports such as football, basketball, volleyball, sprinting and other activities that require quick, propulsive muscle responses. Plyometric exercises fine-tune your flexibility and strength to

Single vs. multiple sets

Are you confused about how many sets of strength training exercises you should be doing? Here's a simple answer. For most people, completing one set of eight to 12 repetitions, with the 12th repetition being difficult, is adequate. To progress, you simply increase the resistance. However, for someone who is looking to increase muscle mass and perhaps increase strength even more, adding a second set may be more effective.

Goal	Intensity	Volume
Strength	Moderate-to-high	Low — One set of 8-12 repetitions
Toning	Low-to-moderate	High — Multiple sets of 15-30 repetitions or work for 1-2 minutes at a time
Bulk	Moderate	Moderate-to-high — Multiple sets of 8-12 repetitions

generate large forces in short periods of time to do things such as jump, change direction and throw balls.

In order to successfully perform plyometric motions, you must have adequate flexibility and strength. Consequently, plyometrics are considered advanced exercises that carry a relatively high risk of injury if not performed properly. The most common plyometric exercises include various hops and jumps that train the legs and lower body to absorb shock and generate force to jump, turn sharply and accelerate. Find examples of plyometric exercises starting on page 185.

Regardless of the method of strength training you choose, try to work all of your major muscle groups, including arms, shoulders, abdomen, chest, back and legs at least twice a week. Working each of these muscle groups regularly is important to avoid posture problems and strength imbalances.

You can perform a combination of exercises, but avoid exercising the same muscles two days in a row. Instead, plan to rest at least one full day between exercising each muscle group. This gives your muscles a chance to rest and recover from the workout.

Start with a weight you can lift comfortably eight times and build up to doing 12 repetitions. *Repetitions* refers to the number of times you lift the weight or push against the resistance, if you're using a machine.

Once you have the appropriate weight, lift or push it into place as you count slowly to three. Hold the position for one

Breathing while strength training

Breathing is something you do without a second thought. When you're strength training, however, you *should* spend some time thinking about your breathing.

Breathe normally through each exercise and don't hold your breath or huff and puff from too much strain. In addition, follow this simple guideline:

- Breathe out (exhale) as you lift, pull or push.
- Breathe in (inhale) as you relax.

For example, if you're doing biceps curls, breathe out as you lift the weight and breathe in as you lower it. It will get easier as you practice.

Strength training and women

Some women may be worried about beginning a strength training program because they don't want to end up with large, bulky, bodybuilder muscles. But because of genetics, hormones and women's natural body types, this is unlikely.

Simply put, the average woman doesn't have near the testosterone of the average man and can't build as much large muscle. Even so, women can experience a 20 percent to 40 percent increase in strength after just a few months of strength training. As their strength grows, most women will experience a small increase in muscle mass. If this is a concern, a qualified trainer can modify a resistance program with lower weights and more repetitions to avoid or minimize this effect.

second, then lower the weight as you slowly count to three. Your movements should be unhurried and controlled.

The weight you use should be heavy enough so that on the 12th repetition, you're just barely able to finish it with good form. For most people, a single set of 12 repetitions with the proper weight can build strength just as efficiently as

three sets of 12 repetitions. You don't have to do multiple sets of each exercise to get the benefits.

If you're a beginner, you may discover that you're able to lift only 1 or 2 pounds or less. That's OK. Once your muscles, tendons and ligaments grow accustomed to strength exercises, you'll be surprised at how you progress. Avoid increasing

Aerobic and strength training: A benefits comparison

The table below shows the relative benefits of aerobic and strength training for a number of basic health functions. A plus sign (+) indicates one positive unit of beneficial effect, while dashes (- - -) indicate a unit of neutral effect.

	Aerobic	Strength
Bone mineral density	+ +	+ +
Body composition		
Percent fat	+ +	+
Lean body mass	- - -	+ +
Strength	- - -	+ + +
Glucose metabolism		
Insulin response to glucose challenge	+ +	+ +
Basal insulin levels	+	+
Insulin sensitivity	+ +	+ +
Serum lipids		
HDL*	+ +	+
LDL**	+ +	+
Resting heart rate	+ +	- - -
Heart stroke volume	+ +	- - -
Blood pressure at rest		
Systolic	+ +	- - -
Diastolic	+ +	+
Aerobic capacity (maximal oxygen intake - VO2 max)	+ + +	+
Endurance time	+ + +	+ +
Physical function	+ +	+ + +
Basal metabolism	+	+ +

*High-density lipoprotein cholesterol, the "good" cholesterol

**Low-density lipoprotein cholesterol, the "bad" cholesterol

weight beyond what you can lift with proper form.

You can develop a plan for working specific muscle groups on given days. For example, on Mondays and Thursdays you work your chest, shoulders, quadriceps and triceps — muscles that push. On Tuesdays and Fridays you can work your back, hamstrings and biceps — muscles that pull. Consider these exercises when putting together your strength program:

Exercise	Muscle group
Leg press/squat	quadriceps, gluteals
Hamstring curl	hamstrings
Chest press/push-up	pectorals
Lat pull-down/row	latissimus dorsi
Lateral raise	deltoid
Triceps extension	triceps
Biceps curl	biceps
Crunch	abdominals

As you do your strength training exercises, whether with free weights, weight machines or resistance bands, keep these guidelines in mind:

- Complete all movements slowly and with complete control. If you're unable to maintain good form, decrease the weight or the repetitions.
- Maintain normal breathing patterns, exhaling as you lift and inhaling as you lower the weight. Avoid holding your breath.
- If an exercise causes pain, stop.
- Stretch your muscles before and after your workout. When stretching before strength training, take a few minutes to

warm up your muscles first. For instance, do some light walking while swinging your arms.

- Keep a progress log. Record your maximum strength every few weeks. This is a great motivator.
- Maintain optimal posture at all times with head over shoulders, shoulders over hips, normal low back curve.

Once you've mastered your starting program and you can comfortably lift a weight 12 times to the point of fatigue and do it in good form, you're ready to progress to the next level. A progressive program enables you to gradually increase your muscle strength and size. Here's how to progress:

- **Step 1.** Increase the weight you're lifting by 10 percent, or just enough so that you can lift it only eight times with good form. If you're working with resistance bands, it may be difficult to use this formula. Successive tubes or bands often have resistance differences greater than 10 percent. If you find that making the jump to the next highest band is too difficult, don't force it. Stay with the lower resistance and do more repetitions. You can try to move to the next resistance level later.
- **Step 2.** Once you've mastered the new weight and can comfortably lift it 12 times, progress to the next level.

Even when you've implemented a regular progression program, you'll reach plateaus when it doesn't feel like your strength is increasing. This is normal. During long-term training, your body

The cost of quitting

Even if you've spent years perfecting your exercise program, you can lose the benefits in a mere 12 weeks if you stop exercising. In fact, three weeks of bed rest can result in a 29 percent decline in fitness. That's almost 10 percent a week. The good news is that you can make up for this loss by restarting your regular exercise program.

Did you know?

Focus on the quality — not the quantity — of your movements when exercising to build core stability.

simply can't improve continuously. In fact, you can expect your progress to plateau about every two months. You can limit these plateaus — and the resulting frustration or boredom — by varying your workout every four to eight weeks. Try different exercises, vary the order of your exercises, change the number of sets and repetitions you do, or alter how long you rest between sessions. See Chapter 6 for specific troubleshooting strategies.

It's important to remember that you can use nothing more than your own body weight to engage in strength training. Exercises such as push-ups, chin-ups, abdominal crunches, lunges and squats use your body's weight for resistance and can be done just about anywhere. See the "Exercise guide" beginning on page 134.

CORE STABILITY TRAINING

Core stability training is a type of strength training. It works the muscles at the center of your body. Added benefits of core stability training can be increased flexibility and balance.

The core of your body — the area around your trunk — is where your center of gravity is located. Your body's core links together your upper body and lower body. When you have good core stability, the 29 muscles in your abdomen, pelvis, lower back and hips work together.

Your core is your body's foundation, linking together your upper body and lower body. Core muscles stabilize the rest of your body and provide support to your spine, whether you're moving, standing or sitting.

Developing a strong, solid core gives you increased balance, controlled movement and a stable center of gravity that will help you improve performance. You use core muscles when you reach up to get a glass off the top shelf, bend down to tie your shoes, or swing a golf club.

A strong core can significantly improve your athletic performance. It's the common link between your lower body, where forces are generated, and your upper body, where forces are applied by the upper limbs. For example, with a strong core you'll be better able to hit golf balls, throw softballs, serve tennis balls and shoot basketballs.

A strong core can also combat poor posture and low back pain, especially as you get older. For many, the prevention of low back pain may be the most compelling argument for exercising core muscles. As a result of sedentary lifestyles, it's estimated that 60 percent to 80 percent of Americans will experience low back pain at least once in life. Seventy percent to 90 percent of these people will develop significant back problems. Core exercises can help prevent and treat this problem.

Target your core muscles as part of your overall fitness program. While regular aerobic and strength training exercises also are important, most of these exercises focus on arm and leg strength without necessarily building a strong foundation of core stability. And exercises aimed at firming your abdomen, such as crunches, don't always reach the deep core muscles.

Examples

Building core stability can be a lot of fun with exercises that can add variety to your standard routine. Whichever core exercises you choose, aim to do them three times a week, or every other day.

Essentially any exercise that uses the trunk of your body without support is a core exercise. For example, a push-up stresses your core more than does a bench press, during which the bench is supporting your trunk. As a result, nearly any exercise can be modified to increase your core activity.

It's a good idea to get some personal instruction as you begin a core training program because pinpointing your core muscles takes some practice. Taking a

class with a certified fitness instructor can help you make sure you're using the correct muscles. In addition, a number of videotapes and DVDs are available to help you learn the various exercises, such as these:

Fitness ball workouts. Fitness balls, which look like large, sturdy beach balls, can be used to work the deep core muscles of your abdomen and back.

If you're stocking a home gym, fitness balls are versatile investments. They're also called stability balls, physioballs or Swiss balls — because they were first used in Switzerland many years ago to help rehabilitate people with stroke-related disabilities. These balls not only work the trunk in almost every exercise they're designed for, but also help with balance and flexibility exercises.

When strengthening your core with a fitness ball, you'll want to create a balance between your abdominal muscles and your back muscles by doing exercises that work each equally. This is because if either your abdomen or your back is significantly stronger than the other, your body will be pulled in that direction. This can lead to pain and poor posture. Practicing the proper exercises with a stability ball can help you develop and strengthen all core muscles, alleviating this problem. See page 120 for more precautions on using fitness balls and how to choose a ball that's right for you.

Pilates. With its recent surge in popularity, you might think that Pilates is a hot new exercise fad. In truth, Pilates is a low-impact fitness technique developed back in the 1920s by Joseph Pilates. Designed specifically to strengthen the body's core muscles by developing pelvic stability and abdominal control, Pilates exercises also help improve flexibility, joint mobility and strength. They can help you develop long, strong muscles, maintain a strong back and improve your posture.

Many Pilates exercises are done with special machines. The earliest Pilates machine, called the Reformer, was a wooden contraption outfitted with cables, pulleys, springs and sliding boards. Using their own body weight as resistance, exercisers used the Reformer to perform a series of progressive, range-of-motion exercises that worked the abdominals, back, upper legs and buttocks.

Although machines are still used, many Pilates programs offer floor-work classes as well, designed to stabilize and strengthen the core back and abdominal muscles. Instead of emphasizing quantity, Pilates focuses on quality, meaning that exercisers do very few, but extremely precise, repetitions. Exercises can be adapted according to a person's own flexibility and strength abilities.

Due to its recent popularity, Pilates classes often can be found at community and senior centers, local health clubs and gyms. Interestingly, trademark restrictions once prevented most Pilates instructors from using the word *Pilates* to promote their classes. Now studios from California to New York can promote their instruction as Pilates, making it easy to find classes.

To examine the Pilates approach before committing to a class, you might want to view a Pilates videotape or DVD.

Floor exercises. Some common exercises that you already may be doing, such as squats, step-ups and push-ups, help strengthen your core muscles. See examples beginning on page 173.

Perhaps the two most important deep core muscles are your transversus abdominis (located along your abdomen), and your multifidus (found in your back). You can find and strengthen these key muscles with the following exercises, which require nothing but your body and the floor.

For your transversus abdominis:

1. Lie on your back on a firm surface. Bend your knees so that your feet are flat on the surface.
2. Rest your hands on your hipbones, fingers in front, thumbs in back.
3. Cough. As you cough, you'll feel your transversus abdominis contract.
4. Relax. Then pull your navel in toward your spine, using your transversus abdominis. If you imagine a dot on your navel and a dot in the middle of your back, the two dots should come closer together. This maneuver is called hollowing, as it creates a slight depression in your lower abdomen.
5. Slide one of your heels away from you until the leg is straight. Feel the contraction in your transversus abdominis.
6. Return the leg to its original position and repeat with the other leg.
7. Repeat five to eight times, breathing normally throughout.

For your multifidus:

1. Lie on your stomach with a pillow under your abdomen and pelvis.
2. Contract your transversus abdominis, as with abdominal hollowing.
3. Slightly raise one leg, just barely off the floor. You should feel your multifidus muscle contract.
4. Hold for eight to 10 seconds.
5. Switch legs. Repeat five to eight times.
6. Build up to two to three minutes total.

When doing exercises to build core stability, focus on proper technique, not on repetitions. Perform the exercises in a slow and controlled manner until you're ready to progress to faster movements, while still controlling each exercise. Your breathing should be slow and steady. When your muscles start to fatigue, stop and change exercises. Your goal should be to gradually work up to performing each exercise continuously for three minutes.

FLEXIBILITY EXERCISE

When you hear the terms *flexible* and *agile,* you may think of Olympic gymnasts or world-class ballerinas. But the truth is that everyone is flexible to some degree, and almost anyone can acquire greater flexibility. Flexibility is the ability to move your joints through their full range of motion.

Like many other fitness indicators, flexibility diminishes as you age. But like other effects of aging and inactivity, flexibility can be regained and maintained.

Increased flexibility, which is achieved by regularly stretching muscles, will help improve your daily performance. Routine tasks, such as lifting packages, bending to tie your shoe and hurrying to catch a bus, are easier and less tiring when your muscles and joints have good flexibility.

Consider this list of flexibility's other notable benefits. Flexibility exercises can help you:

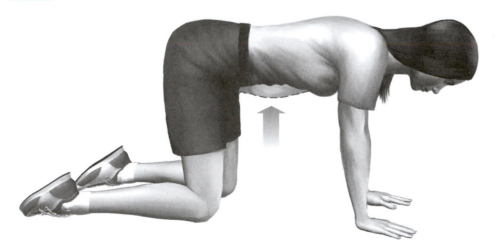

You can exercise your transversus abdominus while lying on your back (described in text), or by getting on your hands and knees as illustrated here. Pull your navel in toward your spine, using your transversus abdominus. Hold, then relax. Repeat five to eight times to build core strength. As described in step No. 4 on page 59, this maneuver creates a depression in your abdomen.

- Relax your body.
- Improve circulation, by increasing blood flow to your muscles.
- Improve your posture. Frequent stretching can help keep your muscles from getting tight, allowing you to maintain proper posture. Good posture can minimize discomfort and keep aches and pains at a minimum.
- Relieve stress. Stretching relaxes tight, tense muscles that often accompany times of stress.
- Improve your coordination. Your movements may be easier and more free, keeping you in better balance and making you less prone to falls.
- Make other activities, such as running or team sports, easier because your body is more prepared for the activity.
- Maintain the flexibility you already have, so you don't become stiffer as you age.
- Reduce your risk of muscle and joint injury. When you improve your flexibility, you can avoid strains and other problems, such as back pain.

Examples

Activities that lengthen your muscles increase your flexibility. Although a regular stretching program is the most common way to increase your flexibility, activities such as swimming, yoga and tai chi also are effective for improving flexibility. Whatever exercise you choose, aim to make flexibility training an integral part of your fitness program.

Yoga, which combines deep breathing,

Fitting stretching into a busy schedule

- Do a few stretches after your morning shower or after you've spent some time in a warm bath. That way, you can shorten or eliminate your warm-up routine because the warm water will raise muscle temperature and prepare muscles for stretching.
- Stretch before getting out of bed in the morning. Try a few head-to-toe stretches by reaching your arms above your head and pointing your toes.
- Sign up for a yoga or tai chi class. You're more likely to stick with a program if you've registered for a class.

Stretching may not be recommended if you have certain types of injuries. For example, strained muscles shouldn't be stretched unless you have been given the OK by your health care professional. If you have an injury or chronic condition, you may need to alter your approach to stretching. Extreme positions or stretches may not be safe for those who've had joint replacement. Talk with your doctor or physical therapist. See Chapter 8 for more information on exercising in the face of medical issues.

Did you know?

- If you have time to stretch only once during exercise, stretch after your workout because then your muscles are warm and more receptive to stretching.
- Do *not* do stretching exercises with your lower body if you have had hip replacement surgery unless your doctor has given approval.

movement and postures, can help reduce anxiety, strengthen muscles, lower blood pressure and help your heart work more efficiently. Yoga's techniques for stretching and strengthening the body can be practiced by people of all ages. Older adults or those with stiff joints may have to adapt some of the traditional poses. If you've had joint replacement surgery, especially hip replacement, some yoga positions may put you at risk of injury and joint dislocation. If you've had such surgery, be sure to talk with your doctor before starting yoga. For more on the different types of yoga, see "Types of yoga" on page 63.

Tai chi. This ancient form of martial arts involves gentle, circular movements combined with deep breathing. Tai chi helps strengthen muscles, improve flexibility and reduce stress. Check martial arts schools for qualified instructors. Health clubs and community centers frequently offer classes with experienced instructors, as well. It's wise to check credentials before taking a class.

Feldenkrais Method. The Feldenkrais Method uses gentle movements to develop increased flexibility and coordination. Though similar to yoga, the Feldenkrais Method doesn't strive for correct positions, but instead aims for more dexterous, painless and efficient body movements. The goal is to create an awareness and quality of movement through your body feedback rather than through pre-defined postures. These techniques often are used in physical and occupational therapies.

In group "Awareness Through Movement" classes, the instructor leads you through a sequence of comfortable, easy movements — sitting in a chair, lying down or standing — that gradually progress with greater range and complexity. In private lessons, called "Functional Integration," the instructor guides these movements through gentle touch.

Certified Feldenkrais practitioners complete a four-year training program approved by the Feldenkrais Guild. To find a certified practitioner, see "Additional resources" on page 344.

Alexander Technique. More than 100 years old, the Alexander Technique is a set of skills that you can use to relieve chronic pain, prevent injury and enhance performance. Like in the Feldenkrais Method, Alexander Technique instructors encourage you to be aware of your movements. But unlike other approaches, such as Feldenkrais, yoga or Pilates, Alexander Technique isn't a set of exercises. Instead, it's a way to heighten awareness of how you move, improve your coordination and become a more intelligent exerciser.

Certified Alexander Technique teachers must complete 1,600 hours of training over a minimum of three years in an approved program. To find a qualified teacher in your area, see "Additional resources" beginning on page 344.

Stretching is a common way to gain flexibility and can be practiced by nearly anyone. It's gentle, easy and can be done almost anywhere. It's truly one of the easiest exercises to work into your routine.

You can stretch:

- Before you get out of bed in the morning
- During work to release tension
- After holding one position for a long period of time, such as sitting at a computer desk
- Whenever your muscles feel stiff or tight

- Whenever the opportunity presents itself, such as when you're reading a book, talking on the telephone or watching TV

Try to incorporate warm-up and cool-down stretches into your aerobic or strength training exercises. A good rule of

Types of yoga

Yoga can be as vigorous or as gentle as you choose, so almost anyone can do it. Although many forms of yoga are slow and calming, other forms are quite strenuous and could be dangerous for beginners. Different styles appeal to different people, depending on their goals and fitness and ability levels.

- **Hatha yoga** is gentle, combining deep breathing with slow stretches and movement through a series of poses.
- **Ashtanga,** also called power yoga, is a fast-paced style designed to build flexibility, strength and stamina. It's an aerobic, athletic form of yoga.

- **Bikram yoga,** also known as hot yoga, is practiced in rooms that can be heated to more than 100 degrees Fahrenheit. It's best practiced by people who are already fit and looking for a new challenge.
- **Kundalini yoga** combines poses and breathing techniques with chanting and meditation.
- **Iyengar yoga** emphasizes mental clarity and precision in doing yoga postures. It uses benches, ropes, mats, blocks and chairs.
- **Svaroopa,** a Sanskrit word that means "bliss," uses postures that focus on the spine and hips.

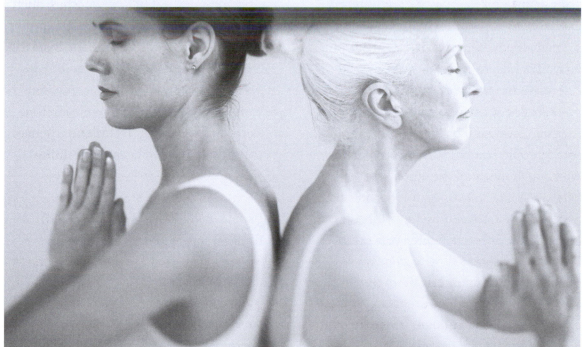

thumb is to spend five to 10 minutes stretching before your workouts and another five to 10 minutes afterward. In addition to stretching before and after aerobic and strength training, you may want to adopt a stretching program. A three-day-a-week program focuses on your body's major muscle groups, including calf, thigh, hip, lower back, neck and shoulder. You may also want to stretch any muscles and joints that you routinely use at work or play. For example, if you frequently play tennis or golf, working in a few extra shoulder stretches loosens the muscles around your shoulder joint, making it feel less tight and more ready for action.

Before stretching, take a few minutes to warm your muscles. Stretching muscles when they're cold increases your risk of injury, including pulled muscles. Warm up by walking while gently swinging your arms, or do a favorite low-intensity exercise for at least five minutes.

Stretching allows you to maximize joint and muscle performance throughout the full range of motion of a joint. Everybody's genetic set-point for flexibility is different, and no matter how hard or often some people stretch, they may not experience much measurable gain in flexibility. With the busy schedules and hectic demands of today, if you have time to stretch only once, do it after you exercise. This is when blood flow to your muscles is increased and the tissues are more flexible.

Stretching techniques are fairly simple and easy to learn. Here are some guidelines to consider:

- Hold your stretches for at least 30 seconds and up to a minute for a really tight muscle or problem area. That can seem like a long time, so use a watch to make sure you're holding your stretches long enough. For most of your muscle groups, if you hold the stretches for at least 30 seconds, you'll need to do each stretch only once or twice.

- When you begin a stretch, spend the first 15 seconds in an easy stretch. Stretch just until you feel a mild tension, then relax as you hold the stretch. The tension should be comfortable, not painful.

- Once you've completed the easy stretch, stretch just a fraction of an inch farther until you again feel mild tension. Hold it for 15 seconds. Again, you should feel tension, but not pain.

- Relax and breathe freely while you're stretching. Try not to hold your breath. If you're bending forward to do a stretch, exhale as you bend forward and then breathe slowly as you hold the stretch.

- Avoid bouncing. This can cause small tears in muscle, which leave scar tissue as the muscle heals. The scar tightens the muscle further, making you even less flexible, and more prone to pain.

- Focus on pain-free stretching. If you feel pain as you stretch, you've gone too far. Back off to the point where you don't feel any pain. That's where you'll want to hold the stretch.

- Avoid locking your joints. Although your arms and legs should be straight, bend joints slightly while stretching.

For more on stretching, see "Stretching, flexibility and when to stretch" on page 78, and the flexibility section of the "Exercise guide" on page 138.

BALANCE EXERCISE

Balance is your ability to control your center of gravity over your base of support. When standing, your base of support is whatever you have on the ground — one foot, two feet or two feet and a cane. Balance is related to your strength, inner ear balance center (vestibular system), vision and sensory input from your feet, as well as muscles and tendons.

Balance is something that you developed when you were a child and practiced when you first learned to walk or ride a bike. The balance required to complete these tasks is often taken for granted in adulthood, but the truth is that if you don't use your balancing skills, you may lose them.

Balance exercises, those activities you do to hone your balance and coordination skills, are beneficial for all people, but especially so for older adults. Poor balance is a major cause of falls, fractures and disability.

As you age, vision problems or conditions such as Parkinson's disease can affect your balance. Arthritis, a disease that often affects older adults, can make you less secure on your feet. A decline in physical activity can result in loss of muscle strength, another factor affecting your

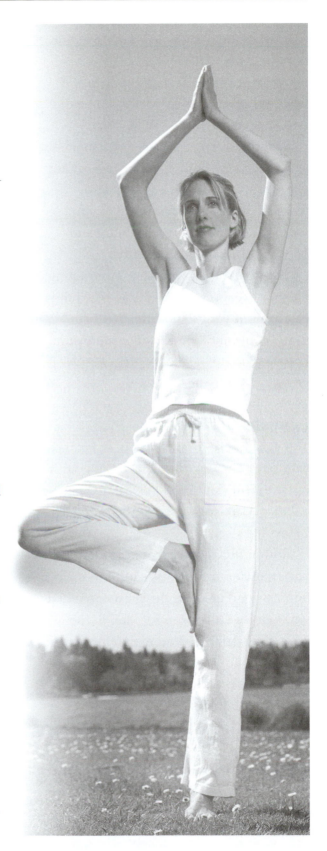

balance. Poor posture and certain medications also may affect your balance. Joint injury or surgery may affect balance. A key part of recovery is performing balance exercises.

Balance exercises can help you maintain your balance — and confidence — at any age. They can help you reduce falls, improve your coordination, give you more confidence in your stability and boost your feelings of security.

When combined with strength training, balance exercises can help you build muscles around your joints, making them more stable and your balance more sure. People who do balance exercises have greater mobility as they age.

Examples

You can choose from a variety of balance exercises. They're often challenging without requiring significant exertion. Specific balance exercises can be found on pages 181 to 184.

Almost any activity that keeps you on your feet and moving is helpful in maintaining good balance. Basic exercises that get your legs and arms moving at the same time can help you maintain your balance in addition to stimulating muscle and nerve communication that increases your coordination.

Muscles and tendons have sensory receptors — called proprioceptors — that play a key role in balance. Proprioceptors sense changes in muscle and tendon tension and pressure and relay that information to the central nervous system.

Proprioceptive training is a specialized form of balance training that deliberately challenges your balance in increments, similar to the way adding more weight challenges muscles in strength training. Proprioceptive training helps increase your ability to balance and to regain your balance. For example, ankle proprioception helps you avoid sprains when hiking on uneven surfaces.

Two-for-ones. One of the best ways to build balance is by walking. So while you're out getting your aerobic exercise with a brisk walk, you're also improving your balance. Walking keeps your leg muscles strong and reinforces your basic balance. The more you walk, the better your balance will be and the more practice you'll get at catching yourself when tripping, changing direction quickly and stepping along uneven trails. No matter how good your balance is, be sure to wear good walking shoes and avoid hazards that may cause falls.

You can also save time by incorporating balance exercises with your strength training. Just add the following variations to strength exercises, such as standing on one leg, using a weight in only one hand, or standing on a pillow or foam pad while performing an exercise. See these exercises beginning on page 181.

For each of these variations, make sure someone is nearby to help you in case you lose your balance, or put yourself in position to hold on to a rail or stable surface if needed.

Tai chi. Tai chi, mentioned earlier as a way to increase flexibility, is also a popular method of improving balance. Tai chi may also help you build stamina and experience greater relaxation.

Tai chi consists of a series of graceful movements that help improve your stance and coordination. You'll learn how to turn your body more slowly. You may also gain more confidence in your movements. Each of these benefits can result in better balance.

Finding an experienced instructor is your best bet for reaping all the benefits of tai chi. If you can't find a class, consider renting or purchasing tai chi videotapes or DVDs. A number of books are available as well, although it may be more difficult to learn the movements that way.

Whether you take a class, rent a video or refer to a book, look for instruction that's geared to your age group or activity level. Start slowly and don't push yourself. Work your way up to trying all of the movements.

Anytime, anywhere. Although it's important to incorporate balance exercises into your regular exercise program, you can also incorporate them into your daily routine. Consider these balance exercises to practice throughout your day:

- Balance on one foot and then the other while waiting for the bus, doing the dishes, brushing your teeth or standing in line at the grocery store.
- Stand up and sit down without using your hands. The nice thing about this exercise is that you'll have a chair right there to catch you if you lose your balance.
- Do the balance walk. Place your heel just in front of the toes of your opposite foot with each step. Make sure your heel and toes touch or almost touch.

Before doing any of these exercises, make sure something steady is nearby that you can use to catch yourself if need be.

THE NEXT STEP

There's a wide variety of exercises from which to choose when deciding what's best for your program. Including aerobic, strength, core, flexibility and balance exercises in your workout can lead to more complete fitness. It may also offer variety that can help you through the occasional slump when you'd rather skip working out. The "Exercise guide" on page 134 has more than 150 exercises with step-by-step instructions.

Creating *your* exercise program

CHAPTER 4

In the first three chapters of this book, you found many examples of why a program of regular exercise can be of great benefit to you. In this chapter, you'll find the help you need to determine how much, how often and what types of exercise may be best for you — and what resources you can use to design a successful fitness plan.

HOW MUCH EXERCISE DO I NEED?

The answer to the question of how much exercise you need varies — and will change over the course of your lifetime. Essentially, the amount of exercise you need is based on some widely accepted guidelines and your specific goals.

Making the decision about the right amount of exercise may seem complicated. Your best friend says her doctor told her that 30 minutes of exercise three days a week is effective. A magazine you picked up last week claims you need to

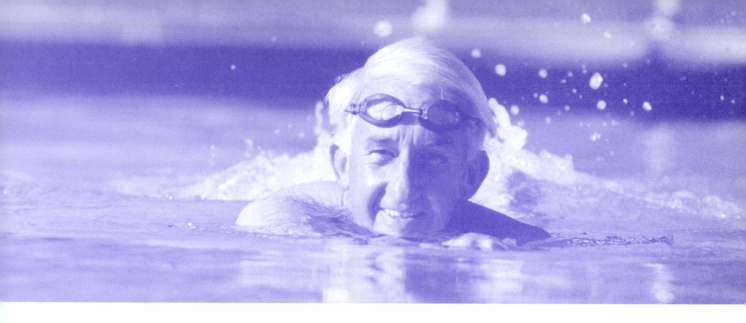

be physically active at least five days a week. And a story on the news last night said everyone should get 60 minutes of physical activity every day. How do you know what to believe?

Clearly this issue can be confusing. Consider the positions of the following reputable sources.

In 1996, the Surgeon General issued a report recommending 30 minutes of physical activity on most days of the week. Most health and fitness agencies agree with this statement. The Department of Health and Human Services says that for general health and well-being, adults should get 30 minutes of moderate activity at least five days a week, or 20 minutes of vigorous physical activity at least three times a week. Children and teens, it contends, should get at least 60 minutes of physical activity a day.

The American Academy of Family Physicians concurs, recommending 30 to 60 minutes of exercise or routine physical activity on most, if not all, days of the week. This exercise can be performed continuously or in smaller increments throughout the day.

Physical activity and exercise — What's the difference?

Though you may hear the terms *physical activity* and *exercise* used interchangeably, they actually mean two different things.

Physical activity is any movement you make that burns calories — from gardening to golfing to taking an afternoon walk.

Exercise is planned, structured and repetitive physical activity that you do to improve your fitness. It may include lifting weights at the gym, taking brisk 45-minute walks each morning or swimming laps at the community center. Plan to do 30 to 60 minutes of moderate physical activity or exercise on most days of the week.

Likewise, the American College of Sports Medicine and the Centers for Disease Control and Prevention state that health benefits can be attained from as little as 30 minutes of moderate-intensity physical activity most days of the week — with greater duration and intensity offering even more benefits.

A bit of controversy occurred in September 2002, when the Institute of Medicine (IOM) issued a report recommending that adults spend at least 60 minutes in moderately intense physical activity every day. Why is the IOM's recommendation higher than others'? The unfortunate trend is that Americans are getting heavier. And evidence shows that 30 minutes of activity on most days of the week may not be enough for some people to maintain an ideal weight and achieve maximum health benefits. The IOM has taken this trend into consideration and factored it into its recommendation.

How intense is it?

How intense is your exercise? Consider this list of generally light, moderate and vigorous activities.

Light (less than 11 on the Borg RPE scale* and 30 percent to 59 percent of MHR**)

Golfing with a cart	Mowing the lawn on a riding mower
Horseback riding	Bowling
Walking slowly at 2 mph	Fishing while sitting
Doing light stretching exercises	

Moderate (11 to 14 on the Borg RPE scale and 60 percent to 80 percent of MHR)

Walking briskly at 3 to 4 mph	Raking leaves
Pushing a stroller 1 1/2 miles in 30 minutes	Shoveling snow
Swimming laps	Washing and waxing a car
Bicycling four miles	Golfing while carrying clubs
Dancing fast	

Vigorous (more than 14 on the Borg RPE scale and greater than 80 percent of MHR)

Chopping wood	Skipping rope
Climbing hills	Surfing
Cycling fast, at more than 10 mph	Playing singles tennis or racquetball
Aerobic dancing	Fishing with waders in a fast-moving stream
Jogging at a 10-minute-per-mile pace	

*Borg ratings of perceived exertion scale. See page 71.

**Maximum heart rate. See "How much aerobic activity is enough?" on page 42 for information on how to calculate your maximum heart rate.

Adapted from Dietary Reference Intakes for Energy Carbohydrate, Fiber, Fat, Fatty Acids, Cholesterol, Protein, and Amino Acids, Institute of Medicine, 2002, and the Surgeon General's Report on Physical Activity and Health

Each of these recommendations tends to support the others. It's apparent that 30 minutes of physical activity most days of the week will deliver health benefits. Getting 60 minutes of activity, on the other hand, will deliver greater benefits — and may be necessary to avoid weight gain.

As you consider these recommendations, keep two things in mind — they're very general in nature, and they pertain primarily to improving and maintaining heart health, general well-being and longevity. If your goals include such things as building muscle mass, improving aerobic fitness and strengthening your bones, you'll need to tailor your program to get the desired results. For example, a good program for building bone mass — and thus preventing or minimizing osteoporosis — combines strength training exercises and weight-bearing activities at least three times a week.

One thing is certain. When it comes to getting the recommended amount of physical activity, establishing a structured exercise program is one of the best ways to do it. A physically active lifestyle is an important component in maintaining your health, but it can be difficult to track. And many activities that you may be tempted to count, such as light housework or walking out to get the mail, aren't intense

Borg ratings of perceived exertion scale

Perceived exertion refers to the total amount of effort, physical stress and fatigue that you experience during a physical activity. It's how hard you feel you're working. A rating of 6 on the Borg ratings of perceived exertion (RPE) scale is the equivalent of sitting in your chair, reading a book. A rating of 20 may be compared to jogging up a very steep hill. Ratings of 11 to 14 constitute moderate-intensity activity.

6	no exertion at all
7	extremely light
8	
9	very light
10	
11	light
12	
13	somewhat hard
14	
15	hard (heavy)
16	
17	very hard
18	
19	extremely hard
20	maximal exertion

For aerobic activity, 11 to 14 on the Borg scale is considered moderate intensity. Copyright 1998 Gunnar Borg.

enough to do substantial good for your body. Plus, studies show that most people overestimate their activity levels throughout the day.

Scheduled exercise, on the other hand, is easier to track. Done for the sole purpose of meeting your body's needs and fulfilling your goals, it's planned, structured and easy to count. You can more easily track your 30-minute walk, your 10-lap swim or your 35 minutes on a stationary cycle than you can your accumulated activity throughout a day's time.

Although a physically active lifestyle is important, for most people a structured exercise regimen is essential to achieving and maintaining optimal fitness. Aim for a minimum of 20 to 30 minutes of vigorous exercise, 30 minutes of moderate exercise or 60 minutes of accumulated moderate activity — including both regular exercise and physical activity — most days of the week.

Physical assessment and exam

For most people, physical activity is perfectly safe. If you're healthy, under 40 and don't have a family history of cardiovascular disease, you can probably begin a regular program of moderate-intensity exercise without a medical examination, even if you haven't been active.

But some people should see a doctor for a physical exam before starting an exercise program. How do you know if you're one of these people? Here's a brief checklist:

- You're a man older than age 40 or a woman older than age 50.
- You have a family history of heart-related problems before age 55.
- You have heart, lung, liver or kidney disease.
- You feel pain in your chest during physical activity.
- You have high blood pressure, high cholesterol, diabetes, arthritis, osteoporosis or asthma.
- You have had joint replacement surgery.
- You smoke.
- You're overweight or obese.
- You're unsure of your health status.
- You're taking medications that may pose problems or need adjustment if you exercise. For example, if you have diabetes, exercise can lower your blood sugar level. As a result, you may need to decrease your medication dose.

If any of the above statements describe you, schedule an exam with your doctor

Warning signs

Moderate activity should cause you to breathe faster and feel like you're working — but it shouldn't cause you pain or exhaustion. If you experience any of the following signs or symptoms during exercise, stop immediately and seek medical attention:

- Chest pain or tightness
- Dizziness or faintness
- Pain in an arm or your jaw
- Severe shortness of breath
- Bursts of very rapid or slow heart rate
- An irregular heartbeat
- Excessive fatigue
- Severe joint or muscle pain
- Joint swelling

before launching an exercise program. Even if none of the statements applies, you may still want to work with your doctor to plan a physical activity program that's right for you.

During your physical exam, your doctor may check:

- **Your height, weight and body mass index (BMI).** Your BMI indicates if your weight is healthy or if you're overweight or obese. (The body mass index chart on page 9 can help you determine whether you're overweight or obese.)
- **Your heart, possibly with an exercise stress test.** This electrocardiogram-monitored exercise test can help identify or verify the presence of heart problems. Most stress tests are done while you exercise on a treadmill. As your heart rate goes up, your doctor measures any abnormalities or signs that may indicate a problem.
- **Your lungs.** It's important to make sure that your lungs are healthy and prepared to handle the task of increased and heavier breathing.
- **Your vision and hearing.** If you plan to exercise outside, you need to be able to detect potential dangers posed by traffic and other environmental factors.

Your doctor will also likely take an exercise history and make exercise recommendations based on your goals and fitness level. If you have access to a health club or fitness center, your doctor may also suggest that you check with an exercise physiologist or other exercise specialist to help you start your program.

Take advantage of this appointment to talk with your doctor about any of your pains, limitations or other health concerns. If you have balance problems, for instance, ask about how they will affect your workout and what you might do to alleviate those problems. Ask about specific types of activities you're interested in to see if you should take precautions.

If your doctor discovers health problems or limitations, you'll probably still be able to exercise. See Chapter 8 for more on exercising with medical problems.

Even if you don't need to make a visit to your doctor before starting an exercise program, it's a good idea to have a physical fitness assessment. You can assess your own fitness by using the personal fitness assessment on page 75. The numbers you record will give you benchmarks against which to measure your progress. To gauge your improvement, retake the personal fitness assessment every 4 to 6 weeks.

If you would like to get a professional fitness assessment, contact a personal trainer, a certified fitness specialist at a local health club, or your doctor. He or she can determine your current fitness level and help you create a plan for improving it.

Begin your assessment

The American College of Sports Medicine recommends that you assess your aerobic fitness, muscular fitness, flexibility and body composition. To do this, you'll need a stopwatch or a watch with a second hand, a cloth measuring tape, a yardstick, masking tape and someone to help you.

Record in a notebook or other convenient place the date you complete the assessment and your scores. Compare your scores every four to six weeks to see how far you've come.

Aerobic fitness — 1-mile walk

Practice counting your heart rate (pulse) before you get started. To find your pulse, turn one hand palm up and place the index and middle fingers of the other hand on the underside of the wrist of your upturned hand. Feel your pulse toward the outside of your wrist below the base of your thumb (see image below). When you feel your pulse, count the number of pulses in 10 seconds. Multiply this number by six to get your heart rate per minute — for example, 13 x 6 = 78 beats a minute. Or simply count your pulse for six seconds and add a zero to the number.

When you're confident of your ability to count your heart rate, it's time to get ready for your walk. Take your pulse before you walk and write down your heart rate per minute. Then start your walk. After you complete a mile, check your watch and record the time

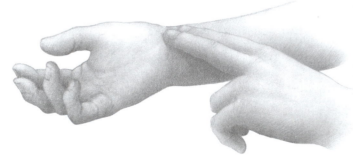

it took in minutes and seconds. Then check your pulse. Record your heart rate per minute.

Muscular fitness — Push-ups

If you're just starting a fitness program, do assisted, or knee push-ups. For instructions on how to do assisted push-ups, see page 158 of the "Exercise guide." Count each time you return to the starting position as one push-up. Using good technique, continue lowering and raising your body until you need to stop for rest. Record how many push-ups you complete.

If you're able, do regular push-ups instead of assisted push-ups.

Flexibility test — Sit and reach

The sit-and-reach test measures the flexibility in the backs of your legs and hips and in your lower back. To get a full assessment of the flexibility (range of motion) of all your joints, you'll need to see a physical therapist or athletic trainer.

Secure a yardstick to the floor, placing a piece of tape across it at the 15-inch mark. Sit upright alongside the yardstick with your legs out in front of you. Place the soles of your feet even with the 15-inch mark. Ask someone to place his or her hands on top of your knees to hold them in place. Then reach gently forward as far as you can, holding the position for two seconds. Write down the distance you reached. Rest. Repeat the test two more times. Record the best of three reaches.

Body composition — Measure your waist

To determine whether you're carrying too much weight around your abdomen, measure your waist circumference at the level of your navel. Record your waist circumference with your other fitness scores. A measurement of more than 40 inches in men and 35 inches in women signifies increased health risks, especially if your body mass index is between 25 and 35.

Body mass index

Your body mass index (BMI) is a measurement based on a formula that takes into account your height and weight in determining whether you have a healthy percentage of body fat. See page 9 for how to determine your BMI.

Make sure you keep track of your progress. Assess and record your fitness scores every four to six weeks. Celebrate your progress.

Personal fitness assessment form

As you begin an exercise program, you'll probably have a few questions. You may wonder what your fitness level is, where you most need to improve and what kinds of exercises will best help you reach your goals.

The personal fitness assessment worksheet below can help you answer each of these questions. Fill in the blanks before the first time you exercise and every four to six weeks after you've started regular activity. Based on your results, you'll be able to get a big picture of your strengths and weaknesses that will help you design an exercise program and set appropriate goals. The purpose of an assessment worksheet is to establish a benchmark as you begin your fitness program and to track your progress over time.

Date	Pulse rate before 1-mile walk	Pulse rate after 1-mile walk	1-mile walk time	Push-ups (number)	Sit and reach (inches)	Waist (inches)	BMI*

*See page 9 for how to determine your BMI.

Setting goals and priorities

You've received medical clearance from your doctor, and you've assessed your current level of fitness. Now you're ready to create your exercise program. The first step is to set some goals. Outlining your goals and establishing exercise priorities will help you shape your program and increase your chance of success.

Both performance and outcome goals are important parts of an exercise plan. Performance goals help you focus on specific activities — such as aerobic, strength training and flexibility — that produce fitness. Outcome goals help you achieve your desired level of fitness — being able to jog a mile or climb the stairs at the office without becoming short of breath.

Reaching your fitness goals

It's great that you've set appropriate fitness goals. But how long will it take you to reach those goals? How fast you improve is largely determined by how fit you are at the start and your current activity level.

When starting an exercise program, if you're relatively unfit, you may experience a dramatic improvement, such as 3 percent a week, during the first month. During the second month, you may improve at about 2 percent a week. You may slow to about 1 percent a week or even less in the following months. This is normal. To fight the boredom you might feel when hitting an exercise plateau, try mixing up your workout with different exercises or set goals for muscle groups that you haven't been using regularly.

Try these goal-setting tips:

- Be specific. Set goals that can be clearly measured. Instead of simply aiming to improve muscular strength, decide to develop a safe strength training program and perform it 30 minutes three times a week for four weeks.

- Set initial goals for a few weeks at a time, and then measure your success based on the specific performance criteria you've set for yourself. If you don't perform at your anticipated level, try to determine what's keeping you from meeting your goals. Perhaps you planned more time than you could realistically commit to, or you needed equipment for which you hadn't planned. These factors are within your control, and you can modify your plans so that you'll increase the chances of meeting your goals in the weeks ahead. For more on reaching your goals, see Chapter 6.

- After you've met your performance goals for several weeks, you may want to consider a big-picture plan. Detail your performance goals for six and 12 months and beyond.

- Write your goals in a journal or on a calendar and experience the satisfaction of crossing them off as you meet them.

YOUR EXERCISE PRESCRIPTION

At the beginning of Chapter 1, you were introduced to the idea of exercise as a drug — something that has many health benefits when taken in regular doses. As a drug, exercise is inexpensive. In fact, getting your regular dose of exercise is one of the least expensive and most important preventive measures you can take to contribute to your good health. Of course, like any drug, exercise must be prescribed appropriately and taken according to your doctor's instructions. Consider the following guidelines:

Prescription. Your prescription can include a range of exercises. For your exercise program, choose activities that you enjoy and will be able to do regularly. You'll be happy to learn that almost anyone can reach his or her goals by doing activities that he or she enjoys. For instance, if running isn't your thing, aerobic dancing may suit you. If you're uncomfortable lifting weights, resistance bands or tubing may be more to your liking. The key is to experiment until you find activities that you enjoy doing regularly.

For many people, variety is the key to a successful program, so don't limit yourself to the same aerobics video or walking trail day after day if you don't want to. For details on training for a particular sport, see Chapter 9.

Your prescription may include exercises from each of the following groups, many examples of which are found in the "Exercise guide," beginning on page 134.

- **Aerobic exercises.** Aerobic exercises use low- to moderate-intensity continuous motion to increase your breathing and heart rate and improve your cardiovascular fitness — the health of your heart, lungs and circulatory system. Aerobic activities cover a range of exercises, including walking, biking, swimming, hiking and aerobic dancing.

- **Strength (resistance) exercises.** Strength exercises build your muscle strength and endurance, which in turn help improve your posture, balance and coordination. These exercises involve working with resistance (pulling or pushing against a force) to increase muscle force-generating capabilities. These exercises can also help build muscle size and improve definition. Activities include lifting free weights, using weight machines, working with resistance bands and using your body weight in exercises like push-ups.

- **Core stability exercises.** A subset of strength training exercises, core stability exercises strengthen and stabilize your trunk muscles. Building strength in these muscles supports your spine, improves posture and balance, promotes better sports performance and may help prevent back injury. Examples of this type of activity include fitness ball exercises and Pilates.

- **Flexibility exercises.** Flexibility exercises increase your range of motion, make your muscles more limber and may help reduce the risk of injury. They also improve your posture and aid in your body's recovery from vigorous activity or exercise sessions. Activities which improve flexibility range from simple stretching exercises to yoga. See "Stretching, flexibility and when to stretch" on page 78.

Stretching, flexibility and when to stretch

Stretching is a way to improve the flexibility of your muscles by lengthening muscle tissues and training your muscles to relax. If you have a tight muscle, increasing its flexibility may improve posture, relieve pain or improve performance.

Stretching can be done in a number of ways, including different types of stretching exercises (static, dynamic and contract-relax), as well as yoga or tai chi. If you have a tight or previously injured muscle, try to stretch before you exercise to balance your body, to promote unrestricted movement and to reduce the chance of overstressing or injuring the muscle. Typically, a short 5-minute aerobic warm-up followed by two to three repetitions of static stretches for that muscle is sufficient. During a static stretch, you move the muscle into a lengthened position until you feel tension of the stretch, then hold it there for 30 to 60 seconds.

Following this, start your activity, being sure to spend the first 5 to 10 minutes slowly increasing the speed and amplitude of your motions. This activity specific warm-up is what's called a dynamic stretch, because it involves a motion rather than holding a position.

Stretching muscles that aren't tight or at increased risk of injury probably isn't necessary. Therefore, focus your pre-activity stretches on muscles that are tight, previously injured or otherwise have been identified as at risk of injury by a qualified health professional.

After your exercise routine, once again stretch the same muscles you did during the warm-up. In addition, it's recommended that you stretch the muscles that were particularly active during the exercise session. For example, if you went for a jog, stretching your calves after the run is recommended.

Most individuals can maintain and improve flexibility with a combination of static and dynamic stretches as discussed above. Contract-relax stretches are more difficult to perform correctly and should be prescribed by a qualified health care professional.

■ **Balance exercises.** Balance exercises help you maintain balance, reducing your risk of falls and injury. They also help improve performance. Activities include tai chi, yoga, weight shift and single-leg balance reach exercises. Many strength training exercises can be modified to improve balance. See the "Exercise guide," beginning on page 134, for examples and illustrations.

Dose. When your doctor prescribes a medication, you receive a certain dose, which indicates the strength of the drug. In exercise, the equivalent is intensity. The intensity at which you exercise reflects the amount of oxygen your body uses to do an exercise and the number of calories you burn while doing it. In aerobic exercise, intensity translates into how hard the exercise feels to you. In strength training, intensity also refers to the amount of resistance that you're overcoming relative to the maximum amount of resistance that you're able to overcome.

As a general rule, moderate-intensity exercise is best. In fact, strenuous exercise doesn't provide many additional fitness benefits, and it may put you at increased risk of muscle or joint soreness or injury. Moderate-intensity activity decreases these risks and may even increase your odds of continuing your exercise program in the long term.

Moderate-intensity exercise should feel somewhat hard for you. How do you determine that you've reached this stage? When it comes to aerobic exercise, you can try one of these three tools — heart rate (pulse), the perceived exertion scale and the talk test.

Heart rate. The more intense your aerobic exercise is, the higher your heart rate will be. When you exercise as hard as you can, your heart beats at its maximum rate. Most people should exercise at a level that puts their heart rate at 60 percent to 85 percent of their maximum. This is called the target heart rate, and you can calculate yours by following the steps on page 42.

If your heart rate falls between 60 percent and 85 percent of your maximum, you're working at a moderate to moderately high intensity.

If you're on certain medications, you may not be able to use your heart rate as an intensity indicator. Talk to your doctor to see if this is the case for you, and, if so, use one of the following rating scales to determine the intensity of your workout:

Perceived exertion scale. Perceived exertion is how hard you feel (perceive) that you're working. It takes into account the total amount of physical effort you experience during an exercise. To help you better gauge your overall feeling of exertion, the "Borg ratings of perceived exertion scale" shown on page 71 helps you give a rating to your total perceived effort.

Talk test. This is the simplest tool for assessing your aerobic exercise intensity. While exercising in the recommended moderate-intensity range, you should be able to carry on a conversation of brief sentences. You want to be able to talk, but not to sing a song.

When it comes to strength training, you're working at a somewhat hard or hard intensity when:

- You're barely able to finish lifting the weight with good form during the 12th repetition.
- You're developing a light sweat.
- You're feeling a sense of strain in your muscles. Note that though you should feel muscle strain, you shouldn't feel muscle pain.

Perhaps the most important thing to remember when it comes to intensity is that exercise doesn't necessarily have to

Exercise terminology

duration. How long a period of time you exercise.
frequency. How many days a week you exercise.
intensity. How hard you work, as measured by percentage of maximum heart rate, Borg ratings of perceived exertion scale and percentage of maximum effort.
mode. The type of exercise — aerobic, strength training, balance, flexibility, core stability.

be vigorous or strenuous in order to be good for you, and it shouldn't be painful. In fact, if you exercise too vigorously, you actually run the risk of overtraining — not unlike overdosing a drug — and succumbing to injuries. Alternate hard, more intense workout days with easier, less intense days. And don't forget to give your body a chance to rest between those more intense activities.

Dosage. If you're over 40, have a chronic condition, are overweight, have recently had surgery or are making a significant lifestyle change, talk with your doctor about the exercise dosage, or frequency, that's best for you. If you don't fit into any of these categories, the frequency that's best for you will depend on your goals, your schedule and the guidelines that follow.

As a general rule, start by exercising three times a week on nonconsecutive days. As you progress, you can increase the frequency of your exercise sessions to four to six times a week to deliver even greater benefits and improvements. If you choose to exercise more than four days a week, alternate between low-intensity and high-intensity exercise from day to day. There's such a thing as too much exercise, and your body needs time to rest, recover and grow stronger. Take at least one day a week of rest from your formal exercise program — though certainly continue your active lifestyle. For more on overtraining, see Chapter 6.

The established guidelines for how often to do each of the recommended five types of exercise are as follows:

- **Aerobic.** Start with three days a week, adding more days when you're ready. When your program is in full swing, you'll be getting at least 30 minutes of aerobic exercise most days of the week.
- **Strength training.** Add strength training to your workout two to three days a week for about 20 to 30 minutes each session. Aim to work your major muscle groups twice each week, including arms, shoulders, back, chest and legs. If you do your strength training exercises on the same day as your aerobic exercises, consider doing the highest priority part of your workout first. For example, if building muscle mass is your primary goal, do your strength training first, then your aerobic workout. This will allow you to put your maximum energy into the strength training portion of your workout.
- **Core stability.** Do this subset of strength training two to three times a week. Aim to target core muscles at the same time you do your other strength training exercises.
- **Flexibility.** If flexibility is a priority for you, make stretching a part of your program. Spend time stretching after a brief aerobic warm-up before you exercise. You may want to do specific stretches for problem areas, followed by a warm-up of about 60 percent effort using the motions you'll use while exercising. In addition, consider stretching problem areas and the muscles you worked during your cool-down after exercise. Consider adding to your week-

ly exercise program yoga or tai chi sessions, which improve flexibility.

- **Balance.** You may not need to schedule individual sessions for balance exercises, unless you want to. You can incorporate them into your aerobic (walking), flexibility (yoga or tai chi) or strength training (certain floor exercises) exercises. Balance exercises also can be included in your daily routine. For example, you might practice standing on one leg while waiting in line at the grocery store, doing the dishes or watching television.

Modifying your prescription when combining different types of exercise. Some activities can be used to fulfill more than one of your basic requirements, which means you can get two or three different types of exercise from a single activity. For example, in addition to being a popular aerobic exercise, walking also builds strength and endurance in your leg muscles and improves your balance. Strength training exercises are also versatile. Exercises that strengthen your core, for example, can also improve your balance. Doing many repetitions of low-intensity strength training exercises can count as aerobic exercise, too. Ultimately, this means you save time — doing in 30 or 40 minutes what might otherwise have taken you 60 or 70 minutes to complete.

DESIGNING A WORKOUT PLAN

It's good to adopt an active lifestyle, but it's also important to develop a regular, scheduled program of exercise. Combine the two, and you can't go wrong. Use this section to help you determine what kinds of activities are best for you and to learn about some important considerations that will help shape how you exercise.

As you've learned by now, a good exercise program incorporates aerobic, strength training, flexibility, balance and core stability exercises. As you choose activities from each of these exercise groups, don't forget some other important considerations, including scheduling enough time to exercise and finding an appropriate location, whether that's your living room or the local health club.

Consider what you want to accomplish. The exercises you choose and how often you do them will depend on your goals and resources. If your goal is to lose weight, you'll need to choose different exercises and intensities than if you're training to run a marathon. Consider these guidelines for different kinds of goals:

- **Attain general health and longevity benefits.** If your goal is to ward off disease, improve your heart health, maintain your healthy weight and have increased energy, you'll benefit from about 30 minutes of exercise or 60 minutes of accumulated activity on most days of the week.
- **Build strength.** Do strength training exercises — lifting free weights, using weight-training machines or resistance bands, or doing exercises using your own body weight for resistance — two to three times a week. Choose a resistance that

Exercise prescriptions for common conditions

	Mode of exercise	Intensity	Duration	Frequency
Cardiovascular disease	Aerobic and strength training	Moderate	30 to 60 minutes	3 or more days a week
High blood pressure	Aerobic and strength training	Moderate	30 to 60 minutes	3 or more days a week
Osteoporosis	Weight-bearing, aerobic and strength training	Moderate	30 to 60 minutes	3 or more days a week
Overweight, obesity	Aerobic and strength training	Low to moderate	60 minutes	5 to 6 days a week

Note: Be sure to see your doctor before beginning any exercise program if you've been diagnosed with any of these or other serious medical conditions.

allows you to complete eight to 12 repetitions in good form. Do at least one set of eight to 12 reps for each major muscle group. Make sure to include at least one day of rest between each session. Once you master a weight — so that you can comfortably lift it 12 times — increase the weight by 5 percent to 10 percent. Continue moving up in weight gradually. For details on toning muscles and adding bulk, see "Single vs. multiple sets" on page 53.

- **Lose weight.** To lose weight, work up to exercising five to six times a week. As you do this, you may want to alternate with different kinds of exercise in order to prevent boredom. As you increase how much time you spend exercising (your training volume), you may need to decrease the intensity of your workouts. For maximum weight loss, aim for a program that combines aerobic and strength training 60 minutes a day five to six days a week. And, of course, pay close attention to your diet.

- **Lower blood pressure.** Regular aerobic exercise can reduce blood pressure by an average of 10 millimeters of mercury (mm Hg), which in turn can reduce the risk of cardiovascular disease and stroke. Therefore, your goal should be to get 30 to 60 minutes of moderately intense activity most, if not all, days of the week. Plan to keep it up, too — you'll achieve these benefits only as long as you keep exercising.

- **Prevent or minimize osteoporosis.** Combine strength training, weight-bearing and flexibility exercises to achieve this goal. Do strength training exercises up to three times a week, weight-bearing exercises, such as walking, jogging or step aerobics, most days of the week, and flexibility exercises whenever you work out. When stretching, focus on the abdominal, chest wall and shoulder muscles, as well as the hamstrings and quadriceps in the legs. If you have osteoporosis, it's important that you talk with your doctor first, before beginning an exercise program (see Chapter 8).

- **Avoid or manage diabetes.** Exercise at least 30 minutes a day most days of the week. Do low- to moderate-intensity aerobic activity, such as walking, bicycling or swimming. Strength training can aid in losing fat and building muscle tissue, which can have a positive effect on blood sugar levels and insulin sensitivity.

- **Overall health.** Finally, when designing your program, take into consideration your age, fitness level, overall health, skills and resources. Thinking ahead and making a well-rounded plan will increase your chance of success.

As you work on developing your own exercise program, spend some time reviewing the following points. From warm-up to recovery time, they'll each play a part in your workout.

Warming up and cooling down

Whatever your physical activity, no training program is complete without a proper warm-up before exercise and a cool-down afterward. Warming up and cooling down help reduce the risk of injuries and muscle damage.

A warm-up prepares the body for exercise. It gradually revs up your cardiovascular system, increases blood flow to your muscles and raises your body temperature.

Start your workout with a few minutes of low-intensity, whole-body exercise, such as walking, light jogging or pedaling on a stationary bike. It's often most convenient to choose a low-intensity version of your planned activity. For example, if you're biking, warm up by cycling at a slow pace.

After this light activity, do any necessary stretches that are appropriate that target problematic areas.

Immediately after your workout, take time to cool down. This gradually brings down the temperature of your muscle tissue and may help reduce muscle injury, stiffness and soreness. Mild activity following exercise also prevents blood from pooling in your legs.

Tight muscles

Muscles get tight for a variety of reasons, including overuse, strain or injury. Even normal, repetitive activity may cause small amounts of damage (microtrauma) in a muscle that can lead to tightness over time. A tight muscle may restrict motion and impair performance, and can cause mild discomfort to significant pain during use. Your doctor may tell you that you have a tight muscle, or you may simply experience it while stretching. In general, you should be able to move all your joints through your desired range of motion without significant muscle resistance or pain. If you can't, then you're tight.

When stretching tight muscles, be sure not to go beyond what's comfortable. And if the tightness persists, see your doctor.

Cooling down is similar to warming up. After your workout, walk or continue your activity at a low intensity for five to 10 minutes. If you've been jogging, walk for about five minutes. If you've been playing basketball, you might cool down by shooting free throws. Follow this with stretching or flexibility exercises that are specific to your sport.

Building in recovery time

When planning your exercise routine, schedule time for recovery — the amount of time your body needs to rest and recuperate after exercise. If you ignore your body's need for recovery, you may wind up with sore or injured muscles and joints, or worse.

As you grow older, you'll likely need more time to recover from strenuous or long-lasting activity. Listen to your body and experiment with schedules that work for you. For more on recovery time, see Chapter 6.

Cross-training

Many people launch their exercise programs with a primary activity, such as walking or biking. This is an excellent first step, but it can pose a couple of challenges down the road. First, you may lose interest. And second, you may overuse or strain the muscles and joints you're using most often. When you use the same muscles and joints every day, you may cause considerable wear and tear while ignoring or underusing other muscle groups. When you cross-train, you select a differ-

Avoiding sore muscles

There's a name for that stiff pain you may feel a day or two after you push a little too hard during exercise. It's called delayed-onset muscle soreness, and it can be avoided. The secret is gradual progression. As you increase the intensity, frequency and duration of your exercise, do so in slow, conservative steps.

For example, those who aren't used to exercising with weights should start with lifting light weights just two times a week for the first month, then gradually build up to heavier weights and more days a week. Likewise, longtime exercisers who are looking to increase their workouts or try something new should begin slowly and work their way up.

ent mode of exercise than you normally use, but something that offers similar benefits. For example, instead of jogging three miles, you might cross-train on an elliptical machine to get a similar aerobic effect without the impact of running. For details on cross-training, see Chapter 6.

GETTING PROFESSIONAL ADVICE

Whether you're a seasoned athlete or a first-time exerciser, calling on the advice of fitness professionals can be a good idea. Whether you're getting feedback from a personal trainer or consulting with a certified instructor at the local YMCA, experienced professionals can help you reach your goals in a safe and efficient way.

Personal trainers

You needn't be rich or famous to have a personal trainer. Trainers can help you achieve your fitness goals, no matter what your age or fitness level.

Personal trainers play many roles. They can help create exercise programs, increase fitness, oversee workouts, provide motivation and even help you lose weight. A personal trainer can work with your doctor to help determine the best program for your needs and to modify that program to fit your resources.

You can choose how often you work with a trainer. Some people prefer to have supervision two or three times a week, while others see a trainer every couple of months — using the time to update their exercise programs or get feedback on their progress.

If you're just beginning to exercise or restarting an exercise program, working with a trainer for just a few sessions may help you get in gear. In just a few hours, you can have a trainer evaluate your fitness level and personalize an exercise program based on that level and your goals.

When you're ready to launch your exercise program, a personal trainer can give you a detailed orientation on the different parts of an exercise program and teach you how to use exercise equipment safely and properly.

Before hiring a personal trainer, find out the answers to these questions:

- Will the trainer provide you a list of references?
- Does he or she have liability insurance?
- What is the cost? Rates typically vary depending on the length of the session and the trainer's experience. Expect to pay $50 an hour or more.
- Does the trainer seem genuinely interested in helping you?
- Can the trainer work with your schedule?
- Is the trainer friendly, positive and likeable?
- Will the trainer assist with special needs?
- Is the trainer certified by a nationally recognized agency, such as the American Council on Exercise, the National Strength and Conditioning Association or the American College of Sports Medicine?

Physical therapists

If you have musculoskeletal problems, such as joint pain, or have recently undergone certain kinds of surgery, you may choose to work with a physical therapist. Physical therapists are trained to teach exercises that will help you overcome injuries and get you back on your feet.

Ask your doctor to recommend a physical therapist if you feel you need one. Ask for at least two names, and then narrow the field by finding the answers to the following questions:

- What are his or her credentials? The therapist and any physical therapist assistants should be licensed.
- Has the therapist treated this problem before? Find a therapist who has experience working with your specific issues. Some specialize in areas of treatment such as orthopedics or geriatrics.
- What will the therapist do for you? A physical therapist should evaluate your

condition, create a treatment program, help you set goals, take the time to answer questions and keep you updated on your progress.

- Will the therapist communicate with your doctor? To get the best possible care, your doctor and physical therapist should provide each other with updates and progress reports.

- What does the therapist's facility include? Take a tour and check for private treatment rooms, an exercise room and convenient — handicapped-accessible, if necessary — parking. Ask to see any equipment the therapist has to help treat your specific injury or problem.

The answers to these questions will help you determine whether you're comfortable with the physical therapist and whether you think he or she is qualified to handle your needs and goals.

SAMPLE WORKOUT PROGRAMS

When it comes to exercise, you can pick from dozens of activities, intensities and lengths to tailor a fitness program to your needs, goals and interests. Consider the sample workout programs on the following pages when you put together your exercise program. Geared to beginners, the programs also work for those who have been active recently. The suggested programs include aerobic exercise, strength training and core exercise that can be combined for a well-rounded fitness lifestyle or used separately to meet specific goals.

Walking program

Walking is an excellent relatively low-impact exercise. It's simple, inexpensive, versatile and requires no equipment other than a good pair of shoes. As you start the program, begin slowly, increasing the pace of your workout over a period of four to six weeks. For the first few weeks, walk on paths over flat, level ground. As you progress, add routes that include hills to increase the intensity of your workout.

In addition, during the first weeks, try to avoid walking on hard surfaces. Instead, walk at a local park, playing fields, golf courses or a running track. Once you're accustomed to the exercise, try designated walking trails, sidewalks or safe, well-lit roads. Note that if you need a nonimpact exercise for your weight loss program, cycling can achieve the same goals.

Use the chart below as a guide to increasing the pace of your walking program.

	Distance	Time
Week 1	1-2 miles	15-30 min./mile
Week 2	1-2 miles	15-30 min./mile
Week 3	2-2 ½ miles	13-25 min./mile
Week 4	2-2 ½ miles	13-25 min./mile
Week 5	2 ½-3 miles	13-20 min./mile
Week 6	2 ½-3 miles	13-20 min./mile
Week 7	3-4 miles	13-20 min./mile
Week 8	3-4 miles	13-20 min./mile
Week 9	4-5 miles	13-20 min./mile
Week 10	4-5 miles	13-20 min./mile
Week 11	5-6 miles	13-20 min./mile
Week 12	5-6 miles	13-20 min./mile

Starter jogging program

Jogging has become increasingly popular in recent years. Many people enjoy the challenge of training for local fun runs and road races, while others enjoy the role it can play in healthy weight management.

Start slowly. When you can comfortably walk two miles in 30 minutes (4 miles an hour), try to alternate walking and jogging — jog one minute, walk one minute — as shown in the chart below.

Don't jog every day. In fact, unless you're a competitive runner, it's recommended that you don't jog more than four times a week — alternating days to minimize joint and muscle discomfort. Because jogging is a high-impact activity, spend one or two days each week cross-training with a low-impact activity. Participating in a lower impact exercise on these days will give your joints a break while keeping your fitness level up.

During the program, it's important that you jog at a comfortable pace and walk briskly. Don't push yourself too hard — you'll be more likely to cause injury to yourself and to enjoy exercising less. Keep within your target heart rate and the ideal perceived exertion range.

Starter jogging training program

Advance one step in this starter program every two to seven days, as you feel able. If you're in step 1, jog for one minute, then walk for one minute. Repeat this until you've jogged and walked for a total of 24 minutes (12 repetitions). When you're comfortable with this portion of the program, move up to step 2. During this phase of the program, you'll jog for two minutes and walk for one minute. Repeat until you have jogged and walked for a total of 24 minutes (eight repetitions). Continue moving up in steps as you're able. By step 10, you'll be able to jog through an entire workout.

The whole program looks like this:

	Exercise time		Repetitions		Total time
	Jog	Walk	Jog	Walk	
Step 1	1 min.	1 min.	12	12	24 min.
Step 2	2 min.	1 min.	8	8	24 min.
Step 3	3 min.	1 min.	6	6	24 min.
Step 4	4 min.	1 min.	5	5	25 min.
Step 5	5 min.	1 min.	4	4	24 min.
Step 6	7 min.	1 min.	3	2	23 min.
Step 7	10 min.	1 min.	2	2	22 min.
Step 8	12 min.	1 min.	2	1	25 min.
Step 9	15 min.	1 min.	2	1	31 min.
Step 10	20 min.	—	1	—	20 min.
Step 11	25 min.	—	1	—	25 min.
Step 12	30 min.	—	1	—	30 min.

Cycling program

Bicycling is a great way to add variety to your workout. Many people enjoy cycling for its speed, its freedom and the opportunity to explore the countryside. Before you start, consider these tips:

- Always wear a helmet. They're available in a variety of colors and patterns. See Chapter 5 for more on choosing a helmet.
- Warm up with easy riding. Save the hills for the middle of your workout.
- Try to keep your perceived exertion at

Cycling training program

Over an eight-week period, your cycling training program might look like this:

	Week 1	Week 2	Week 3	Week 4	Week 5	Week 6	Week 7	Week 8
Monday Ride at a comfortable pace.	30 min.	40 min.	50 min.	40 min.	50 min.	60 min.	70 min.	60 min.
Tuesday Cycle at a brisk pace.	2 x 10 min.*	2 x 15 min.	2 x 20 min.	3 x 10 min.	3 x 15 min.	3 x 20 min.	4 x 10 min.	4 x 15 min.
Wednesday Include hills to build strength and stamina.	15 min.	20 min.	25 min.	20 min.	2 x 15 min.	2 x 20 min.	2 x 25 min.	3 x 20 min.
Thursday Do interval training, pushing harder for brief periods.	3 x 3 min.	3 x 4 min.	3 x 5 min.	3 x 6 min.	4 x 3 min.	4 x 4 min.	4 x 5 min.	5 x 5 min.
Friday Go for distance, but take it easy to help build endurance.	60 min.	70 min.	80 min.	75 min.	90 min.	100 min.	110 min.	120 min.
Saturday	Cross-train. Try a different activity, such as walking, swimming or playing tennis.							
Sunday	Rest.							

*Note: Directions such as 2 x 10 min. mean do two 10-minute brisk intervals during the same exercise session.

the somewhat hard level. (See the Borg RPE scale on page 71.)

- When traveling, make stops for rest and fluids every 30 minutes.

To maintain variety and build your fitness, the eight-week cycling program on page 88 incorporates different kinds of cycling — interval training, hills and different paces — over the course of each week. Each day offers something different. By the end of the program, you can be comfortably cycling up to two hours.

At the end of the program, continue cycling by creating your own routine. Pull elements from this program, work toward a long trip with friends or explore biking trails that introduce new challenges and terrain.

Swimming program

Swimming is a great exercise for building your aerobic capacity without putting strain on your joints. Before beginning the eight-week swimming training program detailed on page 90, assess your skills as a swimmer. You'll need to know how to do a basic swimming stroke and to maintain it for at least 15 minutes. If this seems like it's too much for you right now, take lessons to improve your skill. Then start the program slowly, scaling it down during the first couple of weeks until you're ready to reach the numbers in the chart.

When you have completed the initial swimming program, continue your swimming work-outs by using the kinds of training that you found most enjoyable and rewarding.

Strength training

Strength training increases both muscle and bone strength and reduces the risk of osteoporosis. Complete one set of eight to 12 repetitions, with a weight that works the muscle to the point of fatigue, for each of the muscle groups. Suggested exercises for each muscle group are listed as part of the sample training program on page 91.

Exercise each muscle group two to three days a week, with at least one day of rest between workouts. You can use exercise machines, free weights or a combination of the two. Lift each weight to a count of three, hold for one second, then lower it to a count of three. Breathe out as you lift and breathe in as you relax. When you're able to perform 12 repetitions of an exercise, increase the resistance by 5 percent to 10 percent during your next session. Increase the weight only if you can do the exercise using good form.

Core exercises

Core training targets the abdominal, back and hip muscles. These muscles connect the lower and upper body and are responsible for controlling the transmission of forces and motion from the ground up and vice versa. Core training prepares these muscles both for the rigors of daily activity, such as picking up a bag of groceries, and for sport, such as throwing a baseball. A typical core training program includes exercises that work in different directions — flexion (muscles that bend forward), extension (muscles that bend backward), lateral flexion (muscles that

Swimming training program

Over an eight-week period, your swimming training program might look like this:

	Week 1	Week 2	Week 3	Week 4	Week 5	Week 6	Week 7	Week 8
Monday Swim at an easy pace.	15 min.	20 min.	25 min.	20 min.	25 min.	30 min.	35 min.	30 min.
Tuesday Swim at a faster pace.	2 x 5 min.	2 x 6 min.	2 x 7 min.	2 x 8 min.	3 x 6 min.	3 x 7 min.	3 x 8 min.	4 x 5 min.
Wednesday Swim with arms only then with legs only.	5 min. each	6 min. each	7 min. each	8 min. each	9 min. each	10 min. each	11 min. each	12 min. each
Thursday Swim harder for brief intervals, increasing the pace after four weeks.	3 x 3 min.	3 x 4 min.	3 x 5 min.	3 x 4 min.	4 x 3 min.	4 x 4 min.	4 x 5 min.	5 x 4 min.
Friday Go for distance, but decrease intensity on this swim.	25 min.	30 min.	35 min.	40 min.	35 min.	40 min.	45 min.	50 min.
Saturday	Add variety by trying a different activity or playing water games.							
Sunday	Rest.							

Note: Directions such as 2 x 5 min. mean do two 5-minute intervals during the same exercise session.

bend sideways), and rotation (muscles that twist the trunk). A starting program might look like this:

- Prone bridge
- Prone cobra
- Side bridge
- Standing rotation with resistance band

A more advanced program includes:

- Crunches on stability ball
- Extension on stability ball
- Bird-dog
- Side bridge on ball
- Single arm chop and lift with weight

Sample strength training program*

Muscle group	Monday	Tuesday	Wednesday	Thursday	Friday	Saturday	Sunday
Chest	Chest presses or push-ups	Off		Off	Same as Mon	Off	
Shoulders	Dumbbell presses, or side laterals	Off		Off	Same as Mon	Off	
Back		Off	Lat pull-downs, rows or prone cobras	Off		Off	Same as Wed
Biceps	Curls	Off		Off	Same as Mon	Off	
Triceps		Off	Triceps extensions or kickbacks	Off		Off	Same as Wed
Quadriceps	Leg presses, lunges or squats	Off		Off	Same as Mon	Off	
Hamstrings		Off	Leg curls	Off	Prone cobra	Off	Same as Wed
Core	Crunches	Off	Standing rotation with resistance band	Off	Same as Mon	Off	Side bridge

*This is an example of a typical "push-pull" program in which pushing exercises are done one day and pulling exercises are done another day.

PUTTING IT ALL TOGETHER

This chapter has provided the basic components of an exercise program. By combining aerobic, strength training, flexibility, core and balance exercises that meet your needs, you can become healthier and more fit.

Remember that the exercises listed in this chapter are common examples of what you might consider. It's possible to create a program with many activities not included here. Feel free to try new activities. You may chose from more than 150 exercises listed in the "Exercise Guide," which begins on page 134.

Weekly workout log

Keeping a record of your progress may motivate you to continue with your exercise program. Make copies of this worksheet for future use.

Aerobic training

Day	Exercise type	Pulse before exercising	Pulse while exercising	Perceived exertion	Minutes exercised	Distance (if applic-able)	Comments
1							
2							
3							
4							
5							
6							
7							

Strength training

Day	Exercise type	Intensity	Sets	Repetitions	Rest interval	Comments
1						
2						
3						
4						
5						
6						
7						

Balance training

Day	Exercise type	Duration	Repetitions	Comments
1				
2				
3				
4				
5				
6				
7				

Creating your exercise program **93**

In addition, Chapter 9 provides details on preparing for specific sports. You'll find sample training programs for many common sporting activities.

As is the case with any sample program, the various plans in this book are meant to offer guidelines and suggestions. Don't be afraid to tailor them to your specific needs and goals.

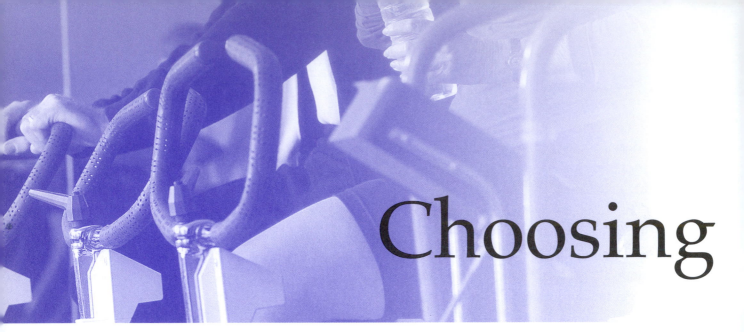

Choosing

CHAPTER 5

You already have the most important and versatile piece of exercise equipment you'll ever need — your own body. It's free and it's accessible — at least most of the time. But beyond this obvious starting point, choosing the right equipment to help you meet your fitness goals can be daunting. Even the most basic gear, such as a good pair of shoes, presents a dizzying array of choices. Some equipment is downright intimidating. For example, you may look at a weight machine and have no clue how to use it.

It's important to remember that you can choose an exercise program that requires little or no equipment. For example, you can set up a plan that uses your own body weight for strength training — doing such activities as push-ups and pull-ups — and get your aerobic workouts from walking or running. You needn't spend hundreds of dollars or more on equipment in order to maintain fitness.

Exercise and fitness equipment can be as simple as athletic shoes suited for your activity or as complex as a state-of-

& using
the right equipment

the-art multistation home gym. What type of equipment is best? The equipment you'll use. There is no one ideal piece of exercise equipment, just as there's no single best exercise. The gear that works best for you will depend on many factors, including your goals, needs, lifestyle and motivation.

Too often, people buy exercise equipment with good intentions — knowing it's good for them — but don't use it. The treadmill ends up as a place to hang clothes, or the exercise bike gets sold at a garage sale. Indeed, nearly 80 percent of exercise equipment purchased in the United States is used for six or fewer weeks, according to the U.S. Public Health Service.

This chapter will help you decide what kind of fitness equipment you're most likely to benefit from and, most important, to use. It offers tips on how to shop for and use a variety of common types of fitness equipment. It also will help you find equipment that's practical, enjoyable and suited for your workouts.

DO YOU NEED EQUIPMENT?

Most forms of exercise can be done without investing a lot of money in fancy gear. You don't need a $3,000 exercise machine for a successful home workout. Your internal drive and motivation are more important than any piece of equipment.

The American Council on Exercise (ACE) asked 36,000 fitness professionals to name their most important exercise items. No. 1 on the list was good shoes. (See "Fitness professionals' top-12 list" on page 96.) Put on that pair of shoes and you're ready to go for a brisk walk, one of the most convenient forms of aerobic exercise. Other simple aerobic options include running, jogging in place and climbing stairs.

Exercises to increase your strength, flexibility and balance can also be done with little or no gear. For example, sit-ups, push-ups and other similar exercises use your body weight as the resistance in order to build muscle strength. You can do yoga using items around your house as props.

Fitness professionals' top-12 list

The American Council on Exercise asked 36,000 fitness professionals what they considered to be the most important exercise items. Their top-12 exercise essentials were:

1. Good shoes
2. Fun or appropriate music
3. Free weights
4. A positive attitude
5. Comfortable clothing
6. Lots of water
7. A supportive sports bra
8. Safe, well-made equipment, such as cardio machines and heart monitors
9. Weight-training gloves
10. Enough time
11. A workout partner
12. Fresh, clean air and sunshine

Source: American Council on Exercise, 2003

It's certainly possible to stay in shape without a roomful of fitness products, but the right equipment can make your workouts more effective and enjoyable. Comfortable, weather-appropriate clothing and good shoes are a must for nearly everyone. Beyond that, the equipment you choose will depend on your fitness goals, budget, space, preferences and personality.

Fitness facility vs. home equipment

Whether you're starting an exercise program from scratch, stepping up your activity level or adding something new to your routine, you may need equipment to achieve your aim. Before you spend a penny, a basic question to ask is whether it makes more sense to join a fitness club or buy equipment for use at home.

Exercising at home is a good choice in these situations:

- You're short on time and can't seem to squeeze in both a drive to the gym and a workout.
- You can't afford the cost of a fitness club membership.
- You live too far from a health club or fitness center or are tired of driving back and forth.
- You can't easily leave the house because of children or other obligations.
- You're self-conscious about exercising in front of others, or you don't like crowds.
- You're motivated to stick to your program without needing much or any outside support.

On the other hand, joining a club may be a better option for you. Fitness facilities usually offer:

- A much greater variety of equipment choices than you could probably afford to buy on your own. Most clubs have the budget to update their machines regularly.

- Fitness professionals who can give advice and teach you proper technique for using various types of equipment.
- Features that you likely don't have at home, such as a swimming pool, running track, basketball court, racquetball court and fitness classes.
- Camaraderie and social interaction.
- Fitness assessments and programs tailored to your goals.

Another factor to consider is your personality and motivation. At a fitness club, you're relatively free from distractions — you're there to work out, and there's not much else to do. For some people, the act of driving to the gym and walking into a roomful of sweating, energized people is a key motivator. It's common to meet a workout partner at the gym, which is a great incentive to get yourself there.

At home, you have to be highly motivated to stick with your exercise program because you'll often be able to find an excuse not to exercise, like the laundry or the dishes. To keep your home workout from getting boring, you may have to get creative, especially if you're on a tight budget.

On the plus side, at home you can work out however and whenever you want. You won't have to wait in line to use machines, and if you feel like watching your favorite TV program or singing at the top of your lungs while you exercise, no one will object.

Of course, you can have the best of both worlds by joining a fitness club and also buying some equipment to use at home.

That way you can vary your workout routine, and you'll be able to stay active at home when you can't make it to the gym.

Factors to consider

Before you can figure out what kind of equipment you need, you have to know your fitness goals, as discussed in Chapter 4. Do you want to concentrate on aerobic fitness, strength training or both? Are you hoping to improve your flexibility and balance, or build core strength? The type of activities you plan to do will help determine what kind of equipment you need. For example, are you interested in sports such as tennis and swimming or activities such as yoga and Pilates?

Other factors to consider include affordability, space and storage issues, and your own commitment.

Affordability

What's your budget for home fitness equipment? If money is no object, you can easily create a top-of-the-line home gym that will serve all your needs. Equipment that's high-quality, reliable and will work for years doesn't come cheap. As a rule of thumb, expect to get what you pay for, which means you may have to spend at least a few hundred dollars, particularly for cardiovascular equipment such as a treadmill or stair stepper. Nonmotorized treadmills, for example, are inexpensive but may feel clunky and awkward or may not move fast enough. Equipment that doesn't "feel" good is a strong de-motivator.

Even on a tight budget you can get the gear that will help you achieve your fitness goals. Some inexpensive items include jump-ropes, resistance tubes and bands, an exercise mat, stability balls (Swiss balls), chin-up bars, free weights and exercise videos. Consider alternatives to high-tech machines and fancy gadgets.

A fitness step or low, sturdy step stool and some step aerobics videos cost far less than does a home stair stepper.

To keep equipment affordable, look for the sturdiest you can find without unnecessary bells and whistles. Some machines cost more because they measure things such as heart rate and calories burned.

Choosing a fitness facility

If you decide that a fitness facility is your best bet, the next step is to find one that meets your needs. Most areas offer an array of choices, from all-purpose gyms to the YMCA to specialized facilities. How do you choose?

As when buying equipment for use at home, your decision will depend on what your fitness goals are. Do you want to work on aerobic fitness, strength training or your tennis game? If your focus is on strength training, then you may not care if there's a swimming pool available. If you prefer to work out on exercise equipment, a wide assortment of classes won't be as important to you.

If you're not sure of your goals or if you want to cover all aspects of fitness, consider joining an all-purpose gym with a large variety of classes and equipment.

When you're ready to begin shopping for a fitness facility, do some research to find out what's available. Call local gyms, ask friends and family for recommendations, or do research on the Internet. You might also want to check with your local Better Business Bureau before entering into any contract with a club. You'll be able to find out if any complaints have been registered against the facility.

Try to visit a few facilities to comparison shop. Most places have regular drop-in hours. You can meet with a staff member, learn what services are available and take a tour. Don't let your tour guide rush you or distract you with a relentless sales pitch. Ask questions — the more information you have, the better prepared you'll be.

Keep in mind these points as you visit each facility:

- **Location.** Is the facility near your home or work? Choose a club that isn't too far out of the way of your daily activities.
- **Hours.** Many fitness centers open early and close late to give early-bird or late-night exercisers some flexibility. Check with the facility to make sure that it will be open at the times you plan to exercise. Ask a staff person what the facility's busiest times are and which fitness areas are most crowded.
- **Environment.** Is the facility clean? Check out the equipment, floors and locker room. Also consider the overall atmosphere — is this a place you'll enjoy spending time?
- **Equipment.** Does the facility have the equipment you want to use? Is it in good condition? Too many "out of order" signs might be a clue to poor maintenance. Ask how often the equipment is replaced.

These features are nice but not necessary. Manual controls often work just as well as programmable machines, which cost more.

If new equipment is too expensive, consider buying used. Look for stores that specialize in used sporting goods and exercise equipment. You can also find pre-owned equipment by checking Web sites, newspaper ads, fitness centers, bulletin boards, and garage and estate sales. Before buying a used machine, inspect it carefully and try it out. Research the price of new equipment so that you know if you're getting a bargain. In addition, check to see what kind of warranty applies in case the equipment is defective.

- **Classes.** If you're interested in fitness classes, find out what kinds are offered and when. It doesn't matter how great the classes are if they're never at a time that you can attend. In addition, find out if class sizes are limited.
- **Friendly, qualified employees.** Do the staffers say hello and smile? Do they circulate around the exercise area, offering tips and encouragement? A caring and friendly staff can go a long way toward helping you stay focused on your fitness goals. Check for a method of certification for staff members who teach classes or instruct members. The American College of Sports Medicine, the American Council on Exercise and the National Strength and Conditioning Association are reputable organizations that provide certification tests for fitness professionals.
- **Cost.** A state-of-the-art mega-gym with a high membership fee isn't necessarily better for you than a smaller, more moderately priced facility that has what you need for your fitness program. Ask how much membership costs and whether any additional fees are imposed, such as for classes or the swimming pool. If membership requires that you sign a contract, review the details carefully. Make sure you understand your obligations, including the length of your agreement, billing procedures and cancellation policies.
- **Amenities.** Does the facility offer amenities such as free parking or on-site child-care services? Is entertainment available, such as televisions or personal music stations? Are members allowed to bring guests?
- **Special needs.** Find out if staff members have training to deal with your needs. This is especially important if you want to take a class that's geared toward a specific condition, such as water exercises for people with arthritis. Also check to see that the building can accommodate any assistive devices you may use.
- **Affiliation with other clubs.** If you travel a lot, consider a large fitness chain or club that's affiliated with other clubs around the country that offer reciprocal membership.

One way to see if a facility is right for you is to try it out before you join. Ask about a temporary pass. Although some places offer free trial memberships, most facilities charge a fee — usually around $10 a day — to try out the club. If you know a member of the facility, you might be able to visit using a guest pass.

If you buy used items online, make sure the cost of shipping won't break your budget. When buying used equipment, also check whether a warranty and service contract are available.

Space and storage

Chances are you don't have an empty room just waiting to be filled with exercise equipment. You'll need to find or clear some space for any gear you get. Having to store equipment or disassemble it every time you use it can quickly squelch your motivation to work out. Before you start shopping, figure out how much space, including ceiling height, you have available and how much you'll need for the equipment you want. How much clearance is required if you're lifting weights, jumping rope or standing on a stair-stepper machine? If your space is limited, you may have to opt for a rack of dumbbells instead of a large multigym machine.

The more comfortable and inviting you can make your workout space, the more likely you'll be to use it. Ideally, the room should have a durable, flat carpet with a good pad for cushioning. Consider putting a mat around the equipment to protect flooring from sweat and spills. You need enough electrical outlets for your exercise machines, a fan to keep you cool, and perhaps a CD player or television. Keep in mind that exercise equipment can be noisy and may bother people nearby.

To determine about how much space you're likely to need for your equipment, use these guidelines:

- Treadmills — 30 square feet
- Stationary bikes — 10 square feet
- Stair steppers — 10 to 20 square feet, with a ceiling height of at least 8 feet
- Elliptical trainers — 10 to 20 square feet, with a ceiling height of at least 8 feet
- Rowing machines — 20 square feet
- Free weights — 20 to 50 square feet
- Multigym — 50 to 200 square feet

Shopping for equipment

The toughest challenge in buying home fitness equipment is choosing from the many options. Before you start shopping, it's a good idea to talk to friends and fitness professionals to see what type of equipment they recommend. You might also want to check out consumer and fitness magazines or Web sites that rate exercise equipment. (See "Additional resources" beginning on page 344.) If you have special health concerns, ask your doctor or physical therapist about equipment that's best for you.

Before buying fitness merchandise, test it out yourself. Wear workout clothes and comfortable shoes to the store so that you can try the equipment long enough to determine whether it feels comfortable to you. Another way to try out exercise equipment is to get a temporary membership or day pass to a fitness or health club. This will let you test many types of equipment to find out which machines you like best.

The equipment should feel solid and durable and operate smoothly. It should be adjustable and easy to learn and use.

Aerobic machines should be able to maintain at least 20 minutes of smooth, continuous motion. Check to make sure parts can be easily removed and replaced. Investigate the cost of repair. A frayed belt on a stationary bike is inexpensive to replace, but a worn belt on a treadmill can run $200.

The feel of the machine is most important. Even if a machine is well-made, you may find it awkward. Pay attention to how your lower back, joints and muscles feel when you're using it. Your body should move safely and in a correct alignment. Does the seat stay comfortable? Are bars, handles and grips easy to use? Are the controls accessible and understandable? Does it have a solid feel to it? Listen to the noise level of the machine while it's running. If you live in an apartment or plan to work out at odd hours, you'll want a machine that's quiet enough that you don't have to worry about disturbing your neighbors or family members.

Buyer beware

Be sure to carefully evaluate advertising and performance claims. If an exercise device promises quick results with little or no effort on your part, save your money. The Federal Trade Commission advises consumers to ignore claims that an exercise product can provide long-lasting, no-sweat results in a short time. The truth is, you can't get the benefits of exercise unless you actually exercise.

Most tried-and-true exercise equipment primarily focuses on just one type of activity. For example, treadmills and ellip-

tical trainers give you a good aerobic workout, and weight machines and free weights build muscle strength. Although infomercials often claim that their products do it all, in reality, they usually focus on a specific activity or body part, such as aerobic exercise, strength training, or working abs, buttocks or thighs.

A 2004 *Consumer Reports* article tested the claims of 12 infomercial products. The report concluded that few of the devices lived up to all of their hype, and those that came closest were the most expensive.

To be a savvy buyer of exercise equipment, keep these tips in mind:

- Be skeptical of claims that a product will allow you to lose several pounds, inches or pant sizes in a short time — for example, "7 inches in seven days" or "six-pack abs in 14 days." It's virtually impossible for most people to achieve major changes in appearance in a few days or weeks.

- Avoid products that promise to tone, trim or spot reduce one particular part of the body, such as your abdominal area, hips or buttocks. There's no such thing as spot reducing. Toning and losing weight in one area of the body requires regular exercise that works the whole body. In general, fitness equipment that works the whole body or major muscle groups helps you burn more calories than do devices that focus on a single part of the body.

- Read the fine print or disclaimers in ads for exercise machines, especially those with testimonials and before-and-after pictures from "satisfied customers." Are those results typical? Or did the person have to restrict calories along with the exercise to achieve those results? One person's success with a product doesn't mean it will work for you, too.

- Do the calculations for payment plans such as "three easy payments" or "only $49.95 a month." The machine may not seem like such a bargain when you realize after a year that it cost you $800. The advertised price of a product may not include shipping and handling fees, sales tax and other costs.

- Be sure any product that you buy offers a warranty. Get details on the warranty, money-back guarantees and return policies.

- Remember that you generally get what you pay for. The *Consumer Reports* test of exercise devices advertised on TV found that as the price decreased, so did quality and effectiveness.

- Check out the company's customer and support services. Call the advertised toll-free number or go online to see how easy it is to reach a customer representative.

- A common advertising tactic used for fitness products is to cast doubt on traditional methods of exercise. For example, an ad for a device designed to work your abs may claim that traditional abdominal crunches are difficult and painful but that using the product is easier and more effective. One treadmill manufacturer even cited a study purporting to show that walking on a treadmill is "better than outdoor walk-

ing," a claim that the details of the study did not support.

- Whenever possible, purchase equipment in person rather than through TV or Web ads. Nothing compares with trying out the gear before you buy it.

TYPES OF EQUIPMENT

You can choose from a variety of equipment for all the major types of exercise, including aerobic, strength, core stability, flexibility and balance. The following pages offer a guide to many of the most popular and common fitness machines and devices. The guide will give you an idea of what to look for and how to use the equipment.

Aerobic

Several types of machines are designed to help you burn calories and increase cardiovascular fitness in the comfort of your home. Each machine has something unique to offer. Some exercise your lower body only, and others work both the upper and lower body. Most equipment that can provide an aerobic workout is bulky and fairly expensive. Exceptions include jump-ropes and exercise videos.

Treadmill

Treadmills are one of the most popular exercise machines on the market. They're easy to use and allow you to adjust the level of impact to your joints as your

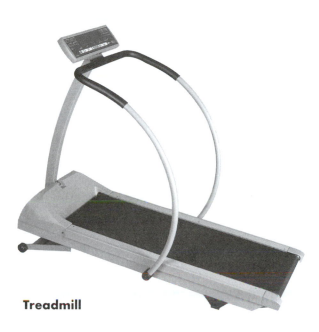

Treadmill

fitness level increases. For example, you can walk, jog or run on a treadmill. The machine helps to build leg strength as well as aerobic capacity.

In one small study, people who used treadmills burned more calories at a given level of exertion than did those who used other indoor exercise machines, such as stair steppers and stationary bicycles. But the study showed that different types of exercise machines were all effective for burning calories and improving fitness. Some research has shown that treadmills are less likely to sit unused than are other machines. And as the market for treadmills has grown and matured, manufacturers have fine-tuned and added features.

Choosing. Most treadmills offer an adjustable degree of incline of up to 15 percent to simulate walking or running up hills. A 15 percent incline is very steep, like climbing an 800-foot hill in a one-mile

walk. Although working out on an incline can bring added benefits, it's not essential for effective training.

A motorized treadmill allows you to adjust the speed for walking or running. It's difficult to walk briskly much less jog or run on a nonmotorized (manual) treadmill. Higher horsepower models generally run more smoothly and are more durable. Look for a treadmill with at least a 1.5 horsepower, continuous-duty motor. If you're going to be running, you'll need 2.0 horsepower or higher.

While the machine is running, stomp your feet on the belt to make sure there's no groaning, grinding or hesitation in the motor. The machine should feel solid, not wobbly, and it should come equipped with an emergency shut-off key, clip or tether. Make sure the treadmill speeds up and slows down gradually and in small increments.

The walking platform or belt should be wide and long enough to let you walk or run comfortably without falling off. Choose a treadmill that's sturdy enough to support your weight, with handrails that are at the right location for you to grip and keep your balance if you need to. If space is an issue, you can choose a treadmill model that folds up.

Many treadmills feature programmed workouts that vary speed and simulated terrain, as well as information on heart rate, speed, calories burned, distance, time and incline. While these features may add variety to your workout, they're not essential to effective training.

In addition, check to see whether the control panel is easy to read and easy to adjust while the treadmill is running. Can you set it for manual use separately from automated programming?

Using. Position your treadmill at least six to eight feet from a wall, window or ledge to avoid injury from falls. Before you get on, experiment with the controls.

Holding the handrails when you're using a treadmill reduces the workout intensity. Once you've mastered the technique, keep your hands off the rails, except when you step on or off the treadmill. Always stand to the side of or straddle the belt while starting the unit. Then step onto the belt one foot at a time when it's moving very slowly.

When walking or running, maintain good posture, with shoulders back, head and chin up, and abdominals tight. Look forward, not down at your feet. When walking or running on an incline, keep your waist bent only slightly. Pay attention to where you are on the treadmill. Avoid drifting sideways or to the back of the belt.

Almost everyone can use a treadmill in some capacity for training. But if you have low back pain or arthritis in the hips, knees or ankles, the impact of running on a treadmill may aggravate your symptoms. In such cases, you may still find a treadmill an effective conditioning tool by walking on it with no incline.

Stationary bike

Stationary (exercise) bikes are another popular option for a low-impact, fairly intense cardiovascular workout. Stationary cycles help build leg strength and improved aerobic capacity. They're generally quiet and space efficient and are relatively inexpensive. For people who have difficulties with balance, an exercise bike may be easier to use than a treadmill.

Choosing. The first decision is whether you want an upright or recumbent seating position. On a recumbent bike, you sit in a chair-like seat with your legs and feet in front of you, rather than under you, as on the upright model. The recumbent position can reduce strain on the lower back, so it may be a safer, more comfortable bike for people with low back pain.

Stationary bike (upright model)

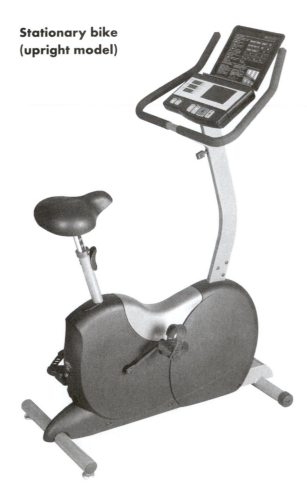

Some exercise cycles have moving handlebars that provide an upper body workout. Known as dual-action bikes, they allow you to burn more calories than with leg action only and may help build upper body strength.

For resistance, stationary bikes use friction belts or wheels, magnets, hydraulics or fans. Avoid bikes that add resistance with rubber pincers that grip the wheel, as these often produce a jerky ride. Bikes with electronic brakes adjust pedal resistance automatically to keep the workload constant at different pedaling speeds. With mechanical brakes, you can increase the resistance and make the workout harder by either adjusting a resistance knob or pedaling faster.

When choosing a bike, make sure you can adjust the handlebars and seat so that you can fully extend your legs and arms. Look for a smooth, steady ride and a comfortable seat. You may also want a bike that offers variable resistance and one that can be programmed for various workouts, such as climbing hills, or for manual workouts. Some models let you pedal backward, which increases the work on your hamstring muscles. Pedal clips keep your feet from slipping and allow your legs to pull as well as push the pedals, working your muscles differently.

Choose a machine that has a covered or protected flywheel or fan. Exposed spokes or holes in the flywheel can be dangerous if you have children in the house.

Using. Your position on a stationary bike is critical to enjoyable and effective cycling. One of the biggest reasons people stop cycling is because of discomfort. Adjust the seat height so that on the downstroke your knee is nearly fully extended — about 10 to 15 degrees of bend. Your hips shouldn't rock back and forth when you pedal. Adjust the handlebars so that you're in a comfortable forward-leaning position. Finally, consider wearing bikers shorts, which are lycra shorts with built-in crotch padding. Such shorts, commonly worn by race cyclists, can reduce discomfort. If you have knee problems, keep the cycle's resistance at a low setting.

Almost anyone, including people with arthritis, can use a stationary bike. If you have back, neck or balance problems, you might be better off with a recumbent bike rather than an upright model. Discuss these issues with your health care professional.

Stair stepper

A stair-stepper machine, also known as a stair climber, helps tone and strengthen your hips, buttocks, legs and lower back, and it provides an effective low-impact aerobic workout. Compared with other exercise machines, stair climbers allow more toning of the gluteal muscles in the buttocks. Some climber models have arm features that give you an upper body workout as well.

If you have knee problems, a stair stepper may not be the best choice for you. A stair stepper can be harder on your knee joints than is a treadmill or exercise bike. If you have knee or hip problems, be sure

Stair stepper

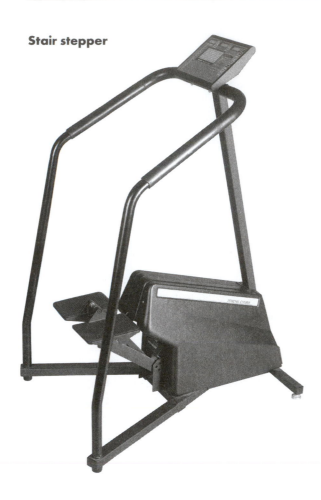

to try a few stair-stepper models to make sure your knees and hips can tolerate them.

Choosing. A nonmotorized machine can be very economical. Many electronic machines, however, offer a variety of programmable workouts that range from basic to sophisticated so that you can change programs to adapt to your changing fitness needs. The more features, options and programs the machine has, the more it will cost. Basic consoles should display calories burned, distance, speed and intensity.

A stair stepper may consist of a moving flight of stairs — like walking up a down escalator — or independent steps that move up and down at various rates or heights. Some models have linked pedals so that pressing down on one forces the other up. Models with independent pedals provide a more natural stepping rhythm. Make sure the pedals work in a smooth, quiet and secure way.

Look for a stepper with easily adjustable resistance, padded handrails, easy-to-use settings and a sturdy steel or aluminum frame. A machine with hydraulic shock absorbers generally will last longer than will an air-filled one.

Using. Stepping height ranges from about 2 to 18 inches. Keep the pedals in the midrange and not touching the floor. The stepping height should feel comfortable on the knees and ankles and should be similar to the stepping action for a normal step.

Stand with upright posture, with your back straight and your knees behind your toes. Bending forward places stress on your back. Keep your feet flat on the pedals as you step. If you're looking down to read, rest your neck every few minutes by changing your head position.

Avoid supporting your body weight with your arms, as this will reduce the amount of work done by your buttocks and leg muscles, and reduce the amount of calories you expend. Hold the handrails lightly for balance, but make your legs do the work. If the machine has moveable arms, use a light grip to help with balance and add upper body movement to your workout.

Trainers and rollers — Bring your outdoor bike inside

If you already have a bicycle and want to cycle indoors during inclement weather, you don't have to buy a stationary bike. An inexpensive piece of equipment called a trainer converts your regular bike to a stationary cycle. A trainer is a compact stand that attaches to the rear axle of your bicycle. You simply lock the back tire into the stand. The rear tire makes contact with a pair of metal rollers, and when you pedal, the tire makes the rollers spin.

Using your own bike with a trainer is not only less expensive than buying a stationary cycle but also is likely to be more comfortable. In addition, a trainer takes up less space than a stationary bike. Most trainer models fold up for easy storage.

Trainers create resistance in one of three ways. The three types of trainers are:

- **Fan.** Also called wind trainers, this type uses a fan that's turned by the rear wheel of the bike. The spinning fan displaces air to create resistance. The faster you pedal, the more resistance you generate. The resistance is much like the wind resistance you experience when riding outdoors. It's smooth and increases gradually. Fan trainers are a good choice for beginners or those who want an occasional workout. They're also great for interval training, which involves alternating higher and lower intensity activity.
- **Magnetic.** "Mag" trainers use magnetic fields to generate resistance by moving a magnetic plate closer and farther from the rollers. Magnetic trainers provide a much wider range of resistance than do fan trainers, allowing you to simulate more intense, anaerobic activities such as sprinting and hill climbing. You adjust the resistance manually or electronically, and it increases according to how hard you pedal. Magnetic trainers are extremely quiet, which makes them a popular choice for people who live in apartments.
- **Fluid.** This type of trainer uses internal fluid to generate hydraulic resistance. A fan is encased in a silicone fluid, and different settings add or drain fluid to and from the chamber holding the fan. Fluid trainers offer more resistance than do the other types of trainers. They give a very smooth, quiet ride that has a realistic road feel.

Another option for indoor training using your regular bicycle is a roller. It consists of a frame holding three revolving cylindrical drums on which you ride your bike. Your rear wheel sits on two drums while the front wheel rotates on one drum. The drums are connected with a large rubber band that keeps them in sync. The same forces that keep you upright while you're riding on the road also keep you upright on rollers, but without the forward motion.

Rollers are trickier to use than are trainers, so they're not a good choice for beginning cyclists. It's harder to keep your balance on rollers than on the road. You have to concentrate on steering, balance and smooth pedaling. For this reason, rollers can help you improve your bike-handling skills and balance, and they can be fun to ride. Rollers are very quiet and cause less wear on your tires than trainers do.

Using a roller takes some practice. The first few times you ride, set yourself up in a doorway or next to a wall so that you don't roll off the edges.

Trainers and rollers can be purchased online or at some sporting goods and bicycle stores. Most manufacturers offer warranties.

Elliptical trainer

Elliptical trainers, like treadmills, are one of the most widely used cardiovascular machines, and they can be just as effective as treadmills. Elliptical trainers combine the motions of stair stepping and cross-country skiing for a low-impact workout. The leg action is elliptical — up and down at an angle. Because ellipticals place less stress on your joints than walking does, they're a good choice for people with knee problems, arthritis or other joint problems.

Many elliptical machines have poles that you can move with your arms as you move your feet, which increases the aerobic benefits. Most machines will allow you to move forward or backward for more variety in your workout.

Choosing. An elliptical trainer may be motorized or nonmotorized. When in use, the machine should be very stable, with no tendency to move or tip over. The side rails should also be sturdy.

Overall fit is important. You should be able to move comfortably and smoothly, with a good upright posture and without your knees bumping into the console. Make sure the pedals are large enough to accommodate your feet. A textured non-slip surface and a ridge around the edge of the pedals will help prevent your feet from sliding around or off.

Some machines allow you to adjust the stride length. Don't buy a trainer if the stride length is too limited for your leg movement range. If the machine has upper body poles or handles, make sure they're easy to reach, with comfortable

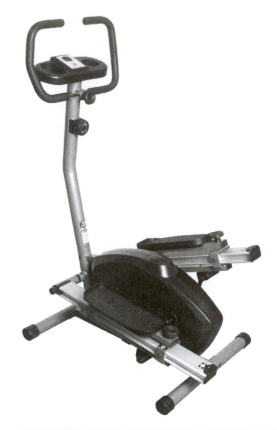

Elliptical trainer

grips. Also make sure that when you exercise without using the poles or handles they aren't crowding or hitting you.

A control panel — helpful but not essential — may display elapsed time, distance, resistance level, calories burned and other information.

Using. When exercising, maintain good posture, with your shoulders back, head up and slightly forward, chin straight and abdominals tight. Look forward, not down at your feet. Don't lean forward or grip the balance bars tightly.

Make sure your lower body supports most of your weight instead of leaning on the handrails. Keep your feet flat on the pedals. You can pedal forward or backward, changing the muscles you target.

Get to know the options that increase the intensity of your workout. For example, most trainers allow you to adjust both the resistance and speed. Adjusting the incline will change the mechanics of your movements, but it will not affect the intensity of your workout or the number of calories burned.

Other cardio gear

Beyond the popular machines just described, other equipment you can use for maintaining or improving aerobic fitness includes:

- **Rowing machine.** In addition to improving aerobic capacity, using a rowing machine puts your entire skeletal muscle system in action. It allows you to work your back, shoulders, stomach, legs and arms at the same time.

    Electric rowers and wind resistance rowers offer the most natural feel. Choose a rower with a seat and oars or

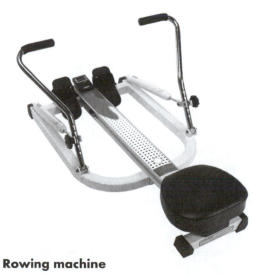

Rowing machine

handles that move smoothly and that provide uniform resistance throughout the rowing motion. Look for footrests that pivot and that keep your feet comfortably in place.

Proper technique is important to avoid back strain. Sit upright, bend forward at your hips, keep your elbows close to your body when pulling and don't overarch your back as you complete each stroke. A proper rowing stroke draws most of its force from your legs and hips.

- **Cross-country ski machine.** Similar in many ways to the elliptical machine, this machine provides a high-intensity aerobic workout, especially if you raise the front of the machine to simulate uphill skiing. Some people find it difficult to master the coordinated arm and leg movements. Look for a machine that offers separate adjustments for upper and lower body resistance, as well as a base that's long enough to accommodate your stride. Most ski machines aren't very wide and may have a tendency to tip from side to side, so be sure to check for stability when testing them.

- **Exercise rider.** This hybrid machine combines rowing and leg-pressing movements to provide a whole-body workout. Highly fit people probably won't get enough intensity from the exercise rider, however it may provide some benefits to people who are less fit. In addition, it offers a relatively low-impact experience. When pulling, straighten to an erect position and avoid arching your back.

- **Jump-rope.** The old-fashioned jump-rope is inexpensive and takes up almost no space. It's also light and easy to pack, so it's a good choice for travel. Today's jump-ropes are made from a variety of materials and feature different grip styles. Choose a lightweight rope with foam grips instead of a weighted rope with heavy handles. To select the right length, step one foot on the center of the rope and bring both handles up to the chest. They should reach about chest-high.

To stay motivated during your workout, turn on some fun, upbeat music. As you jump, keep your shoulders relaxed and your elbows close to your body. Keep your back straight and head up, with your knees slightly bent. Jump low to minimize the impact on your

Self-monitoring tools

People in Japan don't just walk, they keep track of each step. The average Japanese family has three pedometers. The fad hasn't taken off in the United States, but portable exercise devices such as heart rate monitors and pedometers are becoming more popular. They satisfy a demand for sophisticated, customized exercise feedback, which can help with staying motivated, setting goals and tracking progress. Exercise gadgets appeal to those who want to monitor their activity.

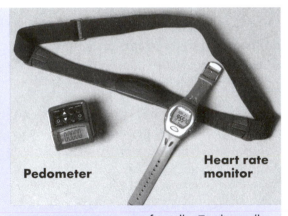

Pedometer   **Heart rate monitor**

A pedometer is an inexpensive device, worn at the waist, that counts the number of steps you take. An internal lever registers each vertical acceleration of the hip, interpreting this as a step. A pedometer can help you keep track of how much activity you're accumulating throughout the day, even when you're not specifically exercising.

Some pedometer models claim to measure distance walked and calories expended, but those measures are less accurate than steps taken. A pedometer that allows you to calculate your personal stride may make it easier to translate steps into distance. Look for a pedometer that's unobtrusive and easy to operate.

Perhaps the most widely used portable exercise device is the heart rate monitor. Technological advances have made heart rate monitors more user friendly. Traditionally, users have worn a chest strap that transmits wirelessly to a wristband monitor, but some new models have eliminated the chest strap. Users check their pulse by pressing their fingertips onto the wrist monitor.

A heart rate monitor tells you if you're exercising at the recommended intensity level, or target heart rate — such as 60 percent to 85 percent of maximum heart rate. (For information on calculating your maximum heart rate, see page 42.) The device is especially useful for competitive athletes who use heart rate information as a training guide, people who have medical conditions and need to stay in a safe aerobic zone, and beginning exercisers who want to learn to set limits and monitor progress.

High-end monitors may have features such as progress trackers, target zone alarms, calorie counters and integrated pedometers.

knees and ankles. To avoid joint injury, jump rope on surfaces that have some give, such as a cushioned floor mat.

- **Walking poles.** Also called walking sticks or trekking poles, they work your arms, shoulders, chest and upper back muscles through a full range of motion as you walk or hike. The arm movement adds intensity to your aerobic workout and fosters balance and stability. Because walking poles take some of the load off your lower back, hips and knees, they're useful for people with arthritis or back problems.
- **Exercise videos.** Using an exercise video is like having a health club aerobics or step class in your own living room. Look for a video that features a certified, experienced instructor who includes a warm-

up and cool-down in the workout. (See "Choosing the best fitness videotapes and DVDs," page 125.)

Strength training

Strength training, also referred to as resistance training or weight training, tones and strengthens the body's muscles. To become stronger, your muscles must push or pull against an opposing force, such as weight or gravity. The resistance can be achieved in many ways — moving or pushing against your own body weight, pulling on an elastic band or lifting weights. For this reason, the term *weightlifting* is not quite accurate. Elastic exercise bands or tubing hardly weigh anything, but they provide enough resistance to strengthen your muscles.

Impact chart

Use this chart to select equipment and activities that are best suited for your joints, especially if you need to avoid high-impact forms of exercise.

	High impact	Medium impact	Low impact
Treadmill (running)	X		
Treadmill (walking)		X	
Stationary or recumbent bike			X
Stair stepper		X	
Elliptical trainer			X
Rowing machine			X
Cross-country ski machine			X
Exercise rider			X
Jumping rope	X		
Water aerobics			X
Step aerobics	X		
Soccer, basketball, racquetball, squash, baseball, softball	X		
Tennis (singles)	X		
Tennis (doubles)		X	

Although it's possible to do a number of resistance exercises, such as push-ups, squats, lunges and isometric exercises, without any equipment, a complete strength training program almost always requires some equipment. The two most popular types of strength training equipment are free weights (barbells and dumbbells) and weight machines. Elastic bands or tubes and stability balls are other options.

If you're new to strength training, the equipment can be intimidating. You may not know the difference between a dumbbell and a barbell, much less how to use them properly. Weight machines may look like a confusing jumble of ropes, pulleys, levers and handles. Where do you start if you want to do strength training at home?

Begin by learning about the different equipment options and evaluating your goals, needs, space and budget. For example, if you want to build larger muscles, you'll probably need more free weights than you'd need if your goal is to develop moderate strength and muscle tone. If you're tight on both money and space, the cheapest and smallest resistance equipment you can get are resistance bands or tubes. A temporary membership to a gym is a good way to try out different types of equipment.

Whatever equipment you choose, it's important to get some instruction if you've never used it before. You'll want to learn proper technique, safety precautions and the various exercises you can do with the equipment. Sign up for a session or two with a certified exercise professional to ensure that you're working your muscles properly. Several organizations, such as the American College of Sports Medicine, the National Strength and Conditioning Association and the American Council on Exercise, provide certification tests for fitness professionals. (For a list of fitness organizations, see "Additional resources," page 344.) If you belong to a gym, check with a fitness specialist there to make sure you're practicing good form and technique. You might also consider a strength training class offered through a community education program, or sign up for a short-term membership at a health club where instruction is available. Some strength training equipment comes with an instructional video. A rule of thumb is to always assume good posture — knees slightly bent, tightened abdominal muscles, shoulders back, chest out and eyes straight ahead — and perform all movements slowly and under control. Breathe out during the exertion or lifting phase.

Free weights

Free weights are free-standing weights that you lift. They're a simple, inexpensive way to build muscle. The two basic types of free weights are dumbbells and barbells:

- **Dumbbells** are individual, hand-held weights. They come in a variety of sizes, shapes and materials, including chrome, plastic, steel, cast iron, vinyl, neoprene and rubber. Plain metal weights may be slightly more durable, but coated weights are quieter. Dumbbells are typically used in pairs, and they can be purchased in different weights, from 1 or 2 pounds up to 150 pounds. Dumbbells are more economical than are barbells or weight machines.

- **Barbells** are long (4 to 7 feet) bars with weights attached at the ends or slots to add weight plates. The bar itself may weigh from 15 to 30 pounds or more, so for a beginner, just lifting the bar may be the first step. As with dumbbells, you can buy barbell plates of different weights. Many stores sell variety packs, often called olympic packs, which include an assortment of weight plates.

Choosing. Both dumbbells and barbells allow you to do dozens of exercises that work every muscle group in your body. Some people consider dumbbells easier to use. They also let you work each arm independently. For some barbell routines, you need a spotter, someone to assist you if you need help completing a set, so using dumbbells is generally safer if you don't have a training partner.

The handles on free weights are important because they provide friction for a good grip. The handle should feel comfortable and stable in your hand. Practice

Dumbbells

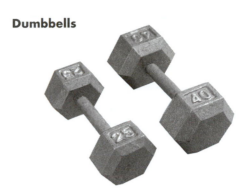

some exercises with the weights before buying them.

An important consideration in buying free weights is how much weight you need. A common mistake is to buy one set of 10-pound weights and use them for every exercise. A salesperson or fitness professional should be able to help you decide how much weight to buy initially. Err on the side of buying too light rather than too heavy. You can add heavier weights as you need them. In addition, make sure that your weights increase in small increments so that you can advance slowly as you build strength.

Weight plates

Barbell

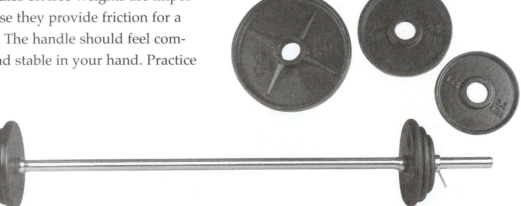

If you're buying free weights, you may also want to purchase a weight bench to add variety to your exercise routine. A weight bench is a sturdy, padded bench that you lie, sit or kneel on to lift weights. It may be flat or vertical. Many benches are adjustable and provide an incline or decline as well as a flat surface. Some benches fold up for easy storage.

You can also buy a rack for storing dumbbells or barbells. Racks save space and keep you from always having to reach down to the floor to pick up weights, but they do add to the expense. Free weights can also be stored on the floor.

One piece of equipment that you don't need is a weightlifting belt. If you go to a gym, you may see power lifters wearing belts to protect their lower backs. Research shows that these belts do little to improve performance or protect the spine. It's better to rely on strong abdominal and back muscles to support you.

Using. Take precautions when you use free weights. Learn the proper technique for each exercise before you do it. Make sure you have a good grip, maintain a stable position sitting or standing, and use proper form. Keep your spine aligned as you perform all exercises. If you're lifting heavy weights, get a training partner to spot you.

Most accidents happen when a weight falls on a body part. When picking up weights from the floor or putting them down, lift with your legs, not your back. Use a clip device, called a collar, to secure weight plates onto your barbell so that they don't fall off. When lifting weights, wear sturdy shoes that have cushioning and ankle support. You might also consid-

Can't afford weights? Make your own

Free weights aren't expensive, but if your budget is slim, you can use household items to make weights:

- Fill empty containers, such as bottled water or dish-washing detergent bottles, with water or sand. Make sure that whatever you use is easy to hold in the palm of your hand. You can gradually increase the weight by adding more water or sand to the containers. Use a household scale to check the weight. Secure the lids with duct tape.
- Canned goods come in a variety of sizes and weights and they're usually easy to hold in your hand.
- Turn a tennis ball into a light dumbbell by cutting a small slit in one side of the ball and filling it with pennies. Once the ball is full, seal it with a strong glue or sealant. You can also fill empty tennis ball cans with sand. Wrap the can with athletic or duct tape to keep the lid from coming off and to prevent spills in case the can cracks.

er using weight lifting gloves to help prevent calluses that can develop with repetitive lifting. Gloves can also help improve your grip as you increase the amount of weight you lift.

Weight machines

Since the debut of the first weight-training machine by the Universal Gym Company in 1957, the number and variety of machines for resistance training have mushroomed, fueled by the fitness boom of the 1970s and the increased popularity of bodybuilding. Today, many such machines are sold for home use.

Weight machines are expensive and take up a lot of space, so it's important to be clear about what your needs are and to understand the pros and cons of various machines. Think about how much space you have available, whether you'll be moving the equipment, what your budget is and whether you're willing to assemble a machine.

Many weight machines are designed to work just one specific muscle group, such as the lower back or chest. Unless you happen to live in an empty warehouse and have an unlimited budget, it's not practical to put an entire line of weight machines in your home. But a home gym that combines multiple weightlifting stations into one frame takes up less space and is more cost efficient. This type of machine is called a multigym. It typically has one or two weight stacks and can accommodate one or two people at a time.

Home weight machines come in many

styles and sizes and use different forms of resistance. Each type has advantages and disadvantages.

- **Weight stack.** Traditional weight machines have a stack of rectangular weight plates, held in place by a vertical bar or track (see image below). A system of cables and pulleys moves the weight. You change the amount by moving a pin that determines how many plates are lifted. *Advantages:* It's fast and easy to change the amount of weight. Resistance feels natural and constant. It's easy to chart progress. *Disadvantages:* It's heavy and bulky, hard to get home, and difficult to assemble and move.

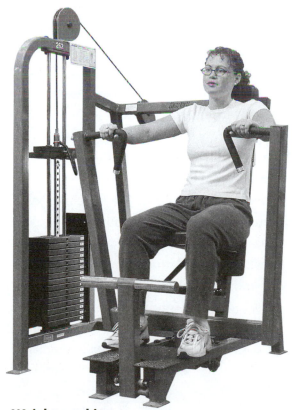

Weight machine

- **Hydraulic pistons.** This particular type of machine works like a car's shock absorber, with a series of pistons that create resistance by pumping fluid or air from one compartment to another. You change the resistance level by changing the point at which the pistons are attached to the levers or by adjusting valves. *Advantages:* It's lightweight and easy to move. *Disadvantages:* The resistance varies with pace and effort. It's harder to chart progress.

- **Flexible rods or bands.** This type of machine uses rods or bands, called weight straps, that stretch to provide the resistance. The rods or bands are attached by cable to a lever that allows you to push or pull the lever arm. You change the resistance by changing the number of rods or bands or the thickness of bands. *Advantages:* It's lightweight, easy to move, and offers a wide variety of exercises. *Disadvantages:* Resistance varies through the entire range of motion and may be hard to control toward the end. It may feel unnatural.

- **User's body weight.** This machine has a movable platform mounted on a track attached to a stand at one end. You sit or lie on the platform and pull on cables to move the platform up or down the track. Your weight provides the resistance, which you can vary by changing the track's angle to the floor. *Advantages:* It's easy to assemble, move and store. You can use it to train different muscle groups easily. *Disadvantages:* It can be

awkward to get into starting position. Resistance is limited to about 50 percent of the user's body weight.

Choosing. Look for a heavy-gauge steel frame, smooth-operating pulleys and sealed bearings. The weight stack should move easily up and down, though most home models don't feel as smooth or solid as health club machines. Make sure the machine can hold enough weight to meet your fitness needs now and as they change. Look for sturdy, thickly padded seats that are covered with a durable, water- and sweat-resistant material.

The best home gym should fit users of different sizes and allow full range of motion in the proper body positions. Try out every exercise station. Some machines — especially those with pulleys — operate smoothly at lighter weights but become wobbly or sticky when you're lifting heavier amounts. The parts should be easy to adjust for different exercises.

Measure the space you have available for a weight machine and check the dimensions of any equipment you're considering. Finally, inquire about free assembly. Otherwise, you may be faced with a large box weighing as much as 240 pounds, with hundreds of parts and complicated assembly instructions.

Using. Follow the machine's instructions for use, and maintain proper body position and exercise technique. Grips that turn your palms away from you are appropriate for presses and pulls. Grips that keep your palms toward you are used for exercises such as biceps curls and rowing and pulling motions.

Make sure your machine is adjusted for your body size and set up on a level surface. A small amount of padding underneath the machine will help to make it more stable and muffle some of the noise. Lift weights from a stable position on the machine's seat or platform. If the machine has a seat belt, fasten it securely. Avoid moving parts and weight plates.

Resistance bands and tubes

Resistance bands and tubes, also known as exercise bands, are elastic rubber bands and tubes that provide resistance when stretched. A variety of upper and lower body exercises can be done with them.

Free weights vs. machines — Which are better?

Ever since strength training machines came on the scene to compete with dumbbells and barbells, people have been debating the merits of free weights versus machines. Both methods of training have pros and cons, but muscle development occurs the same way whether you use free weights or machines. Your muscles don't know or care if the source of resistance is a barbell, a dumbbell, a plate-loaded machine or a bag of groceries.

Here are some of the advantages and disadvantages of free weights and machines:

- Free weights are much cheaper than weight machines.
- Free weights are more versatile. They can be used for just about every muscle in the body, while many machines have more limited functions. In this regard, free weights can be considered a better value.
- Using free weights generally requires more coordination and balance, compared with machines. Accordingly, for people with balance and coordination problems, the risk of injury may be higher with free weights than it is with machines, at least when they're first beginning to lift. Someone who's just starting a strength training program may be better off with a multigym machine, which is safer to use without supervision. However, if you're not at risk, you'll likely get more benefit from using free weights

because they can more closely simulate real-life situations and they present a greater challenge to balance, stability and coordination.

- Free weights generally allow for more freedom of motion and involve several muscle groups at the same time. However, some machines can provide variable resistance, which means that your muscles work harder through a greater range of motion. In addition, some machines accommodate a larger range of motion for certain muscle groups.
- Weight machines enable you to isolate a muscle group, if this is part of your training goal.
- Machines can save you time — you can move quickly from one exercise to another.
- Machines may be easier to use if you're recovering from an injury, have balance or stability problems or would be otherwise challenged by the need to control the free weight while lifting.

Free weights and machines will both do a good job of strengthening and toning your muscles. In the end, personal preference and comfort will likely dictate which type of resistance training you choose. Or you can alternate between the two. Many experts recommend using both free weights and machines.

Bands and tubes are lightweight, portable, inexpensive and versatile. If you can't afford a gym membership or your own set of weights, resistance bands are a cheap way to get a full-body strength training workout. They're also a great option for people who are recovering from an injury, who have a medical condition that limits their mobility, or who travel a lot and want to take their equipment on the road with them. You can use bands anywhere and in comfortable positions, such as lying in bed.

Resistance bands and tubes challenge your muscles in slightly different ways than do free weights or weight machines because the resistance increases in proportion to the stretch of the band or tube. This increased resistance at the end of a motion may limit the available range of motion for an exercise. Some health professionals believe that you can't get as strong using resistance bands and tubes as you might with free weights or machines, although there's no clear proof that this is the case. In addition, it's harder to measure your progress or incrementally increase resistance when using elastic bands, compared with free weights and machines.

Choosing. Resistance bands and tubes are sold under various names at most fitness and discount stores. The bands and tubes are typically color-coded to offer varying levels of resistance, which you select based on your fitness level. Increase resistance gradually by working up to the next level of colored bands.

Make sure you buy bands or tubes that are specifically designed for exercise rather than for some other purpose. Discuss with a qualified health professional what colors are right for you and when and how to move from one color to the next.

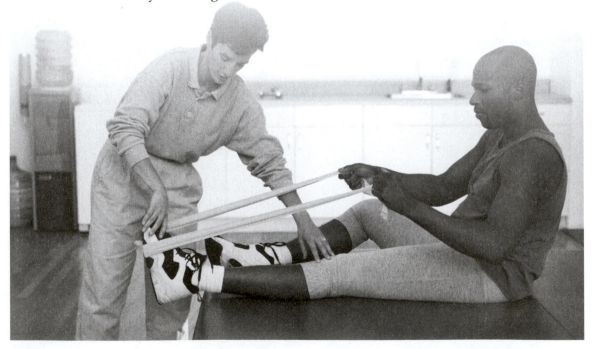

Some bands come as part of a kit that includes accessories such as door anchors and exercise handles, as well as an instruction poster showing different exercises. Many elastic bands and tubes are made of latex. Nonlatex bands and tubes are available for people with latex allergies.

Using. Proper form is key in using bands and tubes. Perform the exercises in a slow, controlled manner both when you pull on the band or tube and when you return to the starting position — don't let the band snap back. Use a relaxed grip. It may help to tie a secure knot in the band to keep it from slipping.

Check your bands or tubing for worn spots before using them. Make sure the equipment is secured underfoot or on an anchor before you begin each exercise. Do your workout on carpeting, a wood floor or grass. Avoid abrasive surfaces such as asphalt or cement, which can tear the elastic.

Maintain good posture while exercising. Exhale when lifting or pulling, and inhale when returning to the beginning position. To change the level of resistance, move to the next color, or simply change the way you hold the band — shortening the length makes the exercises more difficult, while using a longer length makes the exercises easier.

Medicine balls

Once an exercise standard, medicine balls are enjoying a comeback as a way to add variety to a resistance-training program. These leather or rubber balls range in weight from about 1 to 30 pounds. They come in a variety of colors and textures and may be filled with different substances. You can use a medicine ball in a variety of exercises for the upper and lower body. The balls are also good for building core strength by working the abdominal, back and trunk muscles.

Choosing. Medicine balls come in various sizes. You can do many exercises with a ball the size of a tennis ball. But you'll want a larger, heavier ball for exercises that are done with both hands. Choose a lighter weight for exercises that involve throwing the ball.

You can make your own medicine balls using the type of playground balls used for kickball. Pop the plug on the ball and let the air out, then fill it with cold water or sand. Replace the plug.

Using. You can use a medicine ball by yourself, with a partner or in a group. If the ball doesn't come with instructions, consult a book, video or fitness professional for help with learning specific exercises.

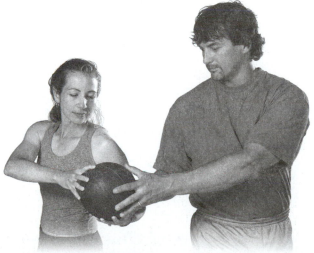

Medicine ball exercises may be done solo or with a partner. They help build core strength.

Other resistance equipment

A pull-up bar, also called a chin-up bar, is a simple, inexpensive resistance tool. This bar can be mounted in a standard door frame and used for pull-ups and chin-ups, exercises that use your body weight for resistance. Both exercises work your biceps and upper back muscles. In a pull-up, you hold the bar with an overhand grip — palms facing away from you — and lift yourself up. In a chin-up, you use an underhand grip to pull yourself up. The chin-up may be easier on the shoulders for some people.

Some equipment isn't specifically designed for strength training but still provides a resistance workout. For example, stability balls can be used to perform resistance exercises and also help you work on balance and flexibility. These balls are discussed in the following section. Another option is resistance equipment that you use in the water. Water workout equipment is discussed on page 123.

Flexibility, core stability and balance exercises

To achieve the other major fitness goals — core stability, flexibility and balance — you can do simple exercises that require nothing more than an exercise mat, comfortable clothes and sturdy shoes. Or you may participate in specialized programs, such as Pilates, that make use of particular equipment. Some equipment can be used for several different types of exercise. (See the "Exercise guide" beginning on page 134 for examples of several of these activities.)

Stability balls

The stability ball is one of the most versatile pieces of exercise equipment — and probably has the most names, including fitness ball, gymnastic ball, yoga ball, Swiss ball, balance ball and physioball. It looks like an overgrown beach ball. It's an oversized, inflatable ball that's designed to improve core stability, flexibility and balance. These fun, adaptable spheres were first used nearly 30 years ago by physical therapists and reached the mainstream fitness world in the late 1980s and early 1990s.

Balancing on a stability ball requires that you use your core muscles for support. These are the muscles of the abdomen, chest and back that stabilize the rest of the body, like a strong column linking your upper and lower body.

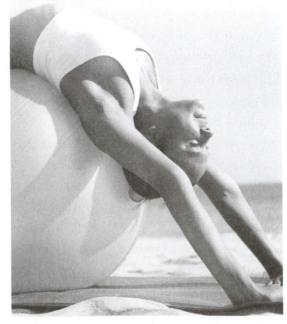

Exercising with stability balls helps to develop and strengthen the core muscles.

Simply sitting on a stability ball and gently bouncing works your abdominal, back and thigh muscles. You can also add arm movements and do exercises such as crunches to get an all-over workout. Research has shown that doing crunch exercises, which are modified sit-ups, on a stability ball instead of a flat surface increases the activity of your abdominal muscles, probably because you have to work them harder to keep from falling off the ball. The curve of the ball also accommodates the curve of your spine, allowing for more range of motion in core exercises.

Stability balls add challenge to the balance component of yoga and Pilates exercises. The balls can also help facilitate stretching. For example, to gently stretch your back muscles and lengthen your spine, you can drape yourself facedown over the top of the ball.

Choosing. Choose a stability ball that's the right size for you. The balls are sized according to their diameter in centimeters, and the appropriate size is based on your height. For most exercises, you'll want a ball that allows your knees to be at a right angle when you sit on the ball with your feet on the floor. Here are some guidelines for buying the right size ball.

Your height	Ball size
	(diameter when inflated)
Under 5 feet	45 centimeters (18 inches)
5 to 6 feet	55 centimeters (22 inches)
Over 6 feet	65 centimeters (26 inches)

Air pressure is another important consideration. The firmer the ball, the more difficult the exercise will be. If you're just starting out, are overweight or older, consider using a larger, softer ball. Most people do best with a slightly deflated 55-centimeter or 65-centimeter ball. You'll need an air pump to inflate the ball.

Stability balls can pop, which can be dangerous if you're lying or sitting on the ball. Look for anti-burst balls.

Using. Several exercise programs using stability balls have been developed for just about every need and body part. Stability balls are specially designed to carry your weight. Don't try the same exercises on ordinary balls, which aren't made to support you. Follow the instructions that come with the ball, or talk to a fitness professional about different exercises.

To keep from rolling off the ball, use a wide-leg stance. Use your ball on a nonslip surface that's free of sharp or irregular objects. Clean the ball regularly, and make sure it's free of cracks, cuts or abrasions. Don't leave a stability ball in the sunlight, which can weaken and warp it.

Pilates equipment

Pilates (puh-LAH-teez) is a system of exercises and body conditioning developed by Joseph Pilates more than 70 years ago. Until recently, the method was used mainly in the dance and performing arts communities, but Pilates classes are now a fixture at health clubs. And more people are trying it with the help of videos.

The Pilates method is designed to strengthen your core muscles — your lower back, hips, abdomen and buttocks. You perform a set of controlled stretches and movements, using your own body for resistance.

Pilates exercises can be done on an exercise mat or with special resistance equipment. Several pieces of specialized equipment are used in a complete Pilates workout. They're known by a variety of names, including Wunda Chair, Cadillac, Spine Corrector, High Chair and Half Barrel. However, these large machines aren't practical for home use.

The most widely used piece of Pilates equipment — and the one that a devoted practitioner might consider buying — is called the Reformer. This apparatus contains straps, springs, pulleys and a sliding carriage and allows you to do more than 100 different exercises. As your body moves in different positions, your muscles work against varying levels of resistance to train every muscle group.

Pilates work can also be done using resistance bands and stability balls, which are more affordable, portable and space-efficient than is the Reformer. You can buy a Pilates kit that includes a how-to video, resistance bands and a fitness ball.

Choosing. If you have the space, budget and motivation to invest in a Reformer, the type you choose will depend on your specific needs. If you're tight on space, consider getting a portable, stackable model.

Look for a Reformer that's built with sturdy, durable, quality materials and has a comfortable, supportive carriage. The equipment should be adjustable and allow for different settings.

An accessory called a box allows you to perform exercises seated on a box rather than on the carriage, which may offer more comfort and better alignment for people who aren't as flexible. You can also drape your legs and upper body over the ends of the box to work through a fuller range of motion and change the direction of resistance to work different muscles.

Using. The Pilates program emphasizes the mind-body connection and, like yoga, requires concentration and focus. The

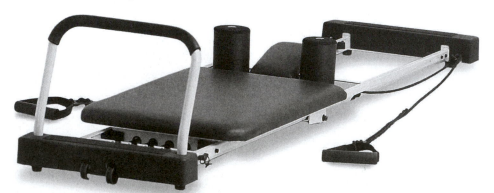

Pilates Reformer. Pilates equipment comes in a variety of designs. Generally, you sit or recline on the unit and place your hands or feet in the handles to perform core strengthening exercises.

training is based on six basic principles — breathing, concentration, control, centering, precision and flowing movement — that are integral to the technique.

Pilates is traditionally taught in one-on-one training sessions. If you can't afford a private session, consider taking a class. Instructional videos that range from beginner to advanced can also show you how to perform the exercises while incorporating the basic principles.

Other equipment

Yoga is a gentle exercise that improves flexibility, balance, strength and muscle tone through physical postures and breathing exercises. The simplest and most basic equipment you need to perform yoga is a sticky mat, an exercise mat with a textured or sticky surface to help keep your hands and feet from sliding as you do postures. Other yoga equipment includes straps and blocks. You can buy a yoga kit that contains everything you need, including a how-to video, sticky mat, strap and block.

Straps, belts, cables and ropes of all sorts can be used for various stretching exercises. Looped stretch cords have loops that you can put your foot in to anchor your stretch. Some are made with several loops of different lengths so that you can adjust as your flexibility level changes.

Water workouts

The pool is not just for swimming laps anymore. Aquatic exercise has expanded to encompass a variety of activities, from water aerobics and water walking or jogging to strength training. Some people are even doing yoga, kickboxing and tae kwon do in the water, and much of the equipment you'd normally find in a gym has an underwater counterpart, including treadmills, stationary bikes, rowers and stair steppers.

Water workouts can provide the benefits of stretching, resistance exercise and cardiovascular training. And aquatic therapy is flourishing as a rehabilitation tool for people recovering from strokes, surgery or injuries, as well as those with disabilities. Water is a hospitable workout environment for just about everyone, allowing people with arthritis and those who are overweight, pregnant or frail to exercise safely and effectively.

Aquatic exercise uses the resistance of water. Water offers 10 to 12 times the

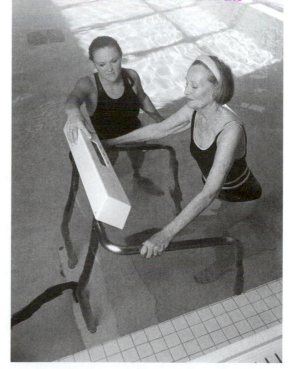

resistance of air, so just walking in water will work your abs and legs. But the right equipment can enhance your water workout. Buoyant equipment enables nonswimmers to participate in aquatic classes and work out in deep water. In shallow water, it provides extra support. Resistance equipment adds to the water's natural resistance to give you a more intense strength-building workout. Other equipment, such as goggles, keeps you comfortable and protected in the water. (Swimwear is discussed on page 133.)

Here's a rundown of some of the equipment you may want to consider for water workouts. These items are generally available at discount and sporting goods stores.

- **Flotation belts.** These help keep you upright and provide back support while you exercise in deep water. Look for a belt that fits comfortably and securely into the small of your back and has a quick-release latch.
- **Buoyancy vests.** Similar to flotation belts, these help hold your body in proper alignment during deep-water walking or jogging.
- **Water shoes.** Also called aqua shoes or aqua runners, these shoes protect your feet and provide traction for shallow-water exercising.
- **Goggles.** Swim goggles help you see clearly when swimming with your head in the water. If you wear contacts, using goggles can help you see under water without losing your lenses. Look for a pair that won't leak, such as a style with foam seals around the eyes.

- **Face mask and snorkel.** These can help you swim laps without having to turn your head to breathe, which is useful if you have back or neck problems. Another option is a hybrid of a snorkeling mask and swim goggle that seals to your face.
- **Hand buoys.** These hand-held buoyant cylinders may be either foam or air-filled and increase your stability and resistance for deep-water workouts.
- **Flotation rings.** These attach to your wrists or legs and create resistance when you push down, strengthening your muscles.
- **Webbed gloves.** These provide added resistance for building upper body and arm strength. The gloves are maneuverable, and you can vary the resistance by changing the angle of your hands.
- **Paddles.** Hand-held paddles have a strap for your fingers to slide through and add resistance for an arm and upper body workout.

Home starter gym

Despite the wide array of exercise equipment available, some of it at considerable cost, you can build a starter gym for under $200. All you need is a stability ball of the correct size, a simple bench on which to do some of your strength training, an assortment of hand weights, and a mat or rug for your floor exercises. With hand weights, start light and add heavier weights as you progress. Resistance bands or tubes can be used to substitute for hand weights.

- **Fins.** Swim fins add resistance when you kick, which helps strengthen your legs and back.
- **Kickboards.** This swimming aid, usually made of coated plastic foam, provides buoyancy and stability. Using a kickboard can improve your body position and can be used for a variety of strength training exercises.

Choosing. All equipment that will be used in a pool must be durable and able to withstand the harsh, corrosive effect of the chemicals added to pool water to keep it free of contamination and infection-causing bacteria.

Using. One way to learn to use aquatic gear is to take a class. Videos are also available on various water workouts.

Choosing the best fitness videotapes and DVDs

If you don't have the time, money or inclination to join a fitness class or facility, another option is to pop in an exercise videotape or DVD. Videos give you the benefits of an exercise class or instructor in the comfort of your own home and on your own schedule. They can also add variety to your regular workout routine and let you stay active on days when the weather is bad.

Like any other piece of equipment, fitness videos aren't one-size-fits-all. Which ones work for you depends on your fitness goals and preferences. Activities that aren't technical and involve minimal risk are probably best for doing at home with an exercise video. It's best to learn programs that focus on weight training or specialized techniques from a qualified instructor before getting a home version.

Before you buy an exercise video or DVD, consider the following:

- **Instructor's credentials.** Read the back of the package for a listing of the instructor's credentials and experience. Look for a certified, experienced instructor who includes a warm-up and cool-down with the workout. Avoid videos that feature a celebrity instructor without support from a trained professional.
- **Fitness level.** Most programs are marked beginner, intermediate or advanced. Start with one that fits your current fitness level, and add to your collection as your ability increases.
- **Workout goals.** Make sure the tape or DVD suits your specific needs. If you want a great aerobic workout, don't buy a tape or DVD that promises to "deflab your abs" or give you "buns of steel." Work toward building a collection that fosters balance and overall conditioning, including aerobics, strength and stretching. Many programs combine these types of exercise.
- **Intensity.** The best programs offer modifications for high- or low-intensity workouts.
- **Space and equipment requirements.** How much room does the workout require? You may feel claustrophobic doing a step routine in a small room. Will you need any special equipment or props, such as steps, barbells, stretch rope or cord, a mat, or a chair?

Cast a critical eye on the hyped marketing that goes along with fitness videos and DVDs. Many often make unsubstantiated claims. Avoid programs that promise quick weight loss or instant results.

One way to ensure you're spending your money wisely is to try before you buy. Find out if a friend, the local video rental store or the library has the program you're interested in.

WORKOUT GEAR

Fitness gear has come a long way since the days of simple cotton sweats, T-shirts and canvas sneakers. Consumers can choose from a vast range of workout clothing and shoes, and chances are they'll be wearing those items for more than just a trip to the gym. Workout wear, from sports bras to athletic shoes to track suits, has entered the fashion mainstream.

The variety of high-tech materials and fancy gear on the market can be overwhelming. But you don't have to bust your budget or spend hours researching fabric blends and fiber technologies to choose the best workout gear. By following some straightforward guidelines, you can find gear that will keep you comfortable, dry and safe.

Shoes

In the American Council on Exercise survey mentioned on page 96, fitness professionals ranked good shoes as the single most important exercise item. That's not surprising because in many physical activities, your feet take the biggest beating. For example, when a 150-pound person runs three miles, the cumulative impact on each foot is more than 150 tons.

Athletic footwear is designed to support your feet, protect them from injury and provide traction so that you don't slip. Doctors who are foot specialists recommend sturdy, properly fitted athletic shoes. They should be the proper width, with cushioning or shock absorption, arch support, a degree of flexibility, and wiggle room for your toes. Depending on your activity, you may want to go with a leather shoe if you want more rigidity and support. A mesh or canvas shoe is lighter and allows your foot to breathe better than a leather shoe does.

Beyond these general guidelines, how do you navigate your way to the correct shoe, considering that you're faced with hundreds of styles and brands to choose from? The multibillion-dollar athletic shoe industry offers so many options that selecting a pair of shoes has become increasingly complicated and confusing.

The most important considerations are the type of activity you'll be doing, your fitness level and the type of foot — normal, high or flat arch — that you have. If you walk or jog a couple of times a week and play some basketball in the driveway from time to time, cross-training shoes, running shoes or walking shoes will all probably meet your needs. But if you participate in a sport or activity three times a week or more, you need a shoe specific to that activity. For example, a runner needs a different type of shoe from a basketball player. Running shoes have more cushioning for shock absorption, and basketball shoes provide more ankle support for sudden stops and starts on the court. Athletic shoes are grouped into several different categories: running, training, walking, court sports (tennis, basketball, volleyball), field sports (soccer, football, baseball), winter sports (figure skating, ice hockey, skiing, snowboarding), track and field, specialty

Anatomy of an athletic shoe

Understanding the basic parts of an athletic shoe will help you sort through the multitude of styles and brands so that you can pick the one that's right for you.

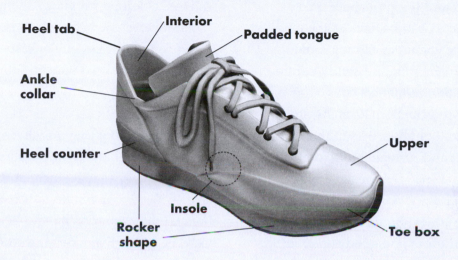

- **Last.** The basic shape of the sole and the footprint that the shoe is built around. The last can be curved, semicurved or straight.
- **Outsole.** Outermost portion of the sole that comes into contact with the ground and is treaded for traction.
- **Insole.** Portion of the sole that fits inside the shoe to provide cushioning and arch support.
- **Midsole.** Padded area between the insole and the outsole that provides comfort, cushioning and most of the shock absorption.
- **Upper.** Top part of the shoe with the laces, fancy designs and bright colors that holds the shoe together and keeps it on the foot. The upper may be made of soft breathable material, leather or synthetic leather, mesh or some combination of materials. A stiffer upper adds support but makes the shoe harder to put on.
- **Heel counter.** Rigid material around the heel of the shoe that provides stability and keeps the heel of the foot in place.
- **Toe box.** Tip of the shoe that provides needed wiggle room for the toes. It should be wide enough for your toes to spread and long enough so that a half-inch space is in front of your longest toe.
- **Ankle collar.** Area around the ankle that's padded for fit and comfort.
- **Heel tab.** Notched area of the ankle collar that reduces stress on the Achilles tendon. Also called Achilles' notch.
- **Reflective tab.** Provides extra visibility at night.
- **Tongue.** Designed to enhance fit. May be padded.
- **Eyelets.** Equalize pressure on foot. Shoe is laced through them.
- **Laces.** Round laces are generally easier to thread and pull through the eyelets, but you may have to double-knot them to keep them tied.

sports (golf, bicycling, bowling, aerobics) and outdoor sports (hunting, fishing).

Here are general guidelines for some of the most common athletic shoes:

- **Running and jogging shoes** are designed to absorb shock as the foot strikes the ground. Features should include cushioning, flexibility, control and stability in the heel counter area, as well as good traction. Running shoes are generally lighter weight than walking shoes and provide more forefoot flexibility. (See "The ideal running shoe" on page 294 for more details.)

- **Walking shoes** should have a comfortable, soft upper and good shock absorption, especially in the heel of the shoe and under the ball of the foot. Look for a rocker sole design, which encourages the foot to roll and push off the toes in a natural walking motion. Half-inch heels can help you avoid overstretching your Achilles tendon. Avoid shoes with thick, spongy soles.

- **Court sports shoes** should provide support for the ankle during side-to-side (lateral) movements. The sole should be stiff but not too thick, and cushioning of the forefoot is important.

- **Aerobics shoes** should have a lot of impact-absorbing cushioning as well as ankle and arch support for side-to-side movement. The soles should allow for twisting and turning.

- **Cross-training shoes** combine features of different athletic shoes so that you can wear them for more than one sport. They have the forefoot flexibility you need for

running, but they also have the lateral support necessary for aerobics or tennis.

- **Cycling shoes** need rigid support across the arch to prevent collapse during pedaling. Look for a heel lift. Toe clips or specially designed shoe cleats help keep your feet on the pedal. For casual bikers, cross-training shoes may be sufficient.

Shopping tips

Before you go shopping for shoes, figure out if your feet have normal, low or high arches. It's easy to tell which kind you have — just wet the bottom of your bare foot and then stand on a piece of cardboard or paper. Examine your footprint. Can you see most of your foot? If so, you probably have low arches. If you see very little of your foot, you likely have high arches. A normal or neutral arch falls somewhere in between. (See "What type of arch do you have?" on page 130.)

Another way to tell is to look at your current shoes to see how they're wearing. Place the shoes on a flat surface, such as a tabletop. Do they tilt inward or outward? If your shoes tilt outward, you likely have high arches, and if your shoes tilt to the inside, you probably have low arches. Check your outsoles. Are the outer edges of your heel and inner edges on the ball of your foot worn down? In that case, you're a heel striker, which suggests that you probably have a neutral-arched foot.

Regardless of the shape of your foot or the style of the shoe, fit is most important. Pay attention to comfort, not fancy looks.

The latest technology won't matter if the shoe hurts your foot in any way.

If possible, purchase your shoes at a store staffed with professional shoe fitters or people experienced in your sport. An experienced salesperson can help you find the right type of shoe for your needs. He or she can also help fit the shoes properly and explain the cushioning and shoe structure. Bring your old shoes with you when you shop for your new pair — most shoe professionals can give you some tips on what to buy based on the wear of your old shoes.

Here are some other tips for buying athletic shoes:

- Go to a sporting goods store or specialty shoe store with a large inventory so that you can try a variety of styles and sizes.

- Have both your feet measured. Your feet may be different sizes, and you'll want the shoes to fit your largest foot. Your feet expand while bearing weight, so make sure you're standing when they're measured.

- Try on shoes after a workout or at the end of the day. Your feet will be at their largest during these times.

- Wear the same type of sock that you'll wear for your sport or activity.

- Try on both shoes and check the fit. Make sure your heel fits snugly in each shoe and doesn't slip as you walk. You should be able to freely wiggle all of your toes. Allow for a half-inch space — approximately the width of your thumb — between your longest toe and the end of the shoe. If you can detect the outline of your toes in the top or on the side of the shoes, try a larger size or wider shoe. Shoes should also feel comfortable through the arch and fit well across the ball of the foot. The widest part of your foot should be in the widest part of the shoe. Your foot shouldn't move from side to side in the shoe.

- Test for comfort by walking or jogging several steps. If the shoes don't feel comfortable right away, try another pair. There should be no break-in period for a pair of athletic shoes.

- Choose shoes for their fit, not according to the size you've worn in the past. Your feet grow larger as you age, so your shoe size may change over time. In addition,

What shoes are the best for walking?

A good pair of shoes is just about all you need to start walking, one of the most popular and convenient forms of exercise. The ideal walking shoe should be stable from side to side, be well-cushioned and allow you to walk smoothly. Many running shoes also fit these criteria. It's fine to wear running shoes even if your primary activity is walking, as long as you're comfortable, stable on your feet and don't experience any pain. Lightweight trail and hiking boots are also suitable for walking.

If you primarily jog or run, steer clear of shoes designed for walking. Your feet sustain a more forceful impact per step when you jog or run, and a shoe specifically designed for running provides extra cushioning to protect your bones and joints.

Which type of arch do you have?

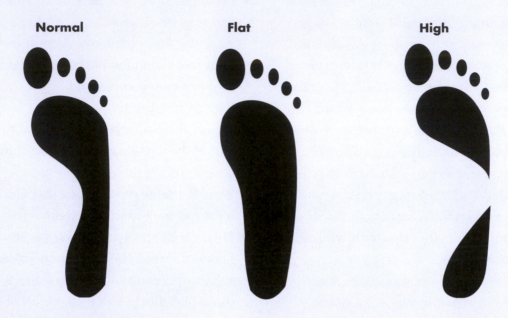

Foot type	What this means	Look for shoes with these features
Normal	You have neutral arches: not too flat, not too high. Your feet land on the ground rolling slightly to the outside of the heel and then roll inward to absorb shock.	Firm midsoles Semicurved lasts Moderate rear-foot stability Medium cushioning
Flat	Your feet land on the outside of the heel and have a tendency toward excessive inward roll (pronation). This common problem may be exaggerated when running. Over time, excessive inward rolling of the foot may lead to overuse injuries.	Firm, stable heel counter Added arch support Straight last Motion control to minimize the natural inward pull of your feet Thick, firm midsole
High	Your feet generally roll toward the outside (supination). This can cause excessive strain on joints and muscles.	Soft midsoles Curved lasts Low rear-foot stability Extra cushioning for shock absorption

slight variations in size may occur due to differences in manufacturing.

- Women with narrow heels needn't get a smaller size just so the heel won't slide. Some companies offer athletic shoes specifically designed for women's feet, with narrower heels.

- Women with wide feet shouldn't shy away from trying a men's or boys' shoe, which is cut a bit larger through the heel and the ball of the foot. A woman's size 10, for instance, equals a man's 8, but the man's shoe is wider.

- Check the shoe's quality — place the shoe on a counter and make sure the heel is straight up when you look at it from the back. The midsole should be well connected to the upper and the stitching complete. Look inside the shoe for any irregular bumps.

- If you have bunions or hammertoes, choose a shoe with a wide toe box.

- Ask the salesperson if you can try the shoes at home without voiding the return policy. Then walk in the shoes for 15 to 20 minutes — on a treadmill, if you have one — to see how they feel.

- Look for a salesperson who understands the different types of feet and who is able to match them with the proper shoe type.

Wear and tear

Athletic shoes wear out. Your shoes may still feel comfortable, but they might not be giving you enough support or shock absorption. Shoes lose their cushioning after three to six months of regular use.

Check the condition of your shoes by placing them on a table or counter and looking at them from the back. If they lean inward or outward, it's probably time to replace them. If the outsole is worn through, it's time for new shoes. Listen to your body. If you experience any new aches and pains, take that as a hint that your shoes may be worn out.

Athletic shoes should be replaced after 300 to 500 miles of running or 300 hours of aerobic activity, or every six months. Your midsoles might be worn down to the point of causing chronic wear-type injuries, but you might not be able to visibly detect any wear and tear. In addition, keep in mind that there's a recovery time for the midsole after each use. If you run every day or are a regular walker, consider getting two pairs of shoes and using one pair every other day.

Clothing

Exercise clothing should keep you feeling comfortable, safe, supported and dry. Your choice of clothing depends on your activity and the weather or place you exercise. Choose comfortable, nonrestrictive items. It's better to underdress than to overdress, because exercise generates a lot of body heat.

Don't overdress in order to increase your sweating as you exercise. This can lead to dangerously high body temperatures. Besides, any weight loss you achieve from sweating is due to water loss, not fat, and will be replaced when you drink.

Today's active wear often uses high-tech performance fabrics such as polypropylene and synthetic blends such as polyester-cotton or nylon-lycra. These are wicking materials, which draw sweat away from the skin to the outer surface of the garment, where it can evaporate more quickly. These fabrics won't stop you from sweating, but they'll keep your skin drier, which can make you more comfortable. Another type of fabric that's designed to promote drying and cooling is mesh. It helps circulate air between your skin and the garment.

In one small study, synthetic fabrics designed for exercising didn't keep people any cooler or more comfortable during and after an exercise session in moderately warm, dry conditions than cotton clothing did. But the cotton clothes retained more sweat than the synthetics 30 minutes after the workout. For this reason, synthetic fabrics can be especially useful in cooler conditions, when sweat may have a greater effect on your body temperature.

Following are some guidelines to consider when choosing workout wear.

Sports bras and briefs. The right underwear gives you the support you need to stay active. For women, an ordinary bra doesn't keep the breasts from bouncing during physical activity. The more vigorous your activity, the greater the bounce. And the larger your breasts, the more vulnerable they are.

Fortunately, you can resolve this problem with a good sports bra. Here are some tips for choosing a sports bra:

- Fit is crucial. The bra should fit firmly enough to control breast motion, but not so tightly as to interfere with breathing. When you try it on, do a few jumping jacks — your entire upper body should move as one unit, with limited breast bouncing.
- Sports bras either have molded cups that support the breasts or they flatten the breasts against the body. Larger breasted women may be more comfortable with molded cups.
- Look for minimal vertical stretch in the fabric. Horizontal stretch is necessary, however, to get the bra on and off easily.
- To help wick away sweat and keep odor in check, choose a blend of at least 50 percent cotton and a breathable material such as lycra mesh or Coolmax. Cotton provides more comfort, reduced stretch and greater support than do synthetic materials.
- Choose wide, nonstretch straps or a wide Y-back panel.
- Avoid seams over the nipple area, which may cause chafing.

For men, sports underwear no longer means just a jockstrap (athletic supporter). Although jockstraps are still used in contact sports such as football — they mainly serve to hold a plastic cup that protects the genitals — more comfortable alternatives are available for other physical activities.

Sports underwear, including compression shorts and runners shorts, provide support and some protection by keeping the genitals close to the body. They also may help keep sweat from accumulating. Compression shorts are made of nylon and spandex. They come in a variety of styles and are usually worn under baggy gym shorts. Runners shorts have two layers sewn into one garment. They can help you stay cool in warm weather but offer little protection from the cold.

Another option some men like is wearing a racing-style swimsuit, which offers the gripping support of a jockstrap without the rubbing and chafing.

Everyday briefs also provide decent support and comfort for many physical activities. Because cotton briefs hold moisture, they may stay wet when you sweat. A blend of 50 percent cotton and 50 percent synthetic works better.

Swimwear. Chlorine and other chemicals in pool water can wreak havoc on swimsuits. Some swimwear manufacturers offer chlorine-resistant lycra that's designed to be stronger than ordinary lycra, which is the material used for most swimsuits.

Fitness activity and intensity. For a high-intensity activity such as kickboxing or running, wicking material and mesh linings are useful. For exercises such as yoga, Pilates and tai chi, clothing that provides support on top (for women) and allows for freedom of movement elsewhere is a good choice. For biking, look for shorts with padding that's designed to eliminate pressure on sensitive anatomical areas. Shorts or cropped pants won't get snagged on the pedals or chains.

Safety. For exercising outdoors at night, on busy roads or in fog or other low-visibility conditions, wear a reflective vest and light-colored clothing. Bikers, in-line skaters, snowboarders and horseback riders should always wear safety devices such as helmets, mouth guards, wrist guards, and knee and elbow pads. The same is true if you're playing contact sports such as soccer and football. Goggles are mandatory for indoor racquet sports.

SUMMARY

With the wide variety of exercise equipment on the market, choosing what's best for you can be a daunting task. Remember that you don't have to spend a fortune on the tools you need to get and stay fit. You can start with the basics and work your way up if you decide you need more gear.

Don't forget exercise videos. They can provide the direction and motivation you need to keep exercising, especially if joining a fitness club isn't an option.

Finally, remember that fitness isn't about the equipment. It's about you.

Exercise guide

There are more than 150 exercises on the pages of this "Exercise guide" to help you improve your fitness. The guide is divided into sections on flexibility, strength, core, balance and plyometrics. Within each section, exercises are arranged in sequence, starting with the head and neck and progressing to the arms and upper body, then down through the lower body, legs and feet. In many cases, several exercises are shown for each part of the body. Choose exercises that work best for you, and periodically switch to add variety to your workout. Advanced exercises that are more challenging are indicated by the advanced symbol. (A)

Note: Before using this guide, check with your doctor about which exercises are safe for you. For your safety, perform advanced exercises in the presence of a qualified health professional before trying them at home.

Although this guide can be used independent of the rest of the book, details about how to perform these exercises, as well as how to integrate them into your overall fitness program, are found in chapters throughout this book.

The exercises in this guide are demonstrated by the book's editors in chief, Diane Dahm, M.D., and Jay Smith, M.D. Keep the following points in mind when selecting and performing these exercises.

Flexibility (pages 138-149)

- Stretches should produce muscle tension, not pain.
- For stretches that are held (static stretches), perform three repetitions, holding each stretch for 30 to 45 seconds. To complete motions as part of a dynamic stretch, perform multiple slow motions into and out of the stretched position, increasing the amplitude of the motion each time.
- Avoid bouncing while stretching. For details on stretching techniques and what may be best for you, see "Flexibility Exercise," starting on page 60.
- Unless otherwise directed by your health care professional, perform the same number of repetitions of your stretches with the left and right side.
- Breathe normally while stretching.

Strength (pages 150-172)

- Isometric exercises are generally held for 10 seconds per repetition, unless otherwise stated.
- For exercises involving motion, each repetition should take five to six seconds, equally divided between the upward (concentric) phase and downward (eccentric) phase.
- Many exercises can be adapted so that resistance may be provided by gravity (squat, push-up), immovable objects (isometric shoulder exercises), weights (arm curls), or resistance tubing or bands (shoulder internal rotation).
- Elastic resistance tubing or bands can be attached to doorknobs, table legs or other immovable objects. Always make sure tubing or bands are securely attached before applying force.
- Exercises shown lying on your back can be done on the floor or on a bench.

- In general, to increase strength, choose resistance to allow one set of eight to 12 high-quality repetitions for each exercise. To increase your muscle mass (hypertrophy), do three or more sets of eight to 12 repetitions. For weight loss or toning, do two or more sets with lighter resistance to allow 15 or more repetitions per set.
- Maintain normal breathing patterns and good posture.
- Almost any strength training exercise can be made easier by lowering the resistance or changing the exercise to provide more support, such as using a pole or chair for balance assistance.
- Strength training exercises shouldn't be painful.

Core (pages 173-180)

- This section is divided into subsections by direction of motion — flexion, extension, lateral and rotation. The exercises in each subsection work your core in a different manner. Variety is key. Be sure to choose core exercises from two or more subsections for any particular workout. Change exercises often to maintain variety and challenge.
- Unless otherwise noted, try to maintain a gentle abdominal hollowing maneuver during all your exercises. See page 60 for information on abdominal hollowing.
- Core exercises involving isometric holds can begin with a goal of holding one 10-second contraction. Over time, increase the holding time to a goal of two to

three minutes each for one to three reps. This will train your core for endurance.
- Exercises involving movement should be done in a slow, controlled manner, maintaining normal neck and back curves.
- Do each core exercise until you're just about to lose perfect alignment. Don't continue training after losing proper alignment or good posture.
- Breathe normally during all exercises.

Balance (pages 181-184)

- This part consists of two subsections — isolated balance and integrated balance. Isolated balance exercises focus primarily on balance and weight shifting. Time how long you maintain each position. Perform two to three repetitions as able, with a goal of at least 30 seconds per repetition. Integrated balance exercises increase or decrease the challenge of common exercises by manipulating balance requirements. Any reduction in the base of support, such as standing on one leg or on a pillow, or lifting an uneven load, such as holding a weight in one hand only, increases balance and core challenges. Increasing the base of support or reducing load does the opposite. Perform one to three sets of eight to 12 repetitions.
- As part of your routine, choose at least one balance exercise appropriate for your ability and needs.
- Integrated balance exercises offer greater challenge, but with greater pay-

off because they simultaneously train strength, core stability and balance. They also require more muscles to work simultaneously, burning more calories.

- Only a few variations of integrated balance exercise are shown. However, virtually any standard exercise can be similarly modified. Use your imagination to create new and challenging integrated balance exercises.

- In general, perform balance exercises at the beginning of a workout because of their high demands.

- Always maintain good form and breathe normally.

Plyometrics (pages 185-187)

- This is a specialized form of strength training involving high loads and velocities that stretch a muscle before contracting it. Plyometrics is an advanced training method with excellent carry-over to sports, but with a higher risk of injury. If you have any doubt about performing plyometric exercises, consult a professional before attempting them.

- Choose one exercise that's most appropriate for your needs. Perform one set of five to 10 repetitions with good form. Rest adequately between sets. These are not endurance exercises.

- If possible, perform these exercises on a padded surface such as a mat or carpet.

Exercise terminology

Here are some terms used in the "Exercise guide" that are helpful to know.

Alignment. The position of the body segments. For the purposes of this book, *alignment* and *posture* are used interchangeably (see Posture).

Core. Muscles of the trunk, including the back, abdominals and buttocks.

Endurance. The ability to maintain muscle force over time. This is particularly important when doing core training to increase resistance to fatigue.

Fatigue. Deterioration in the ability to maintain a muscle contraction or level of work over time. Endurance training involves working for longer periods of time to build up fatigue resistance.

Isometric. A muscle contraction in which the muscle doesn't change length. Therefore, the joints and body segments don't move. Tensing up your thigh muscles is an isometric contraction.

Posture. The position of your body. Optimal posture in standing is when the ears are over the shoulders, the shoulders over the hips and the normal spine curves are maintained.

Proper form. Maintenance of normal alignment and posture during the exercise (see related terms).

Range of motion (ROM). The path of motion through which the body moves to complete an exercise movement.

Repetition (Rep). The completion of one exercise movement or position.

Set. A consecutive sequence of repetitions. For example, a strength-training set may consist of eight to 12 repetitions.

Neck stretches and range-of-motion (ROM) exercises

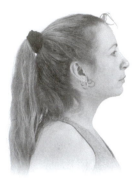 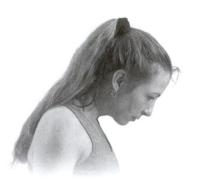 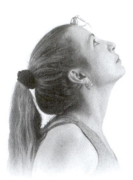

Neutral
1. Start position. Head well-balanced over shoulders, looking straight ahead.

Flexion
2. Slowly look down at your toes. Shoulders stay back, but relaxed. Pause briefly, then return to neutral.

Extension
3. Slowly look up without arching your back. Pause briefly, then return to neutral. Stop if you feel dizzy.

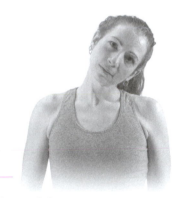 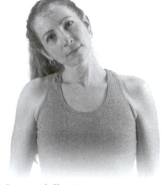

Left lateral flexion
1. Slowly bring your left ear toward your left shoulder. Pause, then return to neutral. Look straight ahead. Don't bend neck forward or backward.

Right lateral flexion
2. Same as left lateral flexion, but move toward your right shoulder.

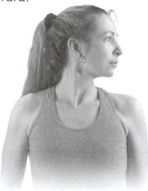 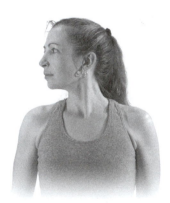

Left rotation
1. Without bending neck, attempt to look over your left shoulder. Pause, then return to forward-facing position.

Right rotation
2. Same as left rotation, but in the opposite direction.

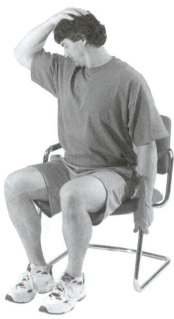

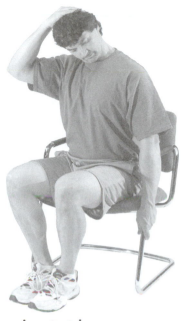

Left levator stretch

Hold chair with left hand to stabilize body. Tuck chin and look down toward right foot. To stretch, pull head down gently with right hand. Repeat on other side.

Left trapezius stretch

Similar to left levator stretch, but look to left foot. To stretch, pull head gently to the right side with right hand. Repeat on other side.

Chest stretches

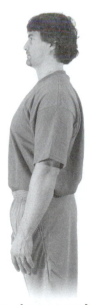

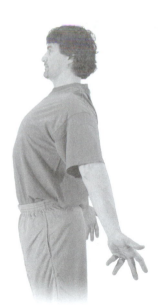

Standing chest stretch

1. Start position. Neutral posture, maintain forward gaze.

Standing chest stretch

2. Move arms backward while rotating palms forward. Squeeze shoulder blades together, breathe deeply, and lift chest upward. Return to start position. Repeat.

Chest stretches (cont.)

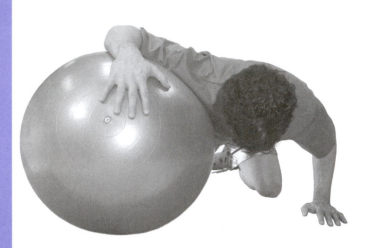

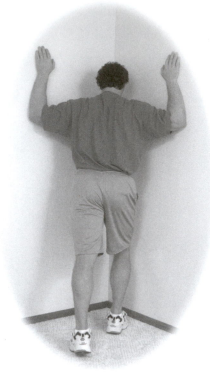

Pectoralis stretch with stability ball
On all fours, with right shoulder resting on stability ball. Trunk stays parallel to floor while you sink down toward floor. Feel stretch in front right shoulder. Repeat on left.

Pectoralis stretch in wall corner
Face corner with arms as shown. Keeping neutral posture, lean toward corner, stretching front chest.

Shoulder stretches

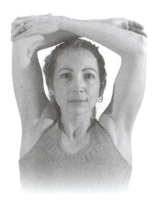

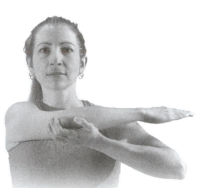

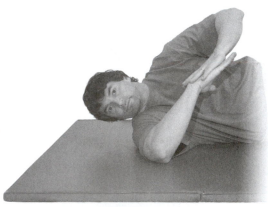

Inferior shoulder stretch
Position as above. Grasp right elbow and gently pull toward right ear. Maintain upright posture. Feel stretch in right armpit. Repeat on left.

Posterior shoulder stretch
Reach right arm across chest as above. Left hand gently pulls elbow farther toward left shoulder. Feel stretch in back of shoulder. Repeat on left.

"Sleeper stretch" for internal rotation
Lie on right side with right arm elevated 80 degrees and elbow bent. Left hand gently pushes right hand toward floor. Feel stretch in back of right shoulder. Repeat on left.

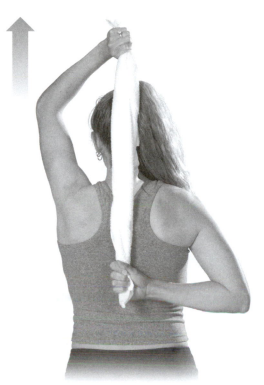

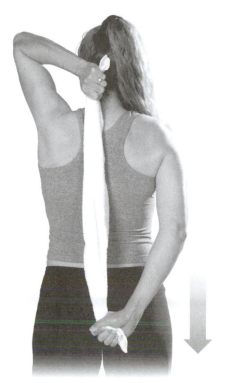

Towel stretch — Right internal rotation
1. Hold towel as above. Slowly straighten left elbow, pulling right hand upward. Feel stretch in right shoulder. Repeat on left.

Towel stretch — Left external rotation
2. Hold towel as above. Slowly straighten right elbow, pulling down toward the floor. Feel stretch in left shoulder. Repeat on right.

Wrist and forearm stretches

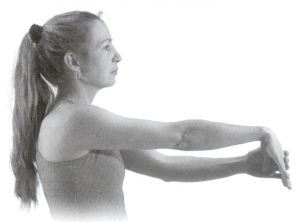

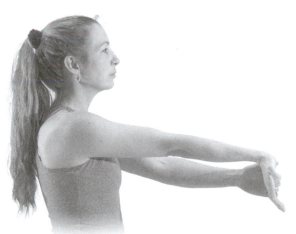

Wrist extensor stretch
Position right arm as above, palm facing the floor. Keeping the elbow straight, gently pull wrist toward your body with other hand. Feel stretch in right forearm and wrist. Repeat on left.

Wrist flexor stretch
Position right arm as above, palm facing up. With elbow straight, gently pull wrist toward the body with other hand. Feel stretch in right forearm and wrist. Repeat on left.

Abdomen and spine ROM exercises and stretches

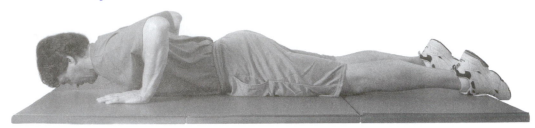

Spine stretch
1. Start position. Palms on floor next to shoulders, legs relaxed.

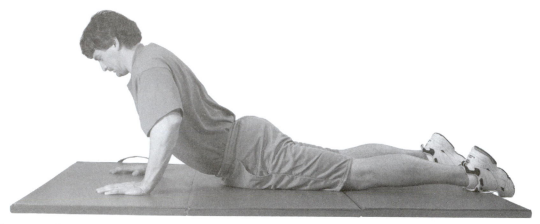

Spine stretch
2. Keeping low back and legs relaxed, gently push upward by straightening elbows until pelvis starts rising from floor. Keep looking at the floor. After completing stretch, return to start position.

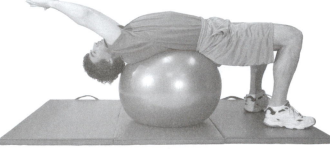

Abdominal stretch on stability ball
Position as above. Reach overhead to feel abdominal muscles stretch. To increase stretch intensity, bend knees to allow buttocks to drop toward floor.

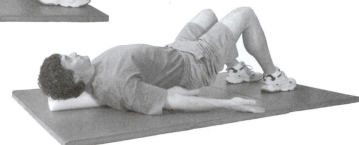

Thoracic spine stretch
Place foam roller or rolled towel along spine. Move arms out to sides, palms facing ceiling. Feel stretch in thoracic spine and chest.

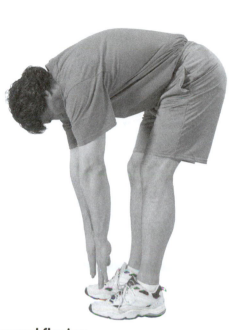

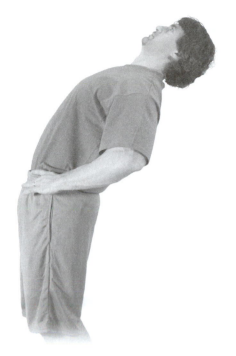

Forward flexion
Slowly bend forward, reaching for your toes. Maintain minimal bend in hips and knees. Avoid bouncing.

Extension
Hands on hips. Slowly lean backward, arching back. Maintain head position as shown. Use caution if you have balance problems.

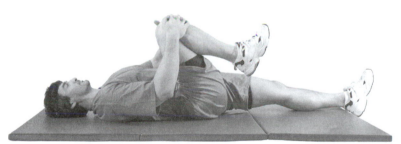

Single knee to chest
Position as above. Slowly pull right knee up toward chest. Keep left leg relaxed. Feel low back and hip stretch. Repeat on left.

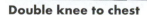

Double knee to chest
Similar to single knee to chest, but pull both knees up toward the chest. This variation usually provides a more intense low back stretch. Note how trunk and head maintain optimal posture.

Spine ROM exercises and stretches (cont.)

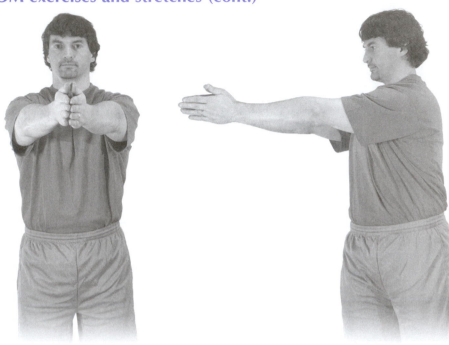

Rotation

1. Stand as above, facing forward with palms together.

Rotation

2. Keeping palms together and feet on floor, slowly rotate to right. Feel stretch in low back and the back of shoulders. Repeat to the left.

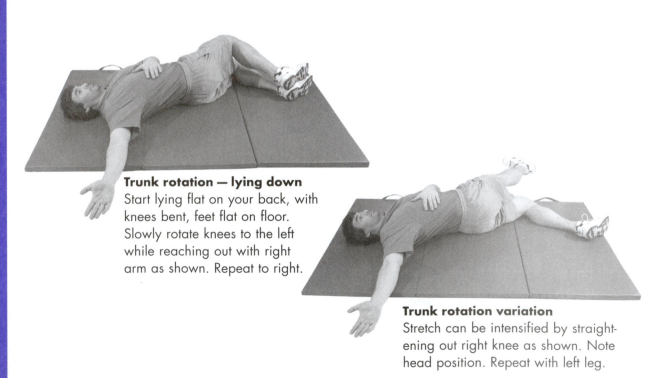

Trunk rotation — lying down
Start lying flat on your back, with knees bent, feet flat on floor. Slowly rotate knees to the left while reaching out with right arm as shown. Repeat to right.

Trunk rotation variation
Stretch can be intensified by straightening out right knee as shown. Note head position. Repeat with left leg.

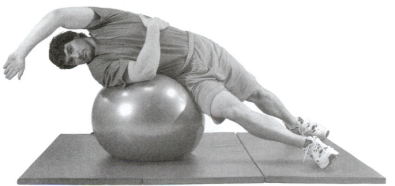

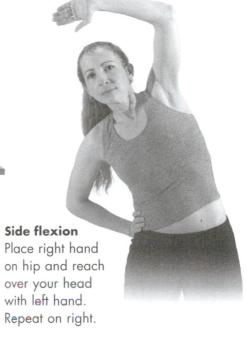

 Side stretch on stability ball
Requires good balance. Lie on right side. Reach overhead with left arm. Don't rotate trunk. Moving ball down toward hips increases stretch. Repeat on other side.

Side flexion
Place right hand on hip and reach over your head with left hand. Repeat on right.

Hip ROM exercises and stretches

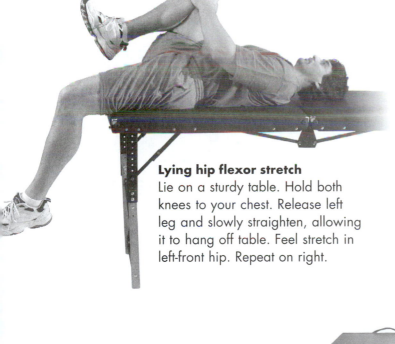

Lying hip flexor stretch
Lie on a sturdy table. Hold both knees to your chest. Release left leg and slowly straighten, allowing it to hang off table. Feel stretch in left-front hip. Repeat on right.

Kneeling hip flexor stretch
Position as above, trunk straight, knees bent to 90 degrees. Pole in left hand provides support. Keeping trunk erect, slowly move trunk forward, feeling stretch in left-front hip. Repeat on right.

EXERCISE GUIDE

FLEXIBILITY

Hip ROM exercises and stretches (cont.)

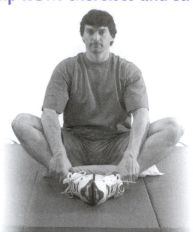

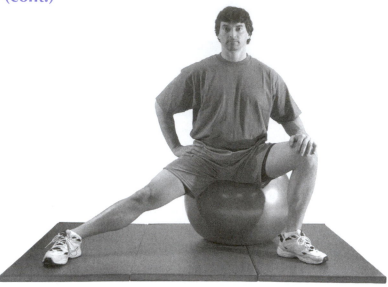

Seated groin stretch
Sit on pillow as above. While maintaining normal arch in low back, gently pull forward with your hands.

Groin stretch on stability ball
Requires good balance. Sit on ball. Maintain normal back arch and straighten right leg as shown. Feel stretch in right groin. Repeat on left.

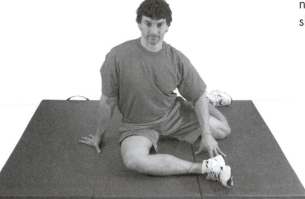

Seated gluteal and groin stretch
Position as above. Arch back and lean forward toward right knee. Feel stretch in right buttock (gluteal) and left groin. Repeat on other side.

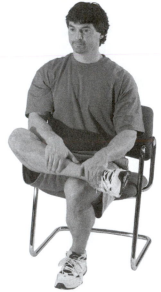

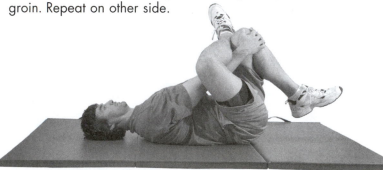

Seated gluteal stretch
Position as above. Lean forward with normal back arch. Feel stretch in right buttock (gluteal) region. Repeat on left.

Lying gluteal stretch
Similar to seated gluteal stretch. Position as above. Wrap hands or towel around left knee and pull toward chest. Trunk stays relaxed. Feel stretch in right buttock (gluteal). Repeat on opposite side.

Knee ROM exercises and stretches

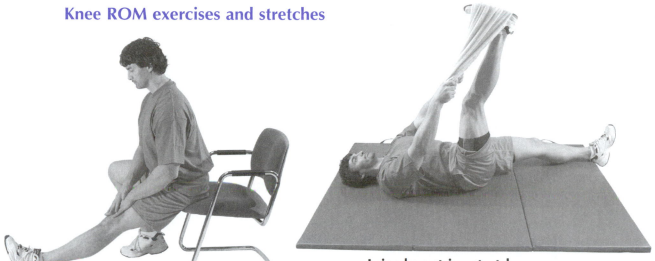

Seated hamstring stretch
Position as above. Maintain normal back arch. Slowly straighten left knee until stretch is felt. May apply gentle downward pressure with hand. Repeat on right.

Lying hamstring stretch
Lie on back with towel around right foot. Raise leg and pull on towel to keep knee as straight as possible. Trunk stays relaxed. Stretches right hamstring. Repeat on left.

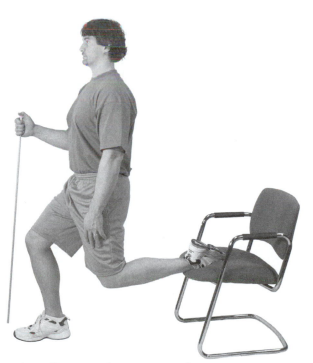

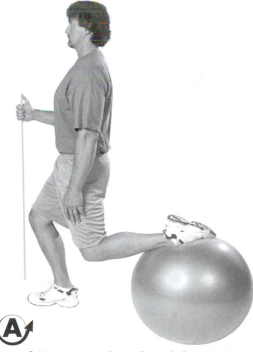

Standing quadriceps stretch
Requires pole for balance assist. Start position as above. Bend right knee while maintaining upright trunk. Feel stretch in left thigh. Repeat on other side.

Quadriceps stretch with stability ball
Similar to standing quadriceps stretch, but requires more strength and balance.

Knee ROM exercises and stretches (cont.)

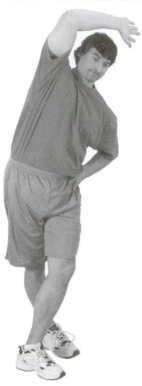

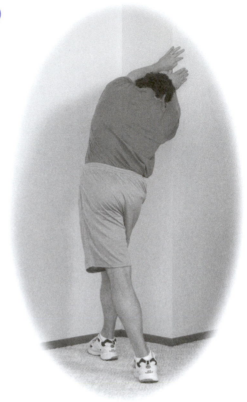

Standing iliotibial band stretch
Stand as shown, crossing left foot over right. Left hand pushes pelvis to right while right hand reaches overhead to left. Feel stretch in right hip and thigh. Repeat on other side.

Trunk iliotibial band stretch
Position as shown. Grasp wall corner for balance. Move left hip forward, then to left. Stretches left trunk, hip and thigh. Repeat on other side.

Ankle ROM exercises and stretches

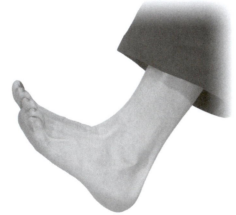

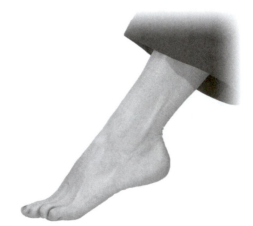

Dorsiflexion
Point toes and ankle upward toward knee, then relax. Do seated (knee bent) or lying down (knee straight). Do both sides.

Plantar flexion
Point toes and ankle downward as shown. Do seated (knee bent) or lying down (knee straight). Do both sides.

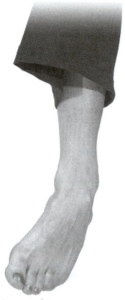

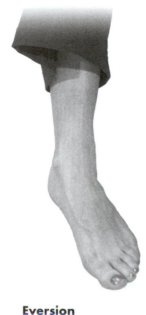

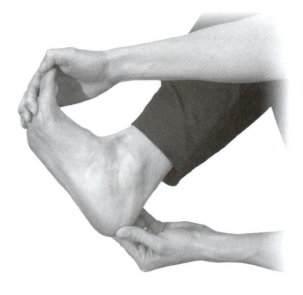

Inversion
Shown for left ankle and foot. Point big toe inward. Perform seated or lying. Do both sides.

Eversion
Shown for left ankle and foot. Point big toe outward. Perform seated or lying. Do both sides.

Plantar fascia stretch
Perform seated with toes pointed upward. Gently pull toes farther upward while maintaining ankle bend to 90 degrees as shown.

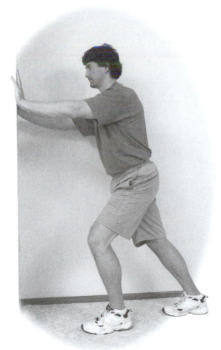

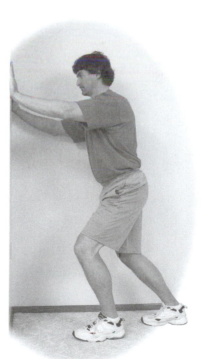

Calf stretch with straight knee
Lean against a wall as shown. While maintaining straight right knee, bend left knee as if to move it toward the wall. Stretches right calf. Repeat on other side.

Calf stretch with bent knee
Similar to calf stretch with straight knee, but with right knee bent. Focuses on deep calf muscle. Maintain upright trunk and face forward. Repeat on other side.

Neck

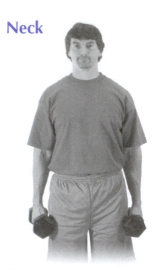

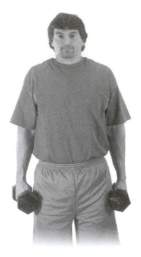

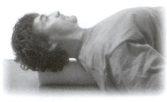

Chin tuck
1. Targets deep neck muscles. Start as above, lying on floor, with foam roller or towel along spine.

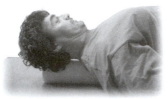

Shrug
1. Targets trapezius and neck muscles. Start as above, with or without resistance.

Shrug
2. While maintaining upright posture, slowly shrug shoulders upward. Keep head and neck erect and straight while looking forward. Return to start position.

Chin tuck
2. Tuck chin directly down toward floor, as if nodding "yes." Don't curl neck upward. Head stays on roller or towel.

Shoulders

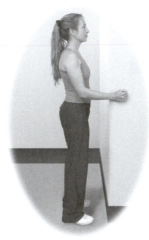

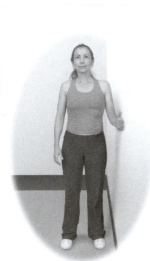

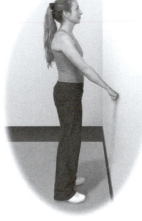

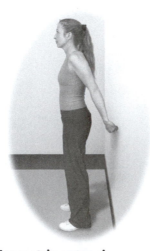

Isometric internal rotation
Targets shoulder and chest muscles. Start as above, facing wall near a corner. Gently press right hand into wall. Repeat on other side.

Isometric external rotation
Targets shoulder muscles, particularly rotator cuff. Start as above. Press back of left hand on wall. Repeat on other side.

Isometric flexion
Targets middle and anterior shoulder muscles. Start as above. Push back of right hand forward and upward on wall as shown. Repeat on other side.

Isometric extension
Targets middle and posterior shoulder muscles. Start as above. Push left hand into wall backward and upward as shown. Repeat on other side.

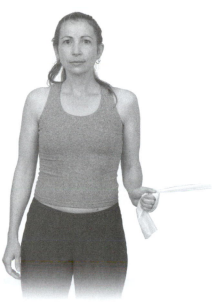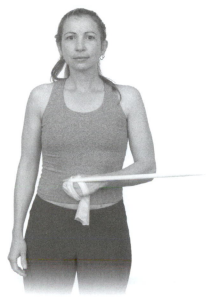

Internal rotation with resistance band
1. Targets chest and shoulder. Start as above with resistance band securely attached. Perform seated or standing.

Internal rotation with resistance band
2. With elbow at side, rotate left hand inward toward right hip. Return to start position. Repeat on other side.

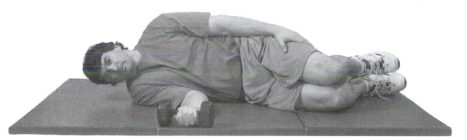

Side-lying internal rotation
1. Targets chest and shoulder muscles. Start as above, with or without resistance. May place pillow under head for support.

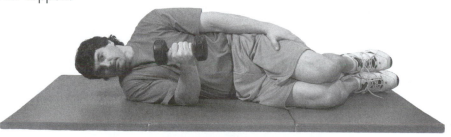

Side-lying internal rotation
2. Slowly move right hand upward and toward your body, while keeping right upper arm tucked against the body. Return to start position. Repeat on left side.

Shoulders (cont.)

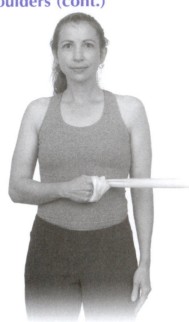 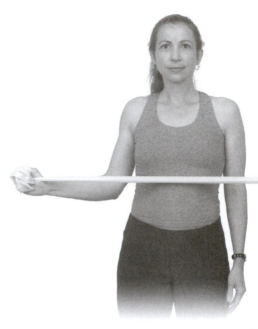

External rotation with resistance band
1. Targets shoulder muscles, particularly rotator cuff muscles. Start as above. Perform seated or standing.

External rotation with resistance band
2. Keeping elbow tucked at side, slowly rotate right arm outward so the back of your hand faces backward. Return to start position. Repeat on left side.

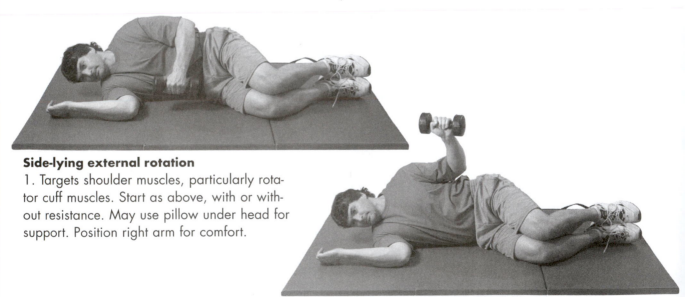

Side-lying external rotation
1. Targets shoulder muscles, particularly rotator cuff muscles. Start as above, with or without resistance. May use pillow under head for support. Position right arm for comfort.

Side-lying external rotation
2. Slowly rotate left hand upward and backward so that the back of your hand faces backward. Return to starting position. Repeat on other side.

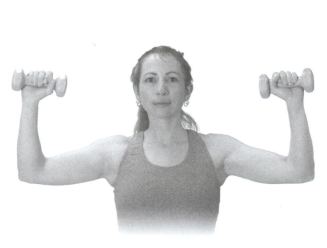

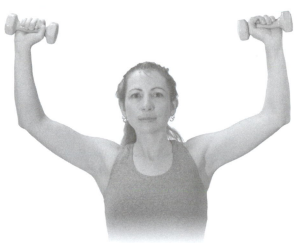

Shoulder press
1. Perform seated or standing. Start as shown, with or without resistance.

Shoulder press
2. Slowly press hands upward, straightening the elbows so that the hands move almost directly upward. Keep head still. Return to start.

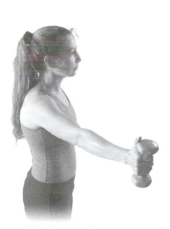

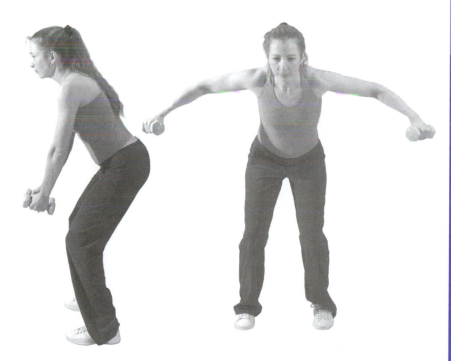

Side-lateral raise
Targets shoulder muscles, particularly rotator cuff. With right arm at side and thumb pointing up, slowly raise arm upward to a point just below perpendicular. Repeat on left.

Bent-over side raise
1. Targets shoulder and upper back muscles. Start position as shown, hips and knees slightly bent, spine curves maintained and shoulders over knees.

Bent-over side raise
2. Slowly move hands outward and backward, squeezing the shoulder blades together. Keep hip, knee and back starting posture. Return to start position.

Shoulders (cont.)

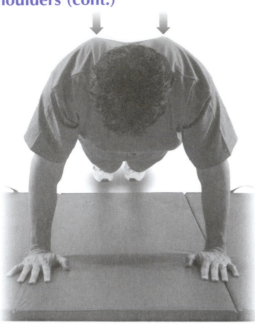

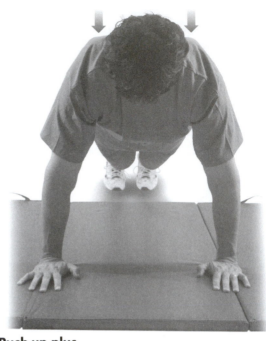

Push-up plus

1. Targets shoulder and chest muscles. Start with a regular push-up and hold the finish position as above. Shoulder blades will be above plane of back (arrows).

Push-up plus

2. Perform plus by pushing more into the floor. Shoulder blades will move forward on rib cage and be less prominent (arrows), raising trunk farther upward. Return to start.

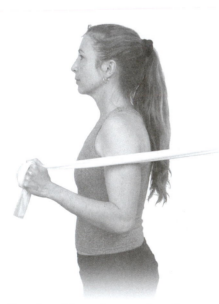

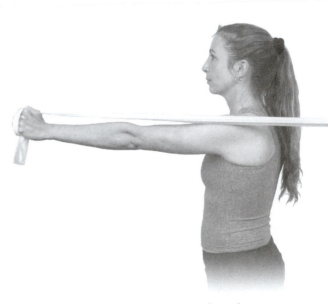

Punch with resistance band

1. Targets chest and shoulder muscles. Perform standing or seated. Attach band securely at shoulder height. Start position as above.

Punch with resistance band

2. Straighten elbow, punching forward. Note that arm position finishes parallel to direction of pull of band. Return to start position. Do both sides.

Back

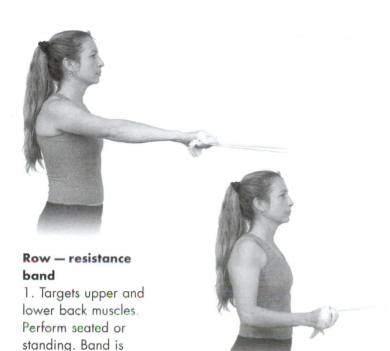

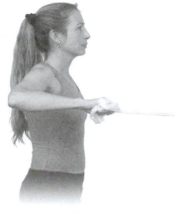

Row — high finish
2B. Pull hand directly back, squeezing shoulder blades together. Hand finishes next to shoulder. Targets upper back. Repeat on left.

Row — resistance band
1. Targets upper and lower back muscles. Perform seated or standing. Band is attached to wall. Start as above.

Row — low finish
2A. Pull hand downward toward right hip, squeezing shoulder blades together. Elbow finishes at side. Targets low back. Repeat on left.

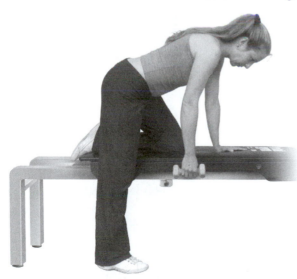

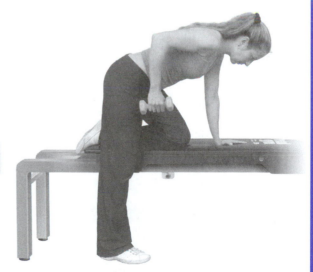

Bench row with dumbbell
1. Similar to row with resistance band, but different start position as above. Bench provides slightly different position for variety and support for balance.

Bench row with dumbbell
2. May pull to high or low (shown) finish, depending on whether targeting upper or lower back. Alternatively, may use resistance band anchored under right foot. Repeat on left.

Back (cont.)

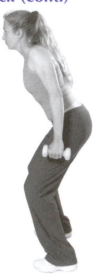
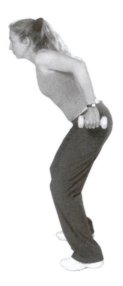
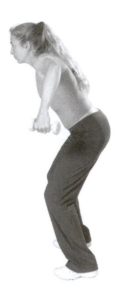

Standing row with dumbbell

1. Targets shoulder and upper back muscles. Start position as shown, hips and knees slightly bent, spine curves maintained and shoulders over knees.

Standing row — low finish

2A. Pull hands backward and upward toward hips, pinching shoulder blades together. Targets low back.

Standing row — high finish

2B. Elbows move up toward ceiling, pinching shoulder blades together. Targets upper back.

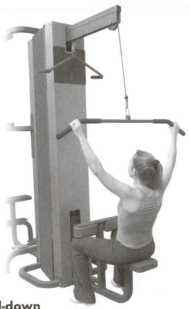
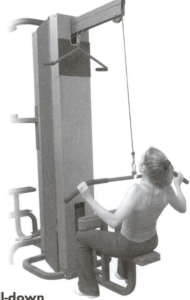

Lat pull-down

1. Targets entire back. Sit as shown above. Grip bar slightly wider than shoulder width.

Lat pull-down

2. Slowly pull bar toward chest, moving elbows toward your back pockets. Keep chest high and pinch shoulder blades together. Finish when elbows reach bottom of range of motion. Bar may not reach chest.

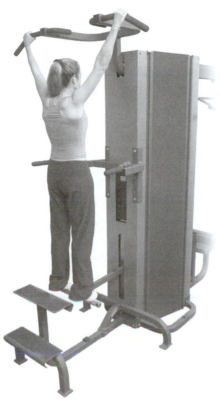

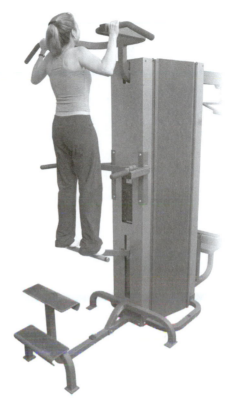

Assisted pull-up

1. Start position as above. Hands spaced slightly greater than shoulder-width apart. Set counterweight (provides assistance) to preference. Pull-ups can be with or without weight.

Assisted pull-up

2. Keeping shoulder blades back and head facing forward, slowly pull upward. Elbows move down and back. Don't arch neck. Return to starting position.

Chest

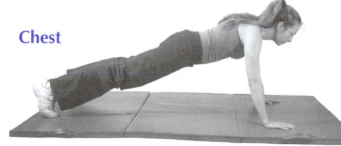

Push-up

1. Start position. Legs and spine in line. Eyes face floor. Hands slightly greater than shoulder-width apart. Foot position to preference. Also a great core exercise.

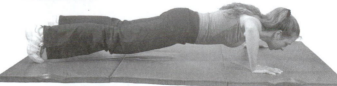

Push-up

2. Slowly bend elbows and lower chest. Maintain starting alignment. Elbows stay wide (elbows closer to sides emphasize triceps). Return to start. Feet close together increases core and balance challenge.

Chest (cont.)

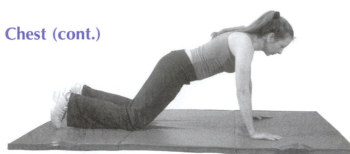

Assisted push-up
1. Similar to standard push-up, but with knees on floor. Bent knees reduces difficulty. Good starting exercise if you're unable to do regular push-up.

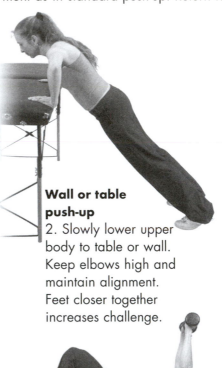

Assisted push-up
2. Slowly bend elbows and slightly straighten knees while lowering chest toward floor. Stop lowering when trunk (core) is parallel to floor. Maintain alignment as in standard push-up. Return to start.

Wall or table push-up
1. Done leaning on table or into wall to reduce challenge. Alignment and motion are similar to regular push-up.

Wall or table push-up
2. Slowly lower upper body to table or wall. Keep elbows high and maintain alignment. Feet closer together increases challenge.

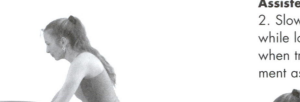

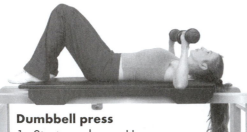

Dumbbell press
1. Start as above. Upper arms almost perpendicular to body, forearms perpendicular to the floor. Head stays neutral and relaxed.

Dumbbell press
2. Slowly press dumbbells upward until elbows are almost straight. Don't lock elbows or push with feet. Return to start.

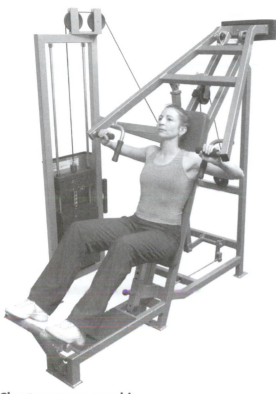

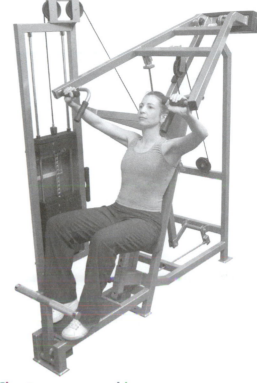

Chest press on machine
1. Start as above. Adjust seat so that hand-grips are at or slightly below shoulder height. Handgrip shown emphasizes chest. Alternative handgrip emphasizes triceps. Machine allows you to push handles forward to start position with feet.

Chest press on machine
2. After slowly releasing weights with your feet, allow handgrips to move toward chest until upper arms are at or slightly behind your body. Then slowly press forward, straightening elbows. Don't arch back or lock elbows. Slowly return to start.

Arms

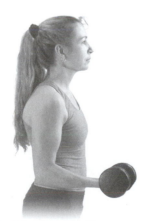

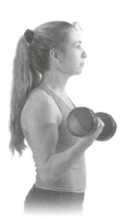

Arm curl with dumbbell
1. Focuses on biceps muscle. Done standing or sitting. Grip weight in hand, palm facing upward. Maintain neutral posture.

Arm curl with dumbbell
2. Slowly curl weight up by bending elbow. Note that upper arm stays aligned with body. Slowly lower weight down to your side. Can be done with one or both arms.

Arms (cont.)

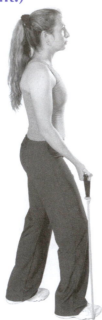

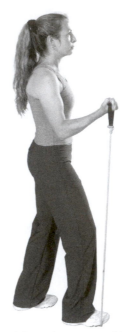

Arm curl with resistance tubing
1. Similar to arm curl with dumbbell. Resistance tubing anchored with foot or other immobile object. Start position as above.

Arm curl with resistance tubing
2. Slowly curl arm upward. Maintain upper arm alignment with body. To avoid injury, make sure handle on tube is secure to avoid having it snap free. Return to start. May also be done with resistance band. Do both arms.

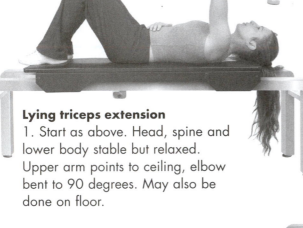

Lying triceps extension
1. Start as above. Head, spine and lower body stable but relaxed. Upper arm points to ceiling, elbow bent to 90 degrees. May also be done on floor.

Lying triceps extension
2. Maintaining body alignment and with upper arm pointing upward, slowly straighten elbow, moving weight upward. Slowly return to start. Do both arms.

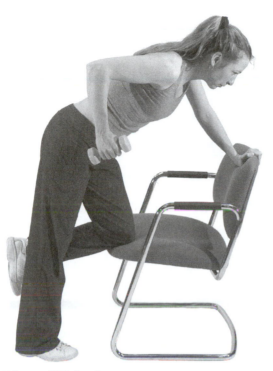

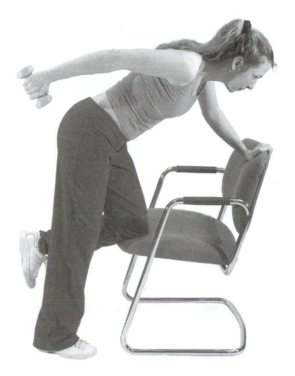

Triceps kickback

1. Slightly different focus on triceps from that of lying triceps extension. Position as above, upper arm parallel to floor, elbow pointing up and back. Left arm and knee give support.

Triceps kickback

2. Maintaining original spine and upper arm alignment, slowly straighten elbow, moving weight up and back. If too challenging, begin with light or no weight. Return to start. Do both arms.

Forearms and hands

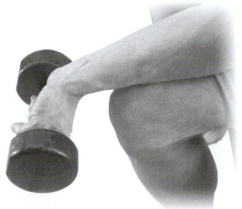

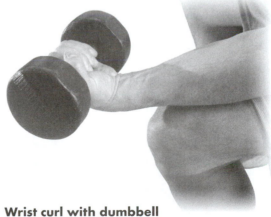

Wrist curl with dumbbell

1. Targets forearms. Start sitting, holding weight, palm facing up, forearm supported on thigh. Let weight move knuckles toward floor. May also be done with resistance band or tubing.

Wrist curl with dumbbell

2. Gripping weight, slowly curl wrist, bringing fingers and knuckles up toward your head. Maintain forearm contact with thigh as shown. Return to start. Do both wrists.

Forearms and hands (cont.)

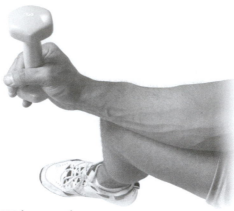

Wrist rotation
1. Targets forearm muscles that rotate hand and wrist. Hold light dumbbell on one end as shown.

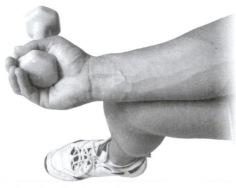

Supination (palm up)
2A. Slowly rotate forearm so palm faces upward. Range based upon comfort. Return to start position. Do both wrists.

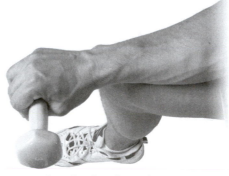

Pronation (palm down)
2B. Slowly rotate forearm so palm faces downward. Range based upon comfort. Return to start position. Do both wrists.

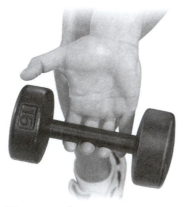

Finger curl
Similar to wrist curl, but targets fingers. Use lighter weight. Curl and uncurl fingers. Can combine with wrist curl. Do both hands.

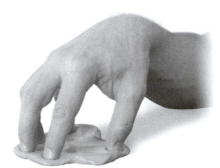

Putty pinch
1. Finger strengthening exercise. Use any semisoft, nontoxic putty. Finger position starts as above.

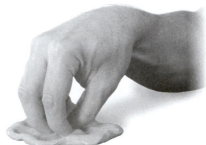

Putty pinch
2. Slowly pinch fingers together, bunching up putty. Downward pressure and putty determine resistance. Do both hands.

Legs

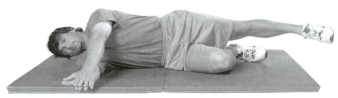

Side-lying hip abduction — left hip
1. Start as above. Right hip and knee bent for stability. May use pillow under head. Arm position for comfort.

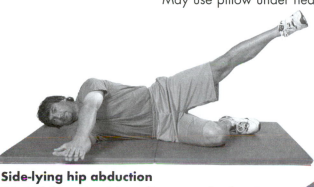

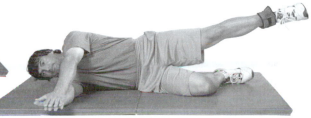

Side-lying hip abduction
2A. While maintaining alignment, slowly raise left leg upward until your trunk starts to move. Hold briefly, then lower leg. Do both sides.

Side-lying hip abduction
2B. Add an ankle weight or other resistance to increase challenge.

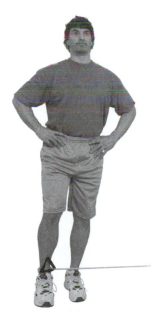

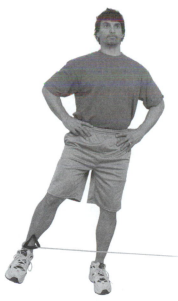

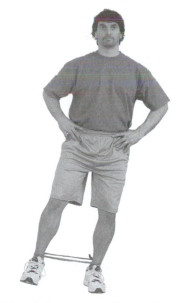

Standing hip abduction with resistance tubing
1. Secure tubing or band to immobile object. Start as shown above. Balance on left leg with right leg slightly off floor.

Standing hip abduction with resistance tubing
2A. Slowly move right leg outward to right, maintaining balance and alignment with left leg. Hold on to stationary object if needed when you first begin. Return to start. Do both sides.

Hip abduction walks with resistance tubing
2B. Alternative exercise. Circle both legs with tubing. Walk sideways, forward or backward, keeping feet apart to work hips in multiple directions. Maintain alignment.

Legs (cont.)

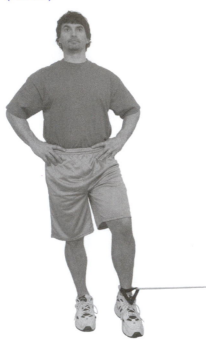

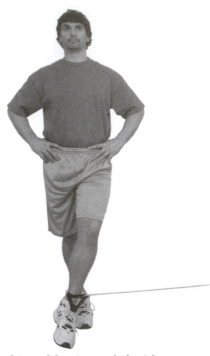

Standing hip adduction — left side
1. Works inner thighs. Similar to standing hip abduction. Balance on right leg, with left leg slightly off floor.

Standing hip adduction — left side
2. Maintaining balance and alignment, slowly move left leg to the right, passing in front of right leg. Return to start. Do both legs.

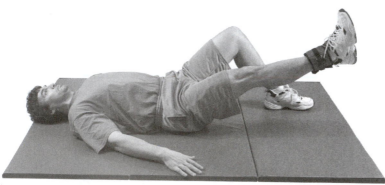

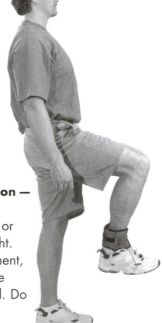

Lying hip flexion — right side
Starting position on back with left knee bent, right leg straight and resting on floor. Slowly lift right leg upward. Return to start. Do both legs. Do with ankle weight (shown here), or without. Move hands inward to increase challenge to core.

Standing hip flexion — right side
Start standing with or without ankle weight. Maintaining alignment, slowly lift right knee upward to hip level. Do both legs.

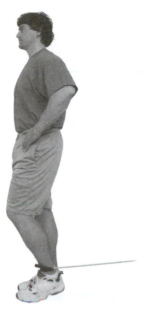

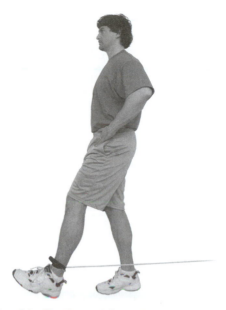

Standing hip flexion with resistance tubing

1. More challenging than lying hip flexion, with added core and balance challenges. Shown for left leg. Start as above, with anchored tubing. Balance on right leg.

Standing hip flexion with resistance tubing

2. Maintaining right leg balance and body alignment, slowly move left foot forward as shown. Return to start. Do both legs.

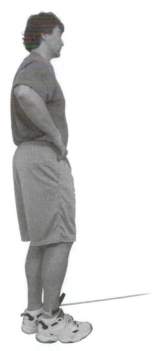

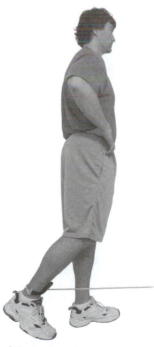

**Standing hip extension
with resistance tubing**

1. Similar to standing hip flexion with tubing, but in opposite direction. Emphasizes gluteals and hamstrings. Shown for right leg.

**Standing hip extension
with resistance tubing**

2. Maintain left leg balance, body alignment, and a firm right knee. Slowly move right foot backward. Return to start. Do both legs.

Legs (cont.)

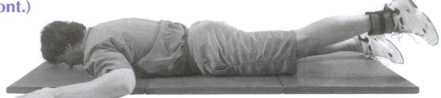

Lying hip extension — left side
Start on stomach, both legs straight, with or without weight. Slowly raise left leg 6 to 8 inches off floor, with toes slightly pointing outward. Don't arch back. Return to start. Do both legs.

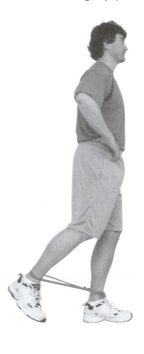

Resisted walking
2. See hip abduction exercises on page 163. Exercises here demonstrate walking motions with a resistance band Shown here is backward walking.

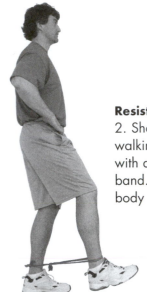

Resisted walking
2. Shown here is walking forward with a resistance band. Maintain body alignment.

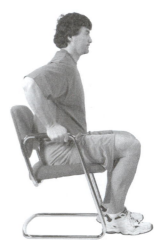

Chair-assisted squat
1. For those unable to perform standard squat. Start as above. Note erect trunk alignment.

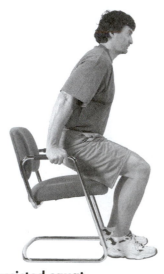

Chair-assisted squat
2. Pushing upward through legs and straightening elbows simultaneously, lift out of chair. Return to start. Reduce arm assist as able.

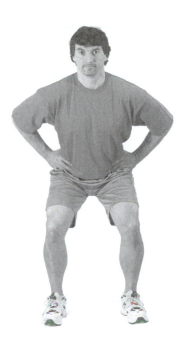

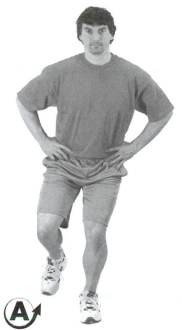

Squat

Start standing with feet slightly greater than shoulder-width apart and toes pointing ahead or slightly outward. Slowly descend, bending through the hips, knees and ankles. Maintain normal back arch. Descend to comfort, but don't bend knees more than 90 degrees. Return to start. May do with or without hand weights

Single-leg squat

Squatting on one leg is advanced and requires more flexibility, balance, and hip and core strength.

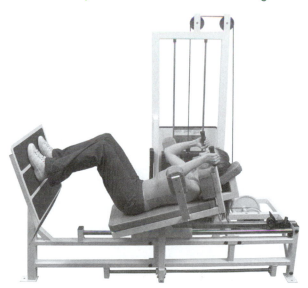

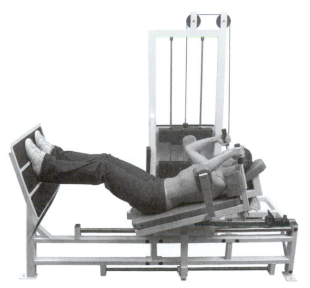

Leg press

1. Start position shown above. Spine and upper body stable, relaxed. Handgrip is for support only. Feet positioned so knee angle is about 90 degrees. Place feet at slightly greater than shoulder-width apart.

Leg press

2. Pushing through your heels, slowly straighten your knees. Maintain alignment. Don't arch back. Keep a slight knee bend at the end of the motion as shown. Return to start. Can also do one leg at a time.

Legs (cont.)

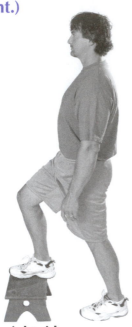

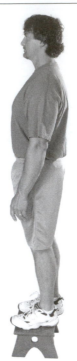

Step-ups — right side
1. Using stairs or a small step stool, start as above. Keep trunk erect, not bent forward.

Step-ups — right side
2. Pushing primarily through right foot, lift your body up onto the step. You can then either step backward to the start position, or forward over the step. Do both sides.

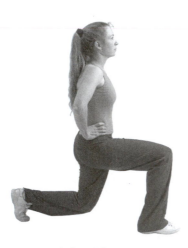

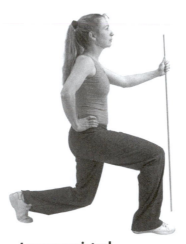

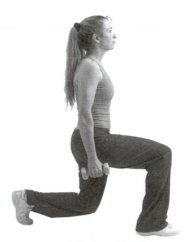

Lunge — right side
1. Start in normal standing position. Step forward with right foot and lower body into position shown above. Keep trunk erect and halfway between front and back foot. Right knee remains behind right foot and is angled 90 degrees. Return to start position. Do both sides.

Lunge-assisted
2A. Easier variation for those just starting or with balance difficulties. Use cane or pole in hand opposite stepping leg for balance assist.

Lunge with dumbbell
2B. For added challenge, use light dumbbells in both hands. For more balance and core challenge, use dumbbell in one hand.

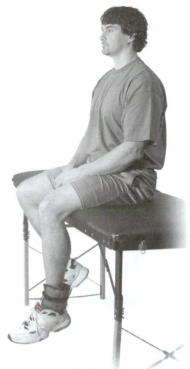

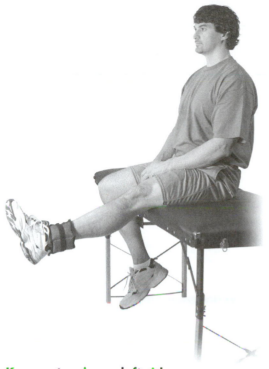

Knee extension — left side
1. Targets front of thighs (quadriceps). Do with ankle weight as shown. Start as above. Spine is neutral.

Knee extension — left side
2. Maintaining alignment, slowly straighten left knee, pause, then return to start position. Do both legs.

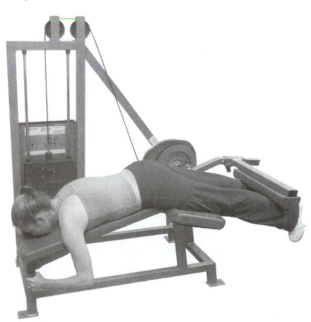

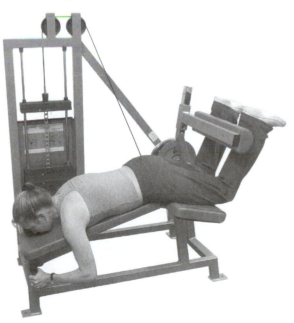

Hamstring curl on machine
1. Start as above. Pad positioned just above ankles. Use a light weight and maintain good form. Keep upper body stable, but relaxed. Handgrip for support only— not for assist.

Hamstring curl on machine
2. Slowly bend knees, pulling feet toward buttocks. Only go as far as you can without feeling your pelvis or spine move. Don't pull with arms, or arch neck or low back. Return to start. May do one leg at a time.

Legs (cont.)

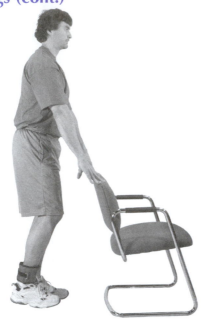

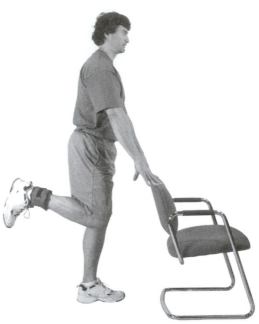

Standing hamstring curl — right side
1. Alternative to machine exercise. Do with or without ankle weights. Balance on left leg with right leg slightly off floor. Use chair for support only.

Standing hamstring curl — right side
2. Slowly bend right knee until lower leg passes just above parallel to the floor as shown. Maintain starting alignment of body and left leg. Return to start. Do both legs.

Ankles and feet

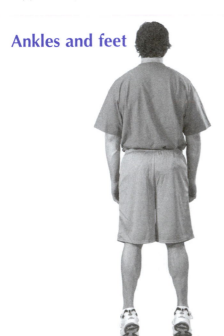

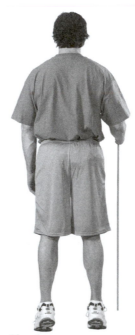

Standing calf raise
Start standing in normal posture, with feet at or slightly greater than shoulder-width apart. Slowly rise up onto your toes as shown.

Assisted calf raise
For those with balance difficulties, a cane, stick or pole can be used for added stability.

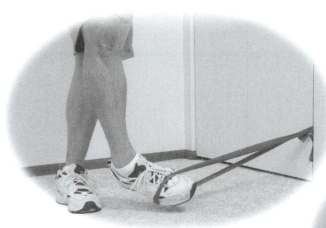

Eversion — right side
1. Start as above, with resistance band solidly anchored. Balance on left leg. May hold on to wall for balance. Foot starts with toes pointing inward.

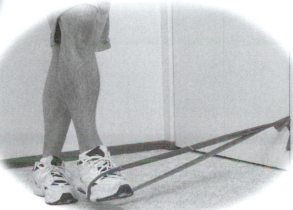

Eversion — right side
2. Moving only through the ankle, move foot outward to right as shown. Motion ends when little toe side of foot is angled upward. Do both sides.

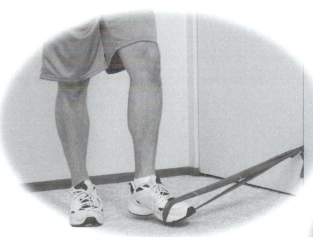

Inversion — left side
1. Similar to eversion, but with a different start position as shown above.

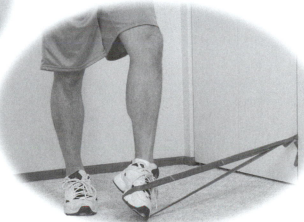

Inversion — left side
2. Moving only through ankle, move big toe inward to right, ending in position as shown. Do both sides.

Ankles and feet (cont.)

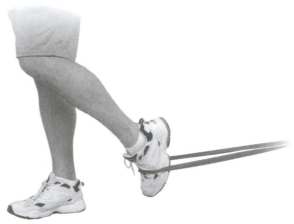

Dorsiflexion — left side
1. Start as above, with resistance band firmly anchored. Hold left knee slightly bent, with band looped over laces of shoe. Begin with toes pointing toward floor.

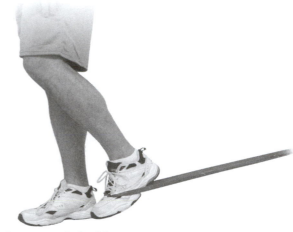

Dorsiflexion — left side
2. Maintaining body and knee alignment, slowly move toes upward — a motion called dorsiflexion. You'll feel the muscles in the front of the shin working. Return to start. Do both legs.

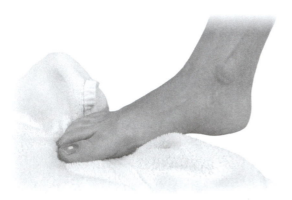

Toe curl
1. Targets toe, foot and ankle muscles, as well as arch muscles. Place towel or thick cloth on floor. Place your toes onto towel in a resting position as shown.

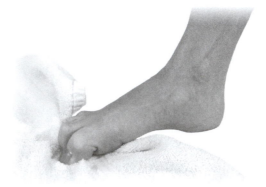

Toe curl
2. Curl your toes, bunching up the towel and pulling it toward you. Emphasize toe curling, not ankle motion. Can place small weights on towel for added resistance. Do both feet.

Core flexion

Targets the front of your core, particularly the abdominal and oblique muscles.

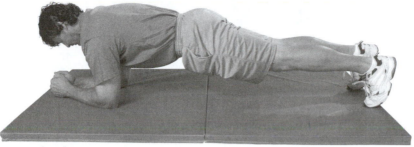

Prone bridge
Start position above. Keep head, core and legs straight and aligned, elbows directly under shoulders. Hold until you feel that you're just about to fatigue and lose form, then stop.

Push-up
1. Start as shown. Legs and spine are in line. Eyes face the floor. Keep hands slightly greater than shoulder-width apart. Feet are hip-width apart.

Push-up
2A. Slowly straighten elbows and push away from floor. Maintain starting spine alignment. Don't lock elbows. Return to start. Place feet closer together to increase core and balance challenge.

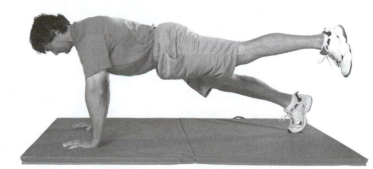

Push-up — advanced
2B. Advanced version calls for raising one leg as you push up from the floor. Maintain core alignment and don't lean toward raised leg. Return to start. Repeat while raising other leg.

Flexion (cont.)

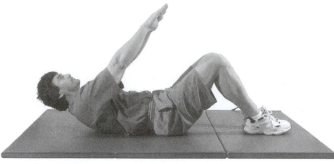

Crunch on floor

Start with head and shoulders on floor and arms straight up. Slowly bring your breastbone toward your pelvis. Finish with feet on floor as shown. Motion is slow and curling. Head and arm alignment are unchanged. Return to start. Repeat.

Ⓐ Crunch on stability ball

1. Start as shown. Ball rests between shoulder blades, with head, trunk and thighs in straight alignment. Keep knees bent at 90 degrees.

Ⓐ Crunch on stability ball

2. Perform same motion as crunch on floor (shown above). More challenging on ball. Return to start.

Leg lowering

1. Start as shown. Breathing normally, gently tighten abdominal muscles by drawing bellybutton up and in. Maintaining low back curve, lower right foot toward floor until you begin to lose alignment. Return to start position. Do both sides.

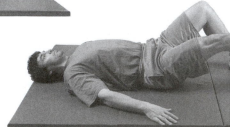

Ⓐ Leg lowering

2. Start position same as with leg lowering at left. However, straighten right knee before lowering leg toward floor. Do both sides.

Core extension

Targets the upper and lower back muscles, buttocks and hamstrings. These exercises may protect the back from injury and improve posture and spine stability.

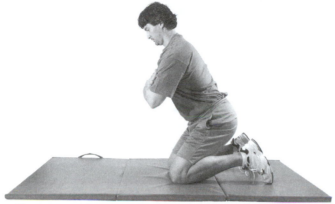

Kneeling extension
Targets low back and hips. Start as above. Use kneepads or mat for comfort. Slowly bend forward at hips, maintaining low back arch. Return to start. Straighten arms to increase resistance.

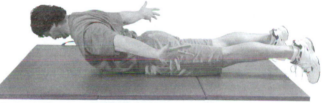

Cobra extension
Excellent posture exercise. Start lying on stomach, facing down, with hands by your sides. Slowly pinch shoulder blades together, rotate arms out so thumbs point up, and arch your back as shown. Keep head in line with trunk.

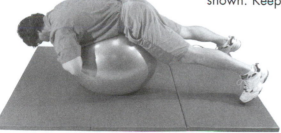

Extension on ball
1. Similar to cobra, but ball increases stability and core challenge. Start as shown above, draped over ball, with top of ball approximately at navel.

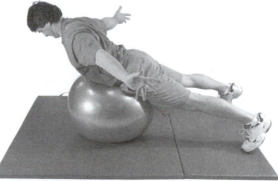

Extension on ball
2. Finish similar to cobra. Note neutral spine alignment, head aligned with body, and arm and foot position. Narrower foot position will increase balance challenge.

Extension (cont.)

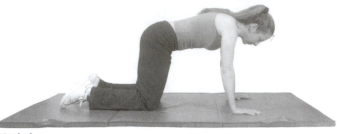

Bird dog
1. Start as shown, knees under hips and hands under shoulders, with head and core aligned.

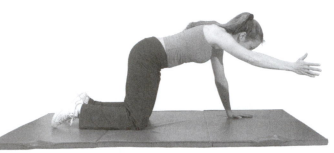

Bird dog — right side
2. Slowly lift right arm upward as shown, thumb pointing up. Maintain trunk alignment as shown. Repeat with left arm.

(A) **Bird dog — advanced**
3. Simultaneously lift right arm and left leg as shown. Maintain core and limb alignment. Repeat with left arm and right leg.

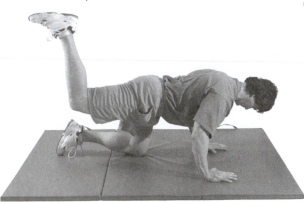

Tripod hip extension
Similar to bird dog (above), but instead of arm, lift one leg at a time. Knee may be straightened for added core challenge. Elbows may be bent to keep core parallel to floor and increase triceps challenge.

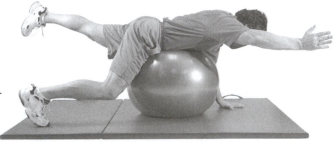

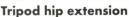

(A) **Bird dog on stability ball**
Targets back and buttocks. Start on all fours with top of ball at navel. Slowly lift left leg and right arm as shown, ensuring that you maintain alignment and that your spine doesn't twist. Other limbs provide balance. Return to start. Repeat with left arm and right leg.

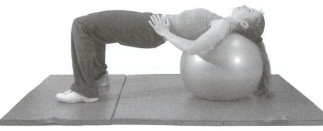

Hip extension on stability ball
1. Start as shown, back and head supported on ball, keeping knees bent at 90 degrees. Note alignment of head, core and thighs.

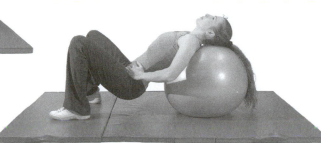

Hip extension on stability ball
2. Slowly let pelvis sink toward floor, controlling motion with hips and core, and keeping core stable. Shins remain upright as shown — at right angles to floor. Push on heels to return to start position. Narrow distance between feet for increased challenge.

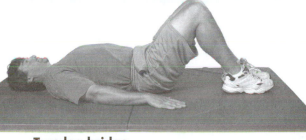

Two-leg bridge
1. Targets back and hip muscles. Start as shown, arms at side for balance support. Tighten abdomen.

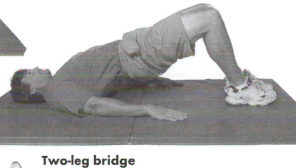

Two-leg bridge
2. Keeping head and shoulders on floor and abdomen tight, slowly push on heels and raise pelvis to form straight line from knees to shoulders. Return to start. Narrower arm position increases core challenge.

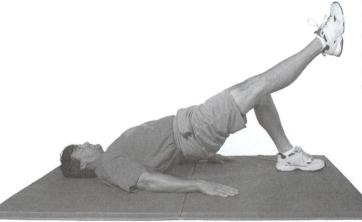

 Single-leg bridge — advanced
3. Similar to two-leg bridge, but in addition, raise right leg off floor and straighten as above. Increases challenges to left hip, leg and core. Do both sides.

Core lateral

Targets sides of core, provides stability and control when bending to the left or right side, or carrying objects in one hand

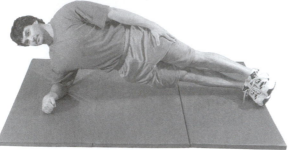

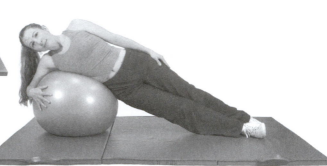

Side bridge — right side
Start position above. Head, core and legs straight and in alignment, and feet together. Right elbow under right shoulder. Hold until you're just about to lose alignment. Do both sides.

 Side bridge on stability ball — right side
Similar to side bridge, but ball provides added balance and core challenge. Start as above, right leg forward and left leg backward for balance. Proceed as with side bridge.

Core rotation

Targets core muscles that control the motion of rotation. Essential for spine protection and athletic function, but more challenging than core extension, flexion or lateral exercises

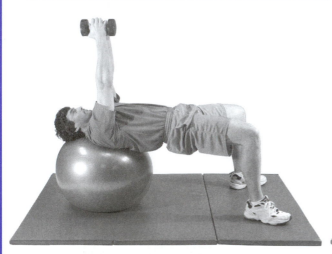

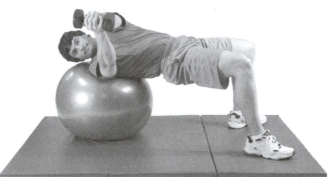

 Rotation on ball — right side
1. Start as above. Keep top of ball between shoulder blades and rest head on ball. Head, core and thighs are aligned parallel with floor. Knees bent to 90 degrees. This is the "tabletop" position.

 Rotation on ball — right side
2. Slowly rotate to right. Move head with trunk. Note pelvis maintains "tabletop" position, and legs move minimally. Control motion through core. Do slowly with or without weights. Return to start. Do both sides.

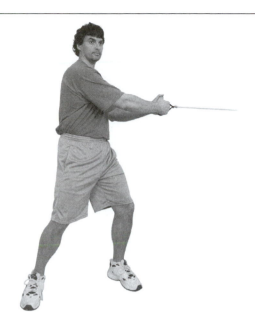

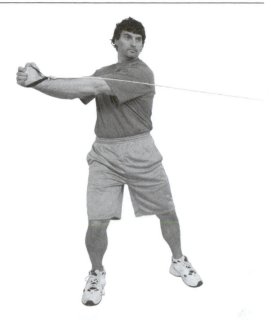

Standing rotation with resistance band
1. Shown for right rotation. Upright position integrates lower body and core in rotation. Start as above with band firmly anchored. Grasp band at nipple height with both hands. Start rotation to right with 70 percent of weight on left foot.

Standing rotation with resistance band
2. Shift weight from left to right foot while simultaneously pulling band directly across in front of you, ending in right rotation as shown. At finish, 70 percent of weight is on right foot. Note leg action. Head faces forward. Do both sides.

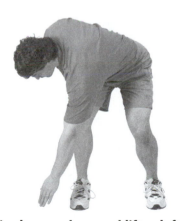

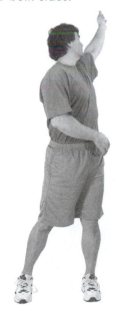

Single-arm chop and lift — left arm
1. Start in normal standing position, but keep knees slightly bent, and avoid locking knees. Reach with left hand to outside of right leg, trying to touch floor. Only go as far as is comfortable. Use caution if you have a history of back pain.

Single-arm chop and lift — left arm
2. Straighten up and reach over your left shoulder as shown. Note how weight naturally shifts to right leg on downward reach, and to left leg on upward reach. Also note lower body action and that head follows hand. Do both sides.

Rotation (cont.)

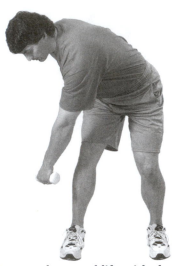

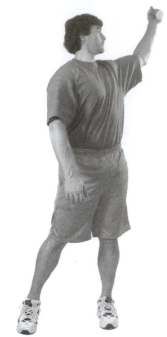

Single-arm chop and lift with dumbbell
1. Same exercise as single-arm chop and lift. Shown for left arm. Weight increases core challenge, but also increases spine stress.

Single-arm chop and lift with dumbbell
2. Because of added weight, individuals with prior or current back problems should perform only with extreme caution and under supervision.

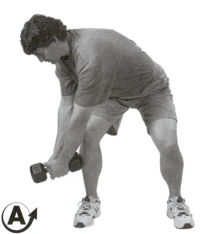

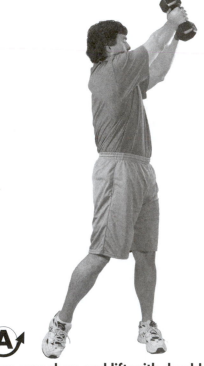

Two-arm chop and lift with dumbbell
1. Similar to single-arm chop and lift. However, this variation involves holding a weight with both hands.

Two-arm chop and lift with dumbbell
2. The two-hand grip will slightly restrict the motion more than a single-hand grip, but will allow use of greater weight.

Isolated balance exercises

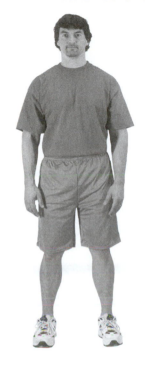

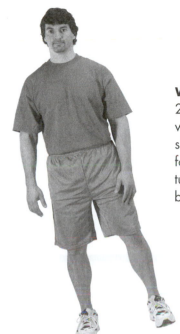

Weight shifts
1. Start in normal standing position as shown with weight equally distributed on both legs.

Weight shifts
2. Slowly shift weight onto right side, then lift left foot off floor. Return to start. Do both sides.

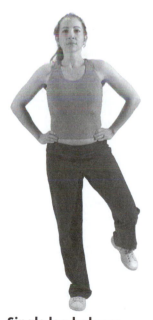

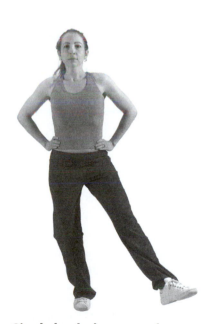

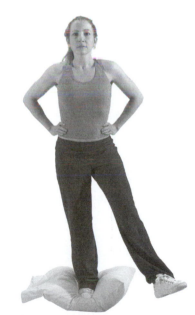

Single-leg balance
1. Shown with left leg. Balance on right leg as shown. Place hands on hips, or hold on to stationary object if needed for balance assistance.

Single-leg balance-reach
2A. Slowly reach out with left foot as far as possible without touching floor. Hold on to stationary object when you first start if needed. Return to start. Vary direction of reach. Do both sides.

Ⓐ↗ Single-leg balance-reach on pillow — advanced
2B. Weight shifts or balance-reach exercises can be done on unstable surfaces for added challenge.

Integrated balance exercises
Biceps curl progression

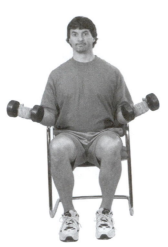
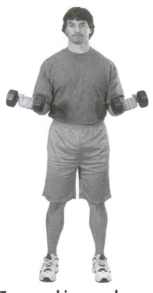
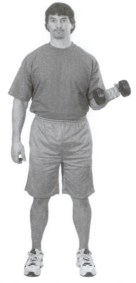

Seated two-arm biceps curl
Similar to arm curl on page 159. Exercise is made easier by sitting.

Two-arm biceps curl
If you have sufficient balance, it's better to do this exercise standing as shown.

Single-arm biceps curl
For added balance and core challenge, use one arm only. Do both sides.

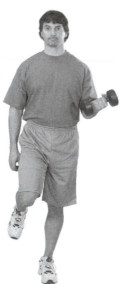
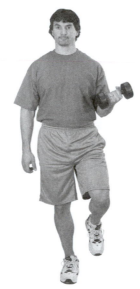
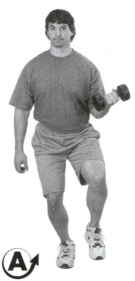
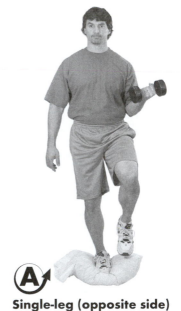

Single-leg (same side) biceps curl
Increase core and balance challenge by balancing on one leg (same side as weight) Keep pelvis in line with trunk. Do both sides.

Single-leg (opposite side) biceps curl
Further increase challenge by balancing on the leg opposite the weight. Keep pelvis in line with trunk. Do both sides.

Single-leg (opposite side) squat biceps curl
Combine with a single-leg squat. Adds hip and lower leg strengthening. Try without weight first.

Single-leg (opposite side) biceps curl on pillow
Further challenge balance and core by standing on an unstable surface. This is a high-intensity exercise, working balance, strength and core. Try without weight first.

Shoulder press progression

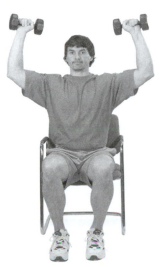

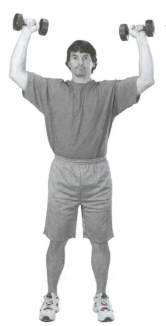

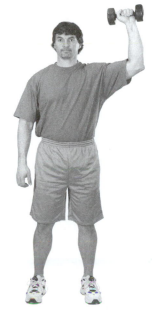

Seated shoulder press
Similar to shoulder press on page 153. Exercise made easier by sitting.

Standing shoulder press
If you have sufficient balance, it's better to do this exercise standing as shown.

Single-arm shoulder press
For added balance and core challenge, use one arm only. Do both sides.

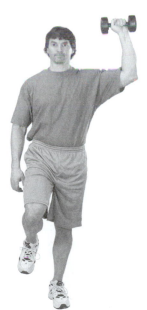

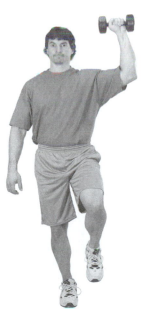

Single-arm (same side) shoulder press with single-leg balance
Increase core and balance challenge by standing on one leg (same side as weight). Remember to keep pelvis in line with trunk. Do both sides.

Single-arm (opposite side) shoulder press
Further increase challenge by standing on the leg opposite the weight. Do both sides.

Integrated balance exercises (cont.)

Shoulder press progression (cont.)

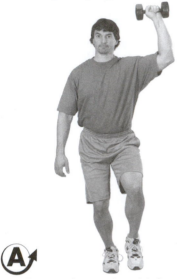

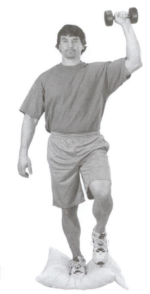

Single-arm (opposite side) squat shoulder press
Combine with a single-leg squat to add hip and lower leg strengthening.

Single leg (opposite side) shoulder press on pillow
Further challenge balance and core by standing on an unstable surface. This is a high-intensity exercise, working balance, strength and core.

Side raise progression

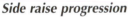

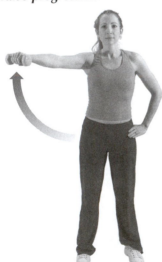

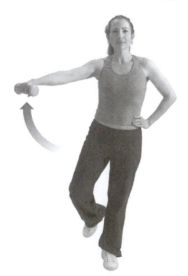

Single-arm side-lateral raise
Variant of side-lateral raise shown on page 153. Using a single dumbbell adds core and balance challenges. Start with dumbbell at your side and slowly raise to the side as shown, not higher than a 90 degree angle. Return to starting position. Do both sides.

Single-arm side-lateral raise with single-leg balance (opposite side)
As with previous progressions, balance and core challenges are increased by standing on one foot, either the same or opposite. Remember to keep pelvis aligned with trunk. You can also add an unstable surface, or squat. Do both sides.

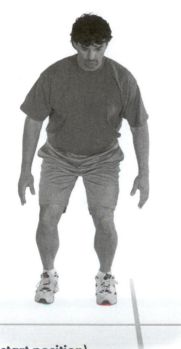

Jump (start position)

1. Begin in partial squat position as shown. It helps to have a piece of tape or other flat object on the floor to jump over. Avoid objects on which you can trip.

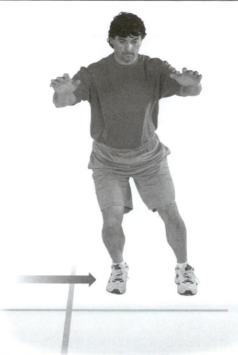

Side jump — two leg

2A. Jump with both feet simultaneously to your left, landing squarely as shown. Jump back to the starting position. Repeat.

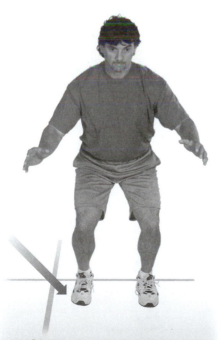

Diagonal jump

2B. From starting position, jump diagonally forward and to your left as shown. Jump back to starting position. Repeat to right side.

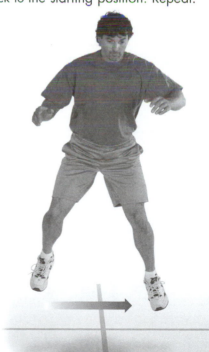

Side jump — one leg

2C. From starting position, push off with your right foot, jump to your left as shown. Landing should be staggered, but stable. Jump back to start position. Repeat to right.

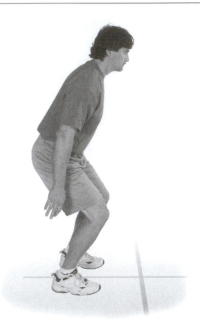

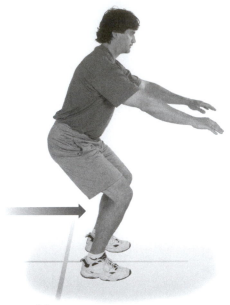

Forward jump

1. Start in partial squat position as shown. It helps to have a piece of tape or other flat object to jump over. Avoid using objects on which you can trip.

Forward jump

2. Push off equally with both feet. Jump forward and land simultaneously and squarely. Maintain position as shown.

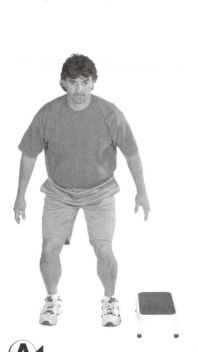

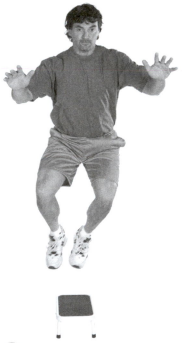

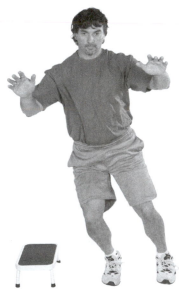

 Side jump over step

1. Caution: If you hit the step, you may fall and injure yourself. Start position as shown.

 Side jump over step

2. Jump to the left with both feet simultaneously. Picture shows midexercise position. Keep body aligned.

Side jump over step

3. Land with both feet simultaneously and equally. Maintain knee alignment over feet as shown. Jump back to right.

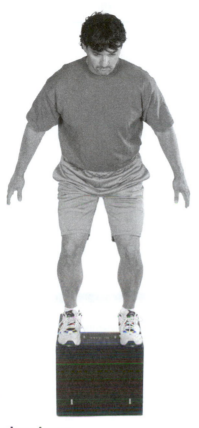

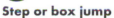

Step or box jump

1. Start on a step or box as shown. This is an intense exercise. Start with low heights and progress as able. Technique is crucial.

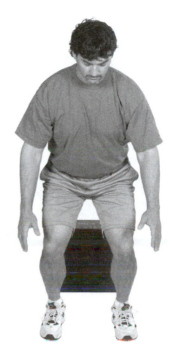

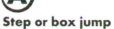

Step or box jump

2. Jump simultaneously with both feet, landing as shown. Note that alignment is maintained with knees over feet, and trunk balanced over hips. Step back up on box. Repeat.

Staying

CHAPTER 6

You've decided on a fitness plan, set reasonable goals and equipped yourself with the right gear. Now the challenge is, as one athletic conglomerate says, to "just do it" — and keep on doing it. Starting a fitness program takes initiative, and sticking with it takes commitment. If you haven't been in the habit of exercising, you'll need to change long-held patterns and behaviors.

Although many people tend to exercise either not at all or too much, a successful fitness program isn't an all-or-nothing proposition. Think of physical fitness as a journey, not a destination. It's not a goal you simply achieve one day and then are done with. Just as with sensible weight management, being a regular exerciser means that you spend time at it for the rest of your life.

As with any journey, you'll encounter some roadblocks and setbacks. For some people, getting started is the hardest step. Others begin with tremendous enthusiasm and go at it so vigorously that they get hurt and stop. In addition, finding

motivated

& troubleshooting your plan

the time to fit in regular physical activity is a challenge for almost everyone. And an occasional cold or the flu can slow you down. Travel, bad weather or a change in lifestyle also can affect your exercise routine.

To have the best chance of success — a lifelong commitment to physical activity — you need to get and stay motivated. By being proactive, you can meet and overcome challenges. To gain the benefits of lifelong fitness, exercising has to be as natural and ingrained a habit as is brushing your teeth or taking a shower.

This chapter helps you understand your own sources of motivation and the barriers that may keep you from being physically active. It offers solutions to many of the obstacles and excuses you'll run up against. It offers practical tips for staying with a fitness program, monitoring your progress, fighting boredom and finding time to exercise. You'll learn strategies for troubleshooting a variety of circumstances that can derail your fitness plan, including plateaus, injuries and illness.

Anyone can get and stay motivated to exercise. If you don't feel motivated right now, it's not because you don't have what it takes. You just haven't identified and activated your own motivational process.

GETTING AND STAYING MOTIVATED

Motivation is at the heart of your fitness plan — it's what gets you going and keeps you at it. But what exactly is motivation, and how do you get it, especially if the idea of exercising excites you about as much as having a root canal?

Motivation is intangible. You can't buy it, and no one can give it to you. It's a mental process that gives you the determination to reach a goal. It connects thoughts and feelings to action and provides a sense of purpose.

Understanding what motivates you

Motivation means different things to different people. By understanding what motivates you, you'll be better able to follow through with your fitness plan.

Research shows that people who are self-motivated are more likely to stick with an exercise program than are those who rely solely on external forms of motivation. If your motivation is internally based, you're doing the activity for yourself — because you enjoy it, because you want to look or feel better or because you want to become healthier. External motivation, in contrast, comes from outside — you're exercising to please someone else or to reach a particular goal, such as a 10-pound weight loss, or reward, such as new clothes. You're more focused on the outcome than the process.

That's not to say that external motivators have no place. An occasional tangible reward, such as a new pair of shoes, may be just the boost you need to keep going. But if you're constantly focusing on such rewards, you may lose some of your intrinsic motivation, exercising less for the enjoyment and more for the rewards. The bottom line is that you'll be more motivated if you can find a way to embrace the activity as something you want to do for yourself over the long term.

Encouragement and support from family, friends, co-workers and others also can be key motivators. Studies show that such social support helps people stick to an exercise plan.

Creating an action plan

For a majority of people, getting started on a fitness program is the hardest step. So if you've been dragging your feet about getting more active, you're not alone.

You may have a million excuses for not exercising. You just don't like to exercise, or you find it boring. You're already too busy and stressed and don't have time for a new activity. Your family and friends want more of your free time. Exercise equipment and health club memberships cost too much.

As you think about the prospect of exercising, you may focus on past failures or bad memories of junior high gym class. You may have tried to exercise in the past and not succeeded, or you may have had a bad experience that soured you on the whole idea.

Chances are that if you examine your habits, you'll find assumptions underlying them. If you haven't been in the habit of exercising, what are the beliefs underlying that behavior? Often, as soon as you start thinking about exercising, a host of negative thoughts pop up: "I don't want to do this." "I know I'll never be able to keep this up." "I don't have time for this." "It's too hard." "I'm not an athlete. I'm just not cut out for it." "I'll hurt my knees."

Lots of people have started from this same place, with the same excuses and the same busy lives, and have come not only to tolerate physical activity but to enjoy it. It's possible to change the beliefs that are keeping you stuck and to mobilize your motivation.

So how can you come up with an action plan for change? Follow these steps.

1. Take some time to recognize what does or doesn't motivate you

Think about your previous experience with changes you've tried to make. What will help you this time around? What can you learn from your past experience?

It may help to make a list of the benefits you want to experience from physical activity. Remind yourself of the many payoffs from physical activity that are outlined in Chapter 1. In addition, list the barriers or potential losses that may be holding you back, such as lack of time or feeling stiff, sore or tired. Target the most important pros and cons.

2. Ask for support

Explain your fitness goals to your friends and family and ask that they buy into your plan. Your odds of success are greater if you have the support of those around you.

Unfortunately, some people in your life may not want you to succeed in getting more active. Your new habits may not include them, which can be upsetting. Be assertive in responding to nonsupportive people, and work on developing friendships with physically active people.

3. Focus on the process and take small steps

Set realistic, attainable goals and continue to evaluate them. It's easy to get frustrated and give up on goals that are too ambitious. For example, if you're currently inactive, the goal of running a marathon in three months isn't realistic.

Your goals should be specific and measurable. Rather than saying something general like, "I will be more active this month," you might set a goal of taking the stairs at work instead of the elevators three times this week.

Some of your goals should be short term, some intermediate and some long term. For example, a short-term goal might be to walk five minutes once or twice a day just to establish a comfortable tolerance level. The intermediate goal might be to work up to 20 to 30 minutes most days of the week. A long-term goal might be to complete a 10-kilometer (10K) race after you complete 12 weeks of training. Other long-term goals may include things like feeling better, looking better, improving your fitness level, losing weight, improving performance in a favorite sport, reducing stress or depression, or toning or strengthening your muscles.

It's also important to evaluate your goals once you're under way. As you accomplish a goal, increase the size of the next step and set new short-term goals. If you're successfully walking 30 minutes at least four times a week, increase the amount of time that you walk. Or add some other activities, such as cycling, strength training or gardening.

Over time your long-term goals may shift. If your initial goal was to get in shape and drop a few pounds for a specific event, you'll want to think about establishing a different goal — perhaps one that's less externally focused — once that event has passed.

Excuse busters

Do you have the perfect excuse not to exercise? Here's the truth about some common "I can't because … " excuses. Yes, you can!

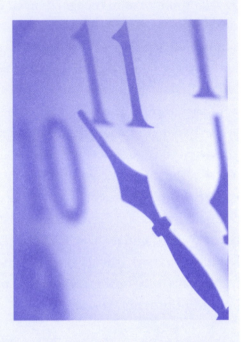

Excuse: I don't have time to exercise.
This is the all-time favorite excuse, but with some creativity and planning, you can make time for fitness. Most people have more free time than they realize. For example, the average American watches more than four hours of television each day. Add to that the time you spend reading the newspaper, surfing the Web and watching videotapes or DVDs, and there's bound to be some time for exercise.

Excuse: I'm too old to exercise.
You're never too old to be physically active, and it's never too late to start. Even moderate physical activity, such as walking or raking leaves, can help prevent or delay age-associated conditions such as heart disease, diabetes, high blood pressure and bone loss. Strength training can help prevent falls and maintain bone density.

Excuse: I'm too tired to exercise.
Maybe that's because you're *not* exercising. Regular physical activity gives you more energy. Fatigue is often more mental than physical and may be related to stress. A brisk walk, tennis game or bike ride can relieve tension and be energizing.

Excuse: I can't exercise because I have a chronic health condition.
This excuse is only valid if your doctor has told you not to exercise. Physical activity can help you better manage symptoms of many chronic conditions. For example, if you have arthritis, proper exercise can help you maintain joint mobility. If you have diabetes, exercise helps lower your blood sugar levels. (See Chapter 8 for more information about staying physically active if you have a chronic medical condition.)

Excuse: I can't exercise because I'm too out of shape.
This doesn't cut it. You may not be able to run a mile, but you can walk a block or two. Start small and gradually increase your activity level. Pretty soon you won't be out of shape.

Excuse: I'm not overweight, so I don't need to exercise.
Being thin doesn't necessarily mean you're fit. Although a healthy weight is important, it's also important that your body get regular exercise. As discussed in Chapter 1, inactivity, even when you're not overweight or obese, is a risk factor for chronic conditions such as diabetes, high blood pressure, stroke and cardiovascular disease.

4. Monitor your progress

Keep track of your progress as you go along. As discussed in Chapter 4, monitoring progress is a great way to reinforce your new habit, feel good about what you've accomplished and help set your goals for the future.

Self-monitoring can help you meet and refine your goals by letting you see the changes you've made — or not made. Try to re-evaluate your progress every few weeks, especially at the beginning of your exercise program.

5. Reward yourself

Work on developing an internal reward system that comes from feelings of accomplishment, self-esteem and control of your behavior. After each exercise session, take a few minutes to sit down and relax. Savor the good feelings that exercise gives you, and reflect on what you've just accomplished. This type of internal reward can help you make a long-term commitment to regular exercise.

External rewards also can help keep you motivated. When you reach a longer range goal, treat yourself to a new pair of walking shoes, a new CD, a massage or tickets to a sporting event. The reward should fit your fitness goals. For example, if you reached a goal of losing 5 percent body fat, an ice cream sundae isn't the most appropriate reward. New clothes, a weekend getaway or a new piece of exercise equipment can reinforce your success without compromising your original goal.

Tips for staying motivated

Even if you've never stuck to an exercise program before, you can do it. The following tips will help you stay motivated for the long haul.

- **Start slowly.** The most common mistake is starting a fitness program at too high an intensity and progressing too quickly. If your body isn't accustomed to vigorous exercise, your joints, ligaments and muscles are more vulnerable to injury. It's often not until the next day that you discover you've overdone it, and the resulting pain and stiffness can be very discouraging.

  It's better to progress slowly than to push too hard and be forced to abandon your program because of pain or injury. You can increase your activity in a deliberate way, but you don't have to be regimented about it. Taking baby steps to increase your activity brings fitness benefits. For example, if you started out walking 10 minutes three times a week and extended each walk just three minutes a week, in three months you would be walking more than 45 minutes on each outing.

- **Make a commitment.** It takes about three months to develop a healthy habit. If you can keep at your fitness program faithfully for that long, you're more likely to stay with it for the long term.

- **Accept some ambivalence.** Everyone who embarks on a major lifestyle change feels ambivalent about it sometimes. Even regular, committed exercisers occasionally have days when they'd rather stay in bed than get up and work out. Ambivalent thoughts don't have to be more than a passing detour.

- **Broaden your definition of physical activity.** Physical activity doesn't just mean working out at the gym for 40 minutes or running several miles. Everyday activities such as walking the dog, biking to the store or taking the stairs at work promote health, too. Doing something daily is what counts. (See Chapter 4 for details on recommended amounts of physical activity.)

- **Choose activities you enjoy.** Boredom is a major reason people stop exercising. If you have to drag yourself to a gym or you find walking on a treadmill mind-numbingly dull, then you're going to seize on any possible excuse to avoid these activities. Instead of beating yourself up about your lack of motivation, find activities you like doing. Consider joining a health club, at least on a temporary basis, so that you can try out many different activities. (Find other tips for battling boredom on page 198.)

- **Choose activities that fit your lifestyle.** Do you like to exercise alone or with a group? If you prefer solitude, consider walking, jogging or biking. If group activities appeal to you, consider enrolling in a yoga or dance class or joining a league or team for golf, basketball or softball. Walk or bike with a group of friends. If you normally watch the evening news, walk on a treadmill, do balance exercises or lift free weights in front of the television.

- **Learn discipline.** To make a permanent change, you have to consciously build your discipline "muscle." Try practicing with small steps. For example, tell yourself you'll use the stairs at work today. Then do it, even if you change your mind and don't feel like it. Eventually, your discipline will pay off in the form of new habits.

- **Plan for exercise.** Reserve a time slot each day for physical activity, and protect that time. If you wait to find the time, you probably won't do it. Schedule an exercise appointment just as you would a haircut appointment or an important meeting.

- **Avoid all-or-nothing thinking.** If you don't have time to run your usual four miles or to spend 30 minutes lifting weights, do what you can — a brisk one-mile walk, some wall push-ups and other at-home strength exercises. When possible, do more. On days when time is tight or your motivation is waning, do less, but do *something*.

- **Remember how good it feels.** When you find yourself dragging your feet, call to mind the thought of how great you feel after an exercise session. Use images of successful experiences that remind you of how good physical activity makes you feel.

- **Savor your transformation.** Many people are amazed to find that the exercise they've been dreading for all these years is actually quite pleasant. Once you've been active for a while, you may find that you're stronger and more fit, which translates to practical benefits like being able to carry more groceries or play with your grandkids.

- **Be patient and flexible.** When you can't perform your usual exercise routine because of illness, injury, travel or demands on your time, don't let guilt paralyze you further. Instead, adapt your exercise program to accommodate your schedule. A brief period of decreased activity isn't a disaster. Just get going again as soon as possible and return to your previous fitness routine.

- **Keep an exercise log.** Record what you do each day. Keep the log in a handy place. It will help you track your progress.

- **Affirm your efforts with words and images.** What you think affects your fitness plan almost as much as what you do. While negative thoughts can keep you from exercising, positive thoughts or affirmations can keep you going. (See "Positive self-talk" below.)

Guided imagery is another technique that can boost your motivation. In a state of concentrated awareness, imagine yourself getting ready to exercise. Picture obstacles that might keep you from working out, and then picture

Positive self-talk

Whenever you think about something, you are, in a sense, talking to yourself. Psychologists refer to this as self-talk. Becoming conscious of what you're saying to yourself and making it more positive can help you break bad habits, boost your self-confidence and encourage you to stick with your exercise program.

Positive self-talk can increase your energy, motivation and positive attitude, while negative self-talk is critical and anxiety producing. Instructional self-talk helps you improve your performance by focusing on technique or how to do something.

One proven technique for overcoming self-defeating self-talk is to replace negative thoughts with positive ones. Here are some examples:

Negative self-talk	Positive self-talk
"I'm so tired."	"I'm going to feel more energized."
"I should be better at this by now."	"I have made some real improvements and am where I need to be."
"Skipping this one walk won't matter."	"Every little bit makes a big difference."
"I'll never stick with this exercise program.	"Just take one day at a time and have fun."
"I'll never recover from this injury."	"Healing takes time. I'll just continue to do something every day."

You can also use self-talk to break old habits and create new automatic responses. If you golf, for example, you can improve your form by saying things such as "Arm straight" or "Head down." Over time, as you reprogram your self-talk, the positive thoughts will be more automatic.

yourself overcoming them. Imagine yourself exercising and enjoying it, feeling energized and reaching your goals.

- **Support your plan with other healthy behaviors.** In addition to exercising, get adequate sleep. Sleep reduces fatigue and helps in recovering from injury and illness. Drink plenty of fluids and eat a variety of healthy foods. Reduce stress and if you smoke, stop.

TROUBLESHOOTING YOUR PLAN

You've made the commitment to regular physical activity and you're sticking with it. You've gained the sense of confidence, well-being and energy that comes from regular physical activity. You're becoming a fitness success story!

Does this mean you're never going to run into problems on your fitness journey? Not a chance. Exercise programs, like diets, have a high relapse rate. That's why fitness clubs traditionally have the highest enrollment rates in January and February, as people try to carry out their New Year's resolutions to get in shape. But many of those new members are nowhere to be seen by late spring.

One of the most important steps in maintaining your success is to anticipate threats to your continued compliance. The key to dealing with such challenges is to plan and prepare for how you will handle them. These obstacles don't have to stop you in your tracks. You can develop strategies for overcoming them.

A solution for every problem

Regular exercisers and nonexercisers all face similar barriers — but regular exercisers have developed realistic solutions for addressing them. In fact, most obstacles to exercise are things that you can learn to control.

See "Overcoming barriers to exercise" on pages 198-199 for a list of common reasons that people give for being inactive. It also provides possible solutions to these problems.

Lack of time

No doubt you're already squeezed for time with work, family and other responsibilities. Many studies have shown that the perception that there aren't enough hours in the day is the No. 1 reason people stop exercising or never start.

Lack of time is usually more a perception than a reality. Often it's a matter of priorities — after all, many people seem to find a few hours a day to watch television. With careful planning, you can find the time. Here are some suggestions for fitting exercise into your life:

- Break your activity into shorter sessions. For example, take three 10-minute walks throughout the day rather than one 30-minute walk.
- Plan physical activity into your daily schedule. Get up early and work out before work, or walk during your lunch hour.
- Think activity rather than exercise. Mow the lawn, climb the stairs, park farther from your destination and walk.

How much time is required for positive results?

One of the main incentives for staying physically active is to reap the benefits of improved strength and fitness, along with increased energy and stamina. But how much time do you have to put in to see these results?

To achieve the full health benefits of exercise, experts recommend that you participate in moderate-intensity physical activity for 30 to 60 minutes on most days of the week. Beyond this general guideline, different fitness goals require different amounts of time. For example, to improve your aerobic fitness, aim for at least 30 minutes of vigorous-intensity activity for three days or more a week. If your goal is to lose weight, try increasing your aerobic activity to 60 minutes five to six days a week. You may need to lower the intensity of your workout so that you can complete longer sessions. For weight loss, you'll achieve better results if you also reduce the number of calories you consume. (For more information, see "Setting goals and priorities" on page 76.)

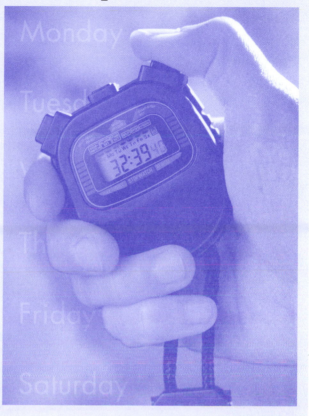

If you're getting the recommended dose of exercise, how soon can you expect to see results? You should notice some changes as soon as the end of the first week of your exercise program, and if you persist, you'll show a little more improvement each week. As your cardiovascular fitness improves, you should find that you're gradually and steadily able to undertake longer, more intense workouts. You'll feel better as you're exercising.

With strength training — especially if you've never done it before — you may see dramatic changes in your strength in the first 12 weeks if you're lifting weights three times a week. In that time, your strength may increase by 10 percent to 25 percent. You'll likely find that you can lift things more easily, and your muscles may start to look more toned and defined. You can continue to build strength by gradually increasing the amount of weight you use. In six months, a person who was previously sedentary can increase his or her strength by 50 percent or more. If you're combining strength training with vigorous aerobic activities, your rate of improvement may increase a bit more slowly.

The initial strength and endurance gains can be impressive and rapid, but they do taper off over time. After you've been exercising for several months, improvements in fitness will occur more slowly. For example, weight loss tends to be slower and steadier after the initial loss. Don't panic — this is normal.

Overcoming barriers to exercise

Potential barriers	**Possible solutions**
Lack of time	■ Break activity into shorter periods of time, such as 10-minute walks. ■ Identify current time wasters, such as TV watching. ■ Plan exercise into your daily schedule. ■ Reframe your concept of exercise to include many everyday activities. (For detailed suggestions, see page 196.)
Boredom	■ Change your routines occasionally. ■ Do a variety of activities rather than just one or two (for example, cross-training). ■ Work out with a friend or in a group. ■ Join a health club or take a fitness class. ■ Listen to music, watch TV or read while you work out. ■ Challenge yourself with new goals. ■ Experiment with interval training. ■ Learn more about technique. ■ Get a new gadget or piece of equipment. (For detailed suggestions, see page 200.)
Inconvenience	■ Work out at home rather than at a club. ■ Choose activities that require minimal facilities and equipment. ■ Incorporate physical activity into your daily routine. ■ Make use of cues or prompts to remind yourself to work out. ■ Choose activities that don't depend on good weather or daylight (For detailed suggestions, see page 202.)
Weather	■ Choose activities that you can do regardless of the weather, such as indoor cycling, aerobics, indoor swimming, stair climbing, dancing or mall walking. (For detailed suggestions, see page 203.)
Lifestyle changes	■ Consider a moderate program of physical activity during stressful times.

Travel	■ Find out what fitness facilities, parks or walking paths are available where you're going. ■ Walk around the airport terminal. ■ Stretch and walk during your flight, or take short walking breaks during a road trip. ■ Work out in your hotel room, and walk the halls and climb the stairs in your hotel. For detailed suggestions, see page 209.
Injury	■ Warm up and cool down when exercising. ■ Talk to your doctor about how to exercise appropriately for your age, fitness level, skill level and health status. ■ Choose low-risk activities. ■ Use the proper equipment, and dress for the weather conditions. ■ If you've been injured, ask your doctor what you can still do. Choose physical activities involving uninjured parts of your body. (For detailed suggestions, see page 211.)
Illness	■ Avoid strenuous exercise when you're sick. But you may be able to work out at a reduced intensity. ■ Don't exercise if you have a fever, chest pain, shortness of breath, generalized muscle aches, a hacking cough, vomiting, extreme tiredness, diarrhea, chills or swollen lymph glands. For detailed suggestions, see page 213.
Overtraining	■ Learn the signs of overtraining. See page 216 for a list. ■ Vary the types of exercises, as well as their order and intensity. ■ Increase the length and intensity of your workouts gradually. ■ Build light workouts and rest days into your schedule. ■ Be sure to get adequate sleep and nutrition.
Lack of facilities or resources	■ Select activities you can do on your own, such as walking, jogging or jumping rope. ■ Identify inexpensive, convenient community resources, such as park and recreation centers or community education programs.

(For more tips, see "Work exercise into your life" on page 19.)

- Do some stretching or strengthening exercises while you watch television. You could also keep a set of weights handy.
- Learn time management skills by taking a class or reading a book on the subject.

Boredom

Even the most dedicated exercisers sometimes get bored with their routines. If your motivation is waning, or you're cutting your workouts short or skipping them altogether, your fitness program may be stale. Consider these suggestions for revitalizing your plan:

- **Change your routines from time to time.** Many people fall into a fitness rut, doing exactly the same activities in the same way at the same time, week after week. While regularity and disciplined consistency can be useful, lack of variation often leads to boredom. Evaluate your current routine to figure out what bores you. A new twist on your favorite

Plateaus

You've been working out for a few months, and you're not seeing the same kind of results as you did in the beginning. What's going on? You may have hit a plateau in your fitness program. This sense of running into a wall is familiar to many exercisers. Unless you update your program regularly, you'll likely come to a plateau at some point along your journey.

Plateaus can happen for several reasons. One is physiologic. After several weeks of working out at the same intensity and duration or lifting the same amount of weight with the same number of reps, your body adapts to that level of activity. You won't see continued improvements unless you alter your routine to reflect the changes in your body.

Sometimes you reach a plateau when you're bored or losing interest in an activity. Or you may hit a plateau if you're overtraining — working out too hard or too frequently.

A plateau doesn't have to be a pitfall. If you find yourself stalling out, first figure out the cause of the plateau and then determine an appropriate solution. If boredom is the problem, review the suggestions on this page (see "Boredom," above) for keeping your program interesting. Are you overtraining? See page 216 for ideas about handling this issue. If you've reached a physiologic plateau, you may need to increase the frequency, duration or intensity of your activity. But doing more may not be an option. For example, you may not have the extra time to commit to exercising. In this case, try the following strategies:

- Gradually increase the intensity of your activity. If you've been walking at a 15-minute-per-mile pace, step it up to 14 or 13. This is a particularly good strategy for strength training. Making your muscles work harder, rather than longer, is the best way to increase strength gains. Be careful to increase the intensity of your activity gradually. Adding too much at once can lead to pain and injury.
- Try interval training. Work out at varying intensities — see page 49 for more information.
- Consider cross-training. Varying your activities can help you avoid plateaus, as can switching the order in which you do your exercises.

activity — such as using free weights instead of working out on machines, or kickboxing instead of step aerobics — may be enough to breathe fresh air into a stale routine. If you've been working out indoors, try jogging, running or biking outside. If you've been working out alone, join a volleyball or soccer team. Change the order of your weightlifting routine or add interval training to your plan.

If you know you're the type of person who's easily bored, plan to make small changes to your routine every month. Any change can be enough to inject some new challenge and enthusiasm. Avoid sudden large changes in exercise intensity, which can put you at risk of injury.

- **Explore new activities.** If tweaking your current routine doesn't do the trick, consider an entirely new activity. If you've always exercised on your own, take up tennis, basketball or another team sport. Explore activities that you've never even thought of doing. Some possibilities might include archery, hiking, rock climbing, jumping rope, kayaking, canoeing, badminton, in-line skating, karate, rowing, dancing (salsa, African, tap, modern, others), yoga, tai chi, cross-country skiing. Have fun!

- **Add variety by cross-training.** Cross-training, or alternating between different activities, is not just for elite athletes. It's a good way for anyone to ward off the exercise blahs. It also improves your overall fitness and reduces your chance of injury from overusing a specific muscle or joint. You can alternate activities — such as walking, swimming, weight training and bicycling — on different days of the week or even in a single workout. Ideally, your program will include aerobic exercise, strength training and flexibility exercises.

- **Work out with a friend or group.** You can socialize while you exercise. You and the people you're with can encourage one another to keep going. Get a group together for a weekend hike and picnic, or have a friend join you for an evening walk. Consider setting an exercise date once or twice a week with someone who's equally committed to physical activity. You're less likely to skip a workout if someone's counting on you to join them.

- **Join an exercise club, health club or fitness class.** Just about every sport or activity has a club. Ask about organized workouts, fun runs and group bike rides or hikes. Health clubs, community centers, parks, schools and gyms offer a variety of fitness classes.

- **Listen to music while you work out.** Upbeat music can rev you up and may increase your pace. One study found that listening to music during exercise made the workout seem easier. It can also make the time pass more quickly.

- **Challenge yourself.** It's great to exercise simply to stay in shape, but you can make your daily workouts more meaningful and exciting by setting a goal that exceeds your current fitness level. For example, if you like to hike, plan to trek through your favorite national park. Consider training for a 10-kilometer (10K) race or triathlon.

- **Try interval training.** Interval training involves alternating short bursts of higher intensity exercise with active recovery, a less intense form of the activity. In a 30-minute workout, for example, you might run for three or four minutes, jog or walk for five, then run again for three or four, and so on. Start by incorporating short bursts of speed into your regular workouts. You could run to the next tree or sprint one lap in the pool.

- **Learn more about technique.** It's easy to fall into a set way of doing your activity. One way to challenge yourself is to learn more about training and technique, as well as alternate approaches to your workout. For example, there are many different ways to train with weights. Explore a new technique.

- **Get an exercise device.** Exercise gadgets such as heart rate monitors and pedometers aren't necessary, but they can add fun and challenge to your routine. Find out what new training equipment is available for your activity.

- **Take an occasional break.** A day off from your routine every now and then can recharge your batteries. Sometimes you really do need time off.

Inconvenience

Many people say they find it inconvenient to exercise. There are several ways to make fitness more convenient:

- If you don't have access to a fitness facility, consider investing in a treadmill, exercise bike, dumbbells or other exercise equipment for use at home. You can also choose activities that require minimal facilities and equipment. All you need to take a walk at home or during your lunch hour at work is a comfortable pair of walking shoes. Other no-fuss options include jogging and jumping rope.

- Incorporate physical activity into your daily routine. Instead of building your life around exercise, build exercise into your life. Activities such as an afternoon of washing your car by hand or weeding your garden will give you some of the same benefits as time spent at the gym. Activities that are at least moderate in intensity — similar to brisk walking — are most effective for improving health and fitness. (See "How many calories does it use up" on page 47.)

- Use cues or prompts in your environment to support your fitness plan. Much of our behavior happens in response to cues in the environment — the way the couch and television can be cues to get a snack. Keep your exercise bag or shoes in sight — in the car, beside your desk at work, by the door — instead of in the closet. Prepare your gym bag for the next exercise session as soon as you get home from the health club so that it's ready to go. Set out your jogging clothes the night before so that you can put them on first thing the next morning. An exercise calendar or self-stick notes on your computer, office door or dashboard can remind you to work out when scheduled. You can even program your computer, cell phone or electronic personal planner to sound an alarm when it's time to exercise.

Weather and climate

It's always a good idea to develop a set of regular activities that you can do regardless of the weather, such as indoor cycling, indoor swimming, stair climbing, dancing and mall walking. Outdoor activities that depend on weather conditions, such as cross-country skiing, can be bonus activities to add as weather permits. Here's how to continue exercising safely when the weather is a challenge.

Hot weather

Exercising on hot days puts extra stress on your cardiovascular system. Both the exercise itself and the air temperature increase your body temperature. To dissipate heat, more blood circulates through your skin. As a result, less blood is available for your muscles, so your heart rate during exercise is higher than on cool days. If the humidity is high, your body faces added stress because sweat doesn't readily evaporate from your skin. As a result, your body temperature rises.

Working out in hot or humid conditions can overstress your body's temperature-regulation system, resulting in an excessive increase in body temperature. Heat-related problems include heat rash, heat cramps, dehydration, heat exhaustion and heat stroke.

To avoid heat-related illness, follow these guidelines:

- **Drink enough fluids.** Your body's ability to sweat and cool down depends on adequate rehydration. During heavy exercise in the heat, you can lose almost 2 quarts of water every hour. Recommended fluids include water, sports drinks and dilute fruit juices. Avoid caffeinated beverages such as coffee, tea and cola, which speed the excretion of water from the body.

  Sports drinks include electrolytes (sodium, chloride and potassium), which are lost through sweating. If you're going to be exercising very intensely or for longer than one hour, you may benefit from fluids containing carbohydrates and electrolytes. Keep in mind that you can't rely on your thirst to signal how much fluid you should drink. Your thirst mechanism underestimates fluid loss in the heat.

- **Wear light-colored, loosefitting clothing made of breathable fabrics.** Dark or nonporous material can increase your temperature and reduce evaporation. Avoid heavy, rubberized clothing, which can be dangerous in any weather. Loose-fitting clothing lets more air pass over the body, providing for sweat evaporation and cooling. A light-colored hat or cap can limit your exposure to the sun.

- **Exercise in the morning or evening instead of the middle of the day.** These are cooler times. If possible, exercise in the shade or in a pool.

- **Wear sunscreen.** Sunburn decreases your body's ability to cool itself.

- **Allow yourself time to acclimate to higher temperatures.** Your body will adapt to the heat, allowing you to exercise with a lower heart rate and lower body temperature. If you're reasonably fit, allow four to five days to become acclimated to higher temperatures. People with chronic illnesses and older adults may need up to 10 to 12 days to adjust. Start with lower duration and intensity and gradually increase effort.

- **Talk to your doctor if you have a chronic medical condition or take medications.** Find out if they affect your ability to work out in hot weather.

- **Stop immediately if you have heat-related problems.** Signs and symptoms of heat exhaustion include cool, clammy and pale skin, a weak pulse, nausea, chills, and dizziness, weakness or disorientation. You may have a headache and be short of breath. Heat stroke is an emergency that can be life-threatening. The skin is flushed, hot and dry. Sweating stops, and the body temperature may rise above 106 F. Confusion and fainting may occur. At the first sign of any of these signs or symptoms, get out of the heat, drink fluids, elevate your feet above your head, either wet and fan your skin or immerse yourself in cool water, and get medical help.

- **Don't exercise outdoors when the conditions are too extreme.** Avoid the high-risk zone for heat stress.

Cold weather

Winter activities can be exhilarating and a great way to enjoy the snow and get some sun. But exercising in very cold weather can be risky. Your body loses heat in a cold environment. Movement exacerbates the heat loss because of wind chill, the combined cooling effect of cool air and wind. Normally, a thin layer of warm, still air insulates you from the outside temperature. Blowing wind removes this protective layer and reduces skin temperature. Cold weather also increases the energy needed to exercise.

In drier winter air, you lose more water through breathing than you do in warmer weather. Very cold air constricts your airways and makes vigorous activity difficult. But while the cold air may make breathing uncomfortable, it won't damage your lungs. Your respiratory system warms and humidifies the air, so the delicate tissues of your lungs are protected.

The human body responds to cold in two main ways — by narrowing the blood vessels, which decreases blood flow to the skin and reduces the rate of heat loss, and by shivering, which increases body heat production. Exercise also generates considerable heat — and is far more effective than is shivering.

Prolonged exposure to low temperatures and high winds puts you at risk of several cold-related injuries, including

Windchill chart

Frostbite of exposed skin occurs in 30 minutes or less.
Frostbite of exposed skin occurs in 10 minutes or less.
Frostbite of exposed skin occurs in 5 minutes or less.

Temperature (°F)

Wind (MPH)	30	25	20	15	10	5	0	-5	-10	-15	-20	-25	-30	-35	-40	-45
5	25	19	13	7	1	-5	-11	-16	-22	-28	-34	-40	-46	-52	-57	-63
10	21	15	9	3	-4	-10	-16	-22	-28	-35	-41	-47	-53	-59	-66	-72
15	19	13	6	0	-7	-13	-19	-26	-32	-39	-45	-51	-58	-64	-71	-77
20	17	11	4	-2	-9	-15	-22	-29	-35	-42	-48	-55	-61	-68	-74	-81
25	16	9	3	-4	-11	-17	-24	-31	-37	-44	-51	-58	-64	-71	-78	-84
30	15	8	1	-5	-12	-19	-26	-33	-39	-46	-53	-60	-67	-73	-80	-87
35	14	7	0	-7	-14	-21	-27	-34	-41	-48	-55	-62	-69	-76	-82	-89
40	13	6	-1	-8	-15	-22	-29	-36	-43	-50	-57	-64	-71	-78	-84	-91
45	12	5	-2	-9	-16	-23	-30	-37	-44	-51	-58	-65	-72	-79	-86	-93
50	12	4	-3	-10	-17	-24	-31	-38	-45	-52	-60	-67	-74	-81	-88	-95
55	11	4	-3	-11	-18	-25	-32	-39	-46	-54	-61	-68	-75	-82	-89	-97
60	10	3	-4	-11	-19	-26	-33	-40	-48	-55	-62	-69	-76	-84	-91	-98

Source: National Weather Service.

frostbite, a dangerously low body temperature (hypothermia) and exercise-induced asthma. But wintry weather doesn't have to keep you stuck inside on the treadmill. Follow these precautions to enjoy outdoor exercising throughout the coldest months of the year:

- **Dress appropriately.** The most common problem for cold-weather exercisers isn't wearing too little clothing but too much. Because exercise raises body temperature considerably, even a moderate workout can make you feel that it's about 30 degrees warmer than it really is. The solution is to wear several layers of loosefitting clothing that protects against not only the cold but also the wind and moisture. Layers provide an insulating barrier of air and can be peeled off if you become too warm. Start opening zippers or removing layers as soon as you start to sweat. When you take off a layer, you can tie it around your waist or put it in a day pack.

Choose fabrics that insulate well, even when wet. Damp clothing conducts heat away from the body faster than dry clothing does. Avoid cotton, which holds moisture next to your skin. Heavy, thick clothing such as a down jacket or vest provides too much insulation, causing you to overheat.

Don't forget your head, feet and hands. Wear a fleece, wool or synthetic cap, hood or headband, or a cap that includes a face mask. Wear boots or shoes that offer good traction and have a little extra space inside to trap heat. Keep your feet warm by wearing an inner sock made of polypropylene and an outer wool sock.

Fluids — How much is enough?

Follow these recommendations for drinking fluids when exercising in the heat:

- **Before exercise,** drink 8 to 20 ounces of water or a sports drink.
- **During exercise,** drink 8 ounces or more every 15 to 20 minutes.
- **After exercise,** drink 8 to 20 ounces.

Another way to determine how much water you need to replace is to weigh yourself before and after your activity. For each pound of weight lost, drink 2 cups (16 ounces) of fluid.

It's possible to drink too much. Forcing fluids well beyond replacement can over time dilute electrolytes — including sodium — in your blood. A deficiency of sodium in the blood — called hyponatremia — is a potentially life-threatening condition.

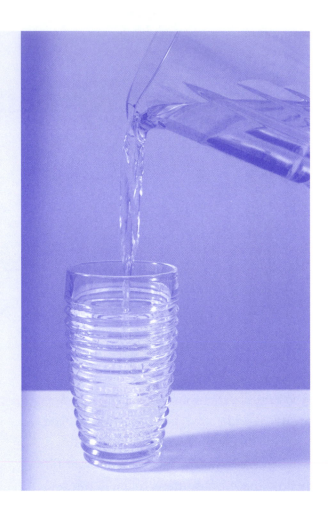

Take care not to wear socks that are so thick that your boots or shoes fit too snugly, which will decrease the blood flow needed to keep your feet warm. Mittens are warmer than gloves are. You can also wear inner glove liners made of polypropylene or another material that draws sweat from your skin.

- **Warm up indoors.** Before going out, do a warm-up indoors by walking, jogging in place, jumping rope or climbing stairs.
- **Drink plenty of fluids.** You need to drink as much in the cold as you do in the heat. It's easy to become dehydrated in cold weather because you lose water from sweating and breathing and because urine production increases. Dehydration increases the risk of frostbite. Drink water or sports drinks before, during and after your workout, even if you're not thirsty. Avoid alcohol and caffeinated beverages.
- **Be aware of wind chill.** The wind can penetrate your clothes and remove the insulating layer of warm air around your body. Fast motion, as when skiing, running, cycling or skating, also creates wind chill, because it increases air

movement past the body. For example, skiing at 20 miles an hour in 10 F conditions and calm air creates a wind chill of minus 9 F. When possible, face away from the wind if you're moving fast. When wind chill is a threat, make sure to cover all exposed skin. (See "Windchill chart" on page 205.)

- **Go out into the wind, return with the wind.** Consider doing the first half of your exercise session going into the wind, especially if you expect to work up a sweat. That way, when you return with the wind at your back during the second half of your workout, you'll reduce the chance of becoming chilled due to excessive cooling.

- **Wear sunscreen and sunglasses.** Snow-covered ground can reflect the sun's ultraviolet rays and burn your face and neck. Wear sunscreen and polarized sunglasses or ski goggles.

- **Eat well to maintain your energy.** Eat nutritious meals before your activity and snacks at regular intervals.

- **Rest and warm up as needed.** Rest when you need to, and stop before you're exhausted. To prevent frostbite, warm your hands and feet every 20 to 30 minutes.

- **Prevent breathing problems.** To avoid problems from breathing cold air, wear a cold-weather face mask or scarf over your mouth and nose. If you're prone to exercise-induced asthma, talk to your doctor about medications to deal with the signs and symptoms. The most common medications for exercise-induced

asthma are bronchodilators, which you take 15 to 30 minutes before exercising. They open up your constricted airways and provide temporary relief.

- **Avoid exercising outdoors in extreme conditions.** When the temperature dips well below zero or the windchill is below minus 20 F, stick with an indoor activity. Get the weather report before you set out. In particular, pay attention to the windchill factor. Be aware of the danger zone for outdoor activity. Wet snow and ice also can be treacherous and put you at risk of falling. In slippery, icy conditions, stay inside.

- **Know the warning signs of frostbite and hypothermia.** Frostbite is most common on the face, fingers and toes. At first it appears as a patch of pale or white skin. Other early warning signs include numbness, loss of feeling or a sharp stinging sensation. After mild frostbite, the skin becomes red and swollen as the blood returns. A severe case may cause the skin to turn purple or black when rewarmed, with excruciating pain.

If frostbite occurs, don't rewarm the affected area if there's any chance it will refreeze. Don't rub the affected skin. If the area won't be exposed to freezing again, you can warm the area, but avoid excessive heat. Seek medical help.

Hypothermia begins with intense shivering and an inability to do complex tasks. Later signs and symptoms include slurred speech, sluggish thinking, mental confusion and memory loss.

Hypothermia is a medical emergency that requires immediate attention.

High altitude

If you've ever traveled to a place that's at a higher altitude than your home is and tried to carry out your normal workout, you were probably huffing and puffing harder than usual. When you get above 5,000 feet, less oxygen is available. Your muscles and other body tissues have to work with a reduced supply of oxygen. This translates to a decline in aerobic fitness and endurance, despite your best efforts.

It takes about three weeks to adjust to a higher elevation, or about one week for each 1,000 feet above 5,000 feet. Once your body has acclimated to the higher altitude, more oxygen will be available to your muscles, but even then your aerobic capacity and endurance will still be less than what they are at lower elevations. Your usual pace will not have the same aerobic effects at higher altitudes.

If you're going to be exercising at a higher than normal altitude, follow these guidelines:

- Start out slowly, giving your body time to adjust.
- Once you've acclimated, go your usual distance or time, but at a slower pace.
- Be aware of the signs and symptoms of acute mountain sickness (AMS). They include headache, progressive shortness of breath, rapid heartbeat, loss of appetite and flu-like malaise within six to 48 hours after ascent. These typically don't appear until you reach 8,000 feet and above. Fluid in the lungs (high-altitude pulmonary edema, or HAPE) is a serious sign of AMS and should be treated as a medical emergency.
- Drink plenty of fluids. You tend to dehydrate more quickly at higher altitudes.

Air pollution

Because a major point of exercising is to improve your aerobic capacity — increasing the volume of air you take into your lungs each minute — it stands to reason that air quality can affect your workout and your health. Unfortunately, air pollution is often a reality for most people who live in or near large cities.

Air pollution can cause problems such as chest pain, coughing, wheezing, watery eyes and respiratory disorders. Air pollution is caused by automobiles, soot, industrial pollutants, and other sources. The two major urban air pollutants are ozone and carbon monoxide. Ozone is produced when sunlight interacts with the nitrogen dioxide in auto and factory emissions. Ozone irritates your airways, causing them to constrict and making it harder for you to breathe.

Carbon monoxide (CO) is an odorless, toxic gas that's created by burning gasoline, wood, coal, diesel fuel and other organic substances. Smoking cigarettes also produces carbon monoxide. When you have higher than normal concentrations of CO in your bloodstream, your athletic performance suffers.

Dust, smoke and pollen in the air — substances referred to as particulates — get trapped in your upper respiratory tract and can irritate the tissues in your lungs. Exposure to these substances can cause coughing and airway restriction, as well as long-term health problems.

To reduce your exposure to air pollutants and keep your lungs healthy no matter where you live, try following these suggestions when exercising:

- **Avoid busy streets and roadways.** Stay at least 50 feet away from heavily traveled roads, especially where cars stop and start frequently. Carbon monoxide levels are highest along busy streets.
- **Avoid rush hour.** Work out at times when traffic is lightest, such as before and after the morning and evening rush hours. At these times, air pollution levels generally are much lower.
- **Be aware of pollution levels.** Many urban television stations provide air quality updates, especially from May through September, when ozone levels are highest. Work out indoors on smoggy days or days when the Air Quality Index is high or when air pollution or pollen warnings are in effect.
- **Choose healthy foods.** Antioxidant foods containing vitamins C, E and beta carotene can help protect your lungs from irritants. Eat plenty of fruits, vegetables and whole grains, and take a daily multivitamin supplement.
- **If you're sensitive to pollutants or allergens, use a dust mask.** Look for a product designed to filter particulate matter. Some masks cut ozone and carbon monoxide exposure, but most can't remove all carbon monoxide.

Travel

Travel doesn't have to disrupt your exercise routine. It's easier than you may think to incorporate physical activity into your trips. And doing so can increase your energy and help you handle stress. With some planning and self-discipline, you'll find that healthy habits travel easily. Here are some tips for staying fit on the road:

- **Plan accordingly.** Call your hotel and ask about fitness facilities on-site or nearby. Ask about parks, running tracks, hiking and walking trails, pools, or tennis courts. Knowing what's available will help you pack the right workout clothes.
- **Walk around the airport terminal.** While you're waiting for a flight, take a walk. Change to your athletic shoes if you're not wearing them. Even a short walk can boost your mood and energy level and help with jet lag if you're changing time zones.
- **Stretch and walk around during your flight.** Get up once an hour to stretch and walk. This will help decrease muscle aches, joint stiffness and swelling. It will also improve blood flow to your legs and can reduce the risk of blood clots (deep vein thrombosis).
- **If you're driving, take frequent breaks to get out and stretch.** Take a short walk around the rest area.

- **Work out in your hotel room.** Pack an exercise band or tubing and a jump rope. (For information about elastic bands and tubes designed for resistance training, see Chapter 5.) You can also do exercises that don't require any equipment. Examples include crunches, push-ups, squats, lunges and balance exercises. You can also walk the hotel halls and climb the stairs.
- **Go sightseeing on foot at a brisk pace.** Or rent in-line skates or a bicycle. Find a local club and go dancing in the evening.
- **Work out at a local gym.** Buy a single-day pass. If you belong to a YMCA or YWCA at home, ask about reciprocal membership agreements.

Aches and pains

Forget the old saying, "No pain, no gain." Exercising shouldn't be painful, nor do you need to suffer to get stronger and more fit. Still, everyone who's physically active is bound to feel some soreness, stiffness or occasional minor aches and pains. And injuries do occur, though you can take steps to reduce the likelihood of getting hurt.

Muscle soreness that follows a day or two after exercise is normal, especially if you've been sedentary or you're starting a new workout routine or trying a new activity. This type of soreness, called delayed-onset muscle soreness, is also common after a bout of heavy exercise, even if you've been regularly active.

The soreness means that your muscles

Muscle cramps

Muscle cramps are a familiar but poorly understood exercise complaint. These sharp, stabbing, cramping or aching pains can range from mild to excruciating. A muscle cramp in the abdomen is sometimes referred to as a side stitch.

Muscle cramps are common among runners, horseback riders, swimmers and people involved in some team sports.

Muscle cramps, though painful, aren't a serious health problem. Popular remedies include stretching, acupressure and, for a side cramp, bending over. Because cramps often occur when you're dehydrated, drinking enough water may reduce your risk.

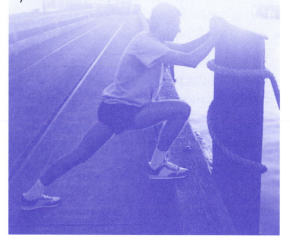

are growing stronger. It's partially caused by structural damage to muscle fibers — a slight tearing of the fibers called hypertrophy. During the repair process, the muscle tissue rebuilds and becomes stronger, a process called adaptation.

If you've been sedentary for a while, you may feel mild discomfort after starting an exercise program. Chances are you haven't injured yourself. It's just your body adapting to a new challenge.

On the other hand, pain during exercise can be a warning sign of impending injury. Excessive exercise can cause severe muscle damage. Severely damaged muscle fibers won't rebuild and recover. Rather, they'll degenerate and will heal only with complete rest.

Many people overdo it when they first start a fitness program. They end up sore because they don't believe exercise is effective unless they feel discomfort. It can be difficult to find a middle road and moderate the amount of exercise you do. Pay attention to what your body is telling you. If you're feeling pain, you're overdoing it.

Gasping for breath and having sore joints are signals to slow down. Muscle stiffness lasting several days means you went too far. If what you're doing hurts, you're overdoing it. Reduce intensity or workload, or try a different exercise.

Another common cause of aches and pains is doing the same activities over and over without variation. Regular exercisers tend to focus on one or two activities. This can lead to overuse injuries, caused by repeated stress on a particular area of the body.

You can still keep working out if you have mild, everyday aches and pains. Try these tips to make it a little easier to deal with pain after a workout:

- Get up and get going. Your muscles need gentle activity to enhance blood flow and promote healing within the muscle. Take a leisurely stroll or ride an exercise bike with no resistance. In addition, getting a proper warm-up before you exercise can help reduce aches and pains after exercise.
- Over-the-counter pain relievers such as acetaminophen or anti-inflammatory medications such as aspirin and ibuprofen are safe for most people. If you regularly use ibuprofen or another anti-inflammatory medication, talk with your doctor.
- Stretch your muscles after your workouts. Gentle stretching reduces muscle soreness when you start exercising.
- Massage can help ease sore muscles.
- Drink plenty of fluids.

Sometimes, your body may be telling you to take a break from exercise. If you have a flare-up of a bone or joint condition, rest until it subsides. If your pain is beyond normal achiness or persists for longer than two weeks, or you have swelling, back off from your fitness activities and consider consulting a doctor. It's also important to know the warning signs that tell you to stop exercising immediately (see page 250).

Injury

Each year, an estimated 7 million Americans receive medical attention for a sports- or recreation-related injury. Although two-thirds of these injuries happen in young people, adults aren't exempt — one-quarter of the injuries occur among 24- to 44-year-olds, and sports-related injuries among people age 65 and older have increased significantly in the last 15 years.

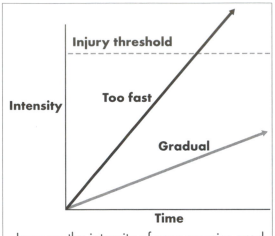

Increase the intensity of your exercise gradually over time to reduce the risk of injury.

Most exercise-related injuries affect the upper and lower extremities — ankles, feet, lower legs, hands, wrists and shoulders. Low back injuries also are common.

Strains and sprains are the most common exercise-related injuries, followed by fractures. These injuries typically occur as a result of a fall, overexertion, hitting something or being hit.

One of the major risk factors for exercise and sports injuries is level of fitness. In general, the less fit you are, the greater

Preventing an injury

Most injuries that occur during physical activity stem from the "terrible toos" — too much, too hard, too fast, too soon, too long. A novice runner who struggles to complete five miles the first time out likely will hurt afterward. The couch potato who comes to life for the annual company softball game is an excellent candidate for a sprain, strain or other injury.

To minimize your chances of getting hurt, follow these guidelines:

- Follow the 10 percent rule. Limit the increases in volume and intensity of your training to 10 percent. For example, if you swim laps for 30 minutes this week, increase to 33 minutes next week, and so on.
- Warm up.
- Start out slowly and exercise at the appropriate intensity.
- Get adequate sleep.
- Keep your muscles conditioned through regular activity. Avoid being a weekend warrior.
- If your muscles are sore, ease up on your exercise routine.
- A previous injury increases your risk of a subsequent one, so if you've been injured before, talk with your doctor about appropriate physical activities.
- Use proper form and technique.
- Wear proper shoes and protective equipment.
- Take appropriate precautions for the weather conditions.
- Drink plenty of water.
- Use pain relievers with caution because they may mask pain that would normally serve to warn you that you're overdoing it.
- Cool down.
- Be aware of warning signs. See page 72.

If you do sustain an injury, first follow the P.R.I.C.E. guidelines on page 213. The acronym *P.R.I.C.E.* is used to describe the first steps in treating any muscle or joint injury.

your chance of getting hurt. Age is another factor. Older adults' muscles and tendons are more susceptible to injury. This is why it's so important to begin any new physical activity or exercise program at low duration (volume) and intensity and build up gradually.

Illness

You were looking forward to your step class today, but now you're feeling tired and achy, with a sore throat. Should you exercise, or stay home with a cup of tea?

The answer depends on what type of illness and symptoms you have. If you have a cold, moderate exercise won't make it worse or prolong it. In fact, working out may temporarily clear a stuffed-up head.

On the other hand, if you have an infection accompanied by fever, exercising increases the risk of dehydration, dangerously high body temperature (heatstroke) and even heart failure. Acute infectious

Treating an injury with P.R.I.C.E.

- **Protect** the injured area from further injury. You can do this in a variety of ways, using anything from braces to crutches.
- **Rest** the injured area. For example, don't walk on an injured ankle. This doesn't necessarily mean complete rest from all physical activity.
- **Ice** the affected area with a cold pack, a slush bath or a compression sleeve filled with cold water to limit swelling. Try to apply ice as soon as possible after the injury.
- **Compression,** as with a bandage or elastic wrap, also helps with swelling.
- **Elevate** the injured area above heart level whenever possible to prevent or limit swelling.

An injury doesn't have to sideline you from all physical activity. Here are some tips for staying conditioned while injured.

- Talk to your doctor about how best to maintain your overall conditioning while your injury heals and what activities you can still do. It's usually possible to work around the injury by doing other activities. For example, if your normal routine includes running but you've got a leg injury that would be aggravated by impact, you could run in water, swim or use a stationary bike. If you've had shoulder surgery and can't participate in your tennis league, try a walking program or stationary bike to stay fit until you can get back on the tennis court. Even with an ankle sprain, you could swim, do an upper body workout with weights or use an exercise bicycle to work your uninjured ankle while resting the leg with the injured ankle.
- Use this time as an opportunity to build up weak parts of your overall fitness program, such as flexibility or strength training. Focus on gentle flexibility and strengthening exercises. Ask your doctor, physical therapist or trainer for guidance.
- Your doctor can help you develop a specific program for rehabilitating the injured area and easing back into your activity. Once you've regained strength in the injured area, work on coordination and balance.

Exercise and immunity

Regular moderate exercise may boost your immune system. Researchers have found a link between regular physical activity and improved immune function. During moderate exercise, immune cells circulate more quickly through your body and are better at destroying viruses and bacteria.

Researchers at the University of South Carolina in Columbia investigated the relationship between different levels of physical activity and the risk of getting a cold (upper respiratory tract infection). The study included 547 healthy adults between the ages of 20 and 70. Those who had a moderate-to-high level of physical activity experienced 20 percent to 30 percent fewer colds than did those whose daily activities were low.

Moderation is key. Some studies have found that intense physical training may lead to a suppressed immune system and increased susceptibility to illness. Running a marathon, for example, may deplete your immune system defenses and leave you vulnerable to colds and other illnesses in the week after the race.

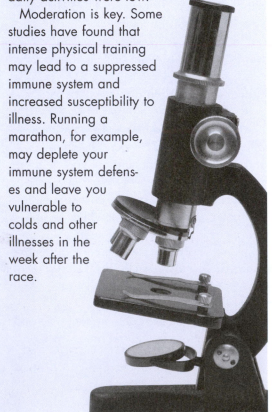

diseases, such as the flu (influenza) and "stomach flu" (gastroenteritis), also result in decreased endurance, strength and concentration.

One common guideline for determining whether you should exercise is to do a "neck check" of your symptoms. If your signs and symptoms are above the neck — a stuffy or runny nose, sneezing or a sore throat — then moderate exercise is generally safe. Start at half speed. If you feel better after 10 minutes, you can increase your speed. But if you feel miserable, stop.

Avoid intense physical activity if your signs and symptoms are below the neck. These include generalized muscle aches, hacking cough, fever, extreme fatigue, vomiting, diarrhea, chills and swollen lymph glands. Exercising with these signs and symptoms can be harmful.

You can start exercising again when your below-the-neck signs and symptoms subside. But ease back into your activity gradually. A good rule of thumb is to exercise for two days at a lower than normal intensity for each day you were sick.

Here are some other guidelines to keep you healthy while maintaining your fitness plan.

- Don't exercise if you have a fever.
- Consider whether you might infect others on your team or league or in your workout area.
- Avoid strenuous exercise when you're feeling sick — work out at a modified intensity.

Detraining — "Use it or lose it"

The beneficial effects of fitness are transitory — when you stop exercising, you'll begin to lose them. This use-it-or-lose-it effect is known as detraining. If you're laid up with an injury or take a break from exercise, some loss of fitness is inevitable. The good news is that you can take steps to avoid or minimize the loss.

How quickly detraining happens depends on how fit you were to begin with, how long you've been exercising and how long you've stopped. It also depends on what activities you were doing.

For cardiovascular activities, people who are extremely conditioned experience a rapid drop in fitness during the first three weeks of detraining, which then tapers off. People with low-to-moderate fitness levels show a more gradual, steady reduction. At any given point during detraining, a more fit person will maintain a higher level of fitness than will a less fit person.

Gains in strength from resistance or weight training may last longer. Newly gained strength may be retained for up to six weeks after you stop training, and you can retain about half the strength you gain for up to a year. Strength declines very slowly in muscle groups that are used regularly.

What's more, when you start strength training again, you'll return to your previous levels of strength with less effort. This is because of muscle memory — the learning that took place earlier.

Your ability to perform a specific sport or activity usually declines if you abandon the activity for an extended time. Some sport-specific skills, such as riding a bike, are easily maintained, while others, such as delivering a powerful and accurate serve in tennis, require well-trained muscles.

To avoid losing the health and fitness benefits you've worked so hard to achieve, cut back on exercise rather than cut it out altogether. If you can't do strength training three times a week, you can still maintain most of your gains by training once a week. If you can't run, try walking, swimming or cycling instead. Maintaining intensity is more crucial than maintaining frequency. Less frequent, similar-intensity exercises will usually do the trick.

■ Don't exercise until checking with your doctor if you have:
  • Chest pain
  • Irregular, rapid or fluttery heartbeat
  • Severe shortness of breath
  • Significant, unexplained weight loss
  • Joint swelling
  • Persistent pain or trouble walking after you've fallen
  • Significantly more fatigue than usual
  • Hernia
  • Blood clot
  • Foot or ankle sores that won't heal
  • Bleeding in the retina or a detached retina
  • Been advised by your doctor not to exert yourself for a given period of time due to surgery or illness
  • Had a cataract or lens implant or laser eye treatment

Reduce risk of infections during cold and flu season by working out during less crowded hours at the gym or by choosing outdoor activities.

If you have a chronic illness such as heart disease, diabetes or arthritis, you may need to take some precautions when exercising. For detailed information about physical activity and major medical conditions, see Chapter 8.

Expecting? You don't have to abandon your fitness plan. See page 268 for tips on exercising during pregnancy.

Overtraining

Overtraining happens when you push your body past the point of full recovery for your next workout. When you exercise hard, you subject your body to some stress and physical trauma. You need sufficient time, rest and nutrition between exercise sessions to allow your body to regenerate and repair itself.

If there's an imbalance between your workouts and rest periods, your performance will decline. If you push too hard before you're ready for the next workout, you run the risk of illness and injury. Studies have found that overtraining results in decreased performance, increased irritability, increases in stress hormones and changes in the immune system. It's the athletic equivalent of jet lag.

About 10 percent of people who work out overtrain during a given year. You can overtrain in any type of activity, including aerobic exercises such as running and resistance exercises such as weightlifting. People who exercise aggressively are most prone to overtraining.

How do you know if you're overdoing it? The most common symptom of over-

training is fatigue. You may feel a cumulative, constant exhaustion that persists even during periods of rest. You feel burned out and stale. Other signs and symptoms may include:

- Lethargy
- Moodiness and irritability
- Loss of interest in working out
- Altered sleep patterns
- An inability to relax
- Depression
- Decreased appetite
- Weight loss
- Persistent muscle soreness and soreness or stiffness in joints and tendons
- Increased frequency of illness
- Menstrual disruptions
- Increased incidence of injuries, such as stress fractures and overuse injuries
- Prolonged weakness
- Decreased performance

If you start to have these signs and symptoms, you may be pushing too hard. Exercise should make you feel better, not worse. If you're feeling worse, you're probably overtraining. If these signs and symptoms persist, see your doctor.

Determining your limits

To avoid overtraining, the most important thing is to listen to your body. Occasionally stop and check your physical and emotional condition. When you're very sore or tired, back off. It's also critical to work out at an appropriate intensity, duration and frequency.

Here are some other suggestions for avoiding overtraining:

- Avoid monotonous training — vary the types of exercise you do, the order in which you do them and the intensity of the activities.

- Keep track of your activity in a log or diary, and learn to detect signs of overtraining. Keeping an exercise log allows you to determine if you moved up your program too fast, didn't take enough days off or worked out too hard.

- Increase your workouts gradually and avoid working out with too much intensity or duration (volume). Be cautious about increasing your workout frequency, adding exercises or exercising longer. Try a cycle of shorter exercise sessions instead of longer sessions. Training volume and intensity should be inversely related. When you train for longer periods, reduce the intensity of your activity, and when you train at a higher intensity, reduce your time.

- Be sure to build in light periods and rest days to your program. This scheduled rest will facilitate recovery, similar to the way elite athletes taper their training before big competitions.

- Make sure you're getting adequate nutrition and sleep.

- Perform high-impact exercise such as running and jumping rope on a surface that has some give to it, rather than always doing these activities on a hard surface. This can improve the recovery time for your lower body.

- If you feel like you're getting sick, rest or reduce your training schedule for a few days.

Recovering

The most basic remedy for overtraining is rest. Rest — both sleep and pure relaxation time — is a vital part of a physically active life. The longer you've overtrained, the more rest you'll need.

You don't have to become totally inactive. It's more important to decrease your activity rather than stop your workouts altogether, which can send you into a crash and burn situation from exercise withdrawal. To recover from overtraining, reduce the volume of your activity by 30 percent to 50 percent. For example, go back to working out three days a week for 30 minutes a session, at a slightly decreased intensity. Do this until you start feeling better.

With reduced training, more rest and good nutrition, you can recover physically and emotionally. By maintaining a reasonable exercise intensity, even with a reduced workout frequency, you typically won't lose your fitness gains.

THE JOURNEY OF A LIFETIME

No one is exempt from challenges, disruptions, low points and occasional setbacks in his or her fitness program. That's the nature of life and exercise. But with the right attitude and the willingness to plan and implement solutions, you'll be able to keep your commitment to being physically active — and fit.

Fitness &nutrition

CHAPTER 7

When it comes to fitness, nutrition and physical activity go hand in hand. To get the most out of your physical activity, a well-balanced, nutritious diet is essential. One basic reason for this is that physical activity requires energy, and energy comes from what you eat and drink. Understanding how your body converts food to energy and how this energy is stored and used enables you to choose the best combination of foods to enhance your well-being and physical performance.

Learning to determine your caloric needs and create a diet that complements your exercise program is an important part of achieving your fitness goals. Being able to evaluate the importance of supplements and other dietary aids aimed at improving physical fitness can also help you build a better fitness plan.

In this chapter, you'll learn how to calculate the amount of energy you expend each day — your basal metabolic rate. You'll also learn about how much energy it takes to do a variety of activities — from just sitting to jogging. You'll also

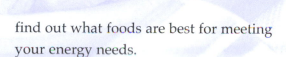

find out what foods are best for meeting your energy needs.

YOUR ENERGY SOURCE

Food is a big part of life, whether you pay a little or a lot of attention to it. When most of us think about food, we think about things like bread, pasta, tomatoes, eggs, beans, potatoes, hamburgers, fish and a host of other items. Food also includes what you drink, such as water, milk, juice, coffee, beer and wine.

Elements of food

Food is made up of several basic elements, including carbohydrates, fats, proteins, vitamins, minerals, water and fiber.

Carbohydrates. Carbohydrates are classified as simple or complex. Simple carbohydrates are sugars, found in fruits (fructose and glucose), milk (lactose) and table sugar (sucrose). Complex carbohydrates are also known as starches and are found primarily in bread, rice, pasta, cereals and vegetables.

Fats. Fats come in various forms. The oils you use for cooking are a form of fat. Fats can be found in foods of animal origin, such as meat, dairy, poultry and fish, and in some foods of vegetable origin, such as avocados, nuts and olive oil.

Proteins. Proteins are composed of building blocks called amino acids. In terms of your health, there are two types of amino acids. Those your body can generate on its own are called nonessential amino acids. Those that can be obtained only from the food you eat are called essential amino acids.

Animal sources of protein, such as meat, poultry, milk and eggs, contain all of the essential amino acids and are therefore considered complete sources of protein. Vegetable sources such as legumes and nuts contain only some essential amino acids, but when they're combined with certain other foods they can provide a complete source of protein. The exception to this is soy, which contains all of the essential amino acids.

Vitamins. Food also contains vitamins, such as A, B, C, D, E and K. Vitamins help your body to process carbohydrates, fats and proteins. They also help produce blood cells, hormones, genetic materials and nervous system chemicals. Fresh foods usually contain more vitamins than do processed foods.

Minerals. Minerals are another component of food. The major minerals found in food include calcium, magnesium, phosphorus, potassium, chloride and sodium. Calcium, magnesium and phosphorus are important to the health of your bones and teeth. Sodium, potassium and chloride, commonly referred to as electrolytes, help regulate the water and chemical balance in your body. Potassium also plays an important role in muscle function. Your body needs smaller amounts of other minerals (trace minerals), including iron, iodine, zinc, copper, fluoride, selenium and manganese.

Water. Water is so common that it almost gets forgotten, but it's an important part of food. Many foods, especially fruit, contain water. Of course, the most direct way to get water is to drink it. Water plays a role in nearly every major body function. It helps to regulate body temperature, carries nutrients and oxygen to cells, and helps carry away waste. Water also helps cushion joints and protect organs and tissues.

Fiber. Fiber is the part of plant foods that your body doesn't absorb. The two main types of fiber are called soluble and insoluble. Foods rich in fiber usually con-

Did you know?

A Snickers bar contains 273 calories. If you set the Snickers bar on fire and burned it completely, the process would produce 273 calories of energy.

Your body also burns calories to create energy, but with a series of chemical reactions rather than with heat. If you're an average-weight person, you would have to run nearly three miles to burn 273 calories.

tain both. Examples of foods high in soluble fiber include citrus fruits, strawberries, apples, legumes, oatmeal and oat bran. Insoluble fiber is found in wheat bran, many vegetables, and whole-grain breads, pastas and cereals. Soluble fiber holds on to water and provides bulk to stool, helping to prevent constipation. Insoluble fiber has a stimulating effect on the colon, which also helps to prevent constipation. In addition, insoluble fiber may help lower blood cholesterol and blood sugar levels.

Measuring food's energy

Another way to think about food is in terms of the energy it contains. This energy is measured in units called calories. Calories are used to measure energy in a wide variety of things, not just food. For example, calories can also be used to measure the energy in gasoline or a piece of wood. Technically, 1 calorie is the amount of energy required to raise the temperature of 1 gram of water 1 C (1.8 F). As a side note, energy contained in food is usually measured in terms of kilocalories (1,000 calories = 1 kilocalorie), even though they're almost always referred to as calories. So in terms of food, calories and kilocalories are often used interchangeably.

Carbohydrates, fats and proteins contain calories and thus are sources of energy. But the amount of energy provided by each is different, as is the mechanism by which each nutrient yields its energy.

Carbohydrates are your body's primary source of energy — what gets used up first. During the digestive process, carbohydrates are broken down into glucose and other simple sugars. Glucose can be used immediately for energy or stored away for later use in the form of long chains of glycogen in your liver and muscles. When your glycogen storage sites are full, excess glucose is converted into fatty acids and stored in fat (adipose) tissue.

Fats are an extremely concentrated form of energy and pack the most calories. When digested, they're broken down into fatty acids, which can also be used imme-diately for energy or for other body processes. When your body absorbs excess fatty acids, a small quantity is stored in your muscles, but most of it is stored in adipose tissue.

Proteins are used mainly to build and repair the structures of your body, produce body chemicals such as enzymes and hormones, carry nutrients to your cells, and regulate your body processes. But proteins can also supply energy for physical activity if your body runs out of carbohydrate power, such as if you consume too few calories or if you're involved in prolonged physical activity.

Vitamins, minerals, water and fiber don't contain calories. Although these don't provide energy, they're important to your overall well-being. A lack of these items in your diet can lead to a number of health problems.

In the following sections, you'll see how carbohydrates, fats and proteins are converted into energy your body can use.

How does food become energy?

For your body to be able to use the energy in food, it must convert calories — in the form of glucose (from carbohydrates), fatty acids (from fats and oils) or amino acids (from proteins) — into a chemical substance called adenosine triphosphate (ATP). ATP is your body's universal energy currency. It's necessary for all of the cellular transactions that occur in your body — from building new cells to transporting nutrients to working your muscles. Whether you're blinking your eyes

Food sources of energy

Fats and alcohol supply more calories per gram than do carbohydrates and proteins combined.

Nutrient	Calories per gram
Alcohol	7
Carbohydrates	4
Fats	9
Proteins	4

or bench-pressing 150 pounds, ATP is always involved.

ATP is in constant production and use. Your body uses three biochemical systems to exchange calories for ATP — the immediate (phosphagen) energy system, the short-term (glycolysis) energy system and the long-term, or endurance (aerobic), energy system. (See Chapter 2 for a complete explanation of these energy systems and how they work.)

YOUR ENERGY ACCOUNT

Imagine that your energy is like a checking account. You have income, and you have expenditures. In the income column is food, with three nutrients — carbohydrates, fats and proteins — providing you with energy. When you eat, you're putting energy into your account.

In the expenditure column, there are three types of withdrawals. The most obvious withdrawal from your energy account is when you exert yourself during physical activity. But your body also withdraws energy for its basic needs, such as breathing, blood circulation, hormone adjustments, and cellular growth and repair. Even while you're in a state of complete rest, such as when you're sleeping, your body is using energy. This energy use at rest is called your basal metabolic rate (BMR). Finally, your body uses energy to take in energy, that is, to digest and absorb food.

Factors that affect your account

If everyone were exactly the same, it would be easy to determine standard energy requirements. But, as is readily apparent, people come in all ages, shapes and sizes, and energy needs vary accordingly. Some of the main factors that influence your basal metabolic rate and your overall energy needs include the following:

Age. Children and adolescents, who are in the process of developing their bones, muscles and tissues, need more calories per pound than do adults. But as hormone levels and body composition change with age, so does a person's BMR. By the time you reach adulthood, your BMR and energy needs begin to decline, generally at a rate of 2 percent a decade.

Body size and composition. A bigger body mass requires more energy, and thus more calories, to operate than does a smaller body mass. In addition, muscle cells burn more calories than do fat cells, so the more muscle you have relative to fat, the higher your BMR. The good news is that based on this principle, you can increase your BMR and the amount of energy you burn by building up your muscle mass through regular physical activity.

Sex. Men typically have more muscle mass than do women of the same age and weight, so they generally have a higher BMR than do women.

Activity level. How much energy you need is also dependent on your activity level. The good news is that you have the ability to increase your energy needs directly through regular exercise.

The thrifty gene theory

Scientists speculate that during the evolutionary process, when food was scarce and its availability unreliable, humans developed genes that became especially good at directing energy storage within the body. When times were good and food was plentiful, the body could take in food and store it so efficiently that when times were bad and food less abundant, the body could draw on those reserves to satisfy its energy needs.

The concern today is that although humans still have great capacity to store energy for future use, food is almost never scarce in most places. So the need to draw on stored energy rarely arises. As a result, people are putting on more and more weight. In industrialized countries, this has been apparent for quite some time. But excess weight and obesity are becoming issues in developing countries as well, sometimes at a faster pace than in industrialized countries.

The World Health Organization (WHO) has declared obesity a global epidemic, reporting more than 1 billion overweight adults worldwide, with at least 300 million of them obese. The WHO attributes this global rise in individual weight to increased consumption of foods high in calories (energy-dense foods), saturated fats and sugars, and reduced physical activity. On a global scale, the energy balance account seems to be tipping heavily toward excess energy storage.

Balancing your account

The result, or physical manifestation, of your energy account balance is your body weight. If you withdraw the same amount of energy that you put in, your weight stays the same. If you withdraw more than you put in, you lose weight. If you withdraw less than you put in, you gain weight. It's all measured in the same way — through calories.

The tricky part often comes in knowing the amount of calories in each of your columns — how many calories you consume on a daily basis and how many you expend. Finding out what these figures are requires a bit of old-fashioned accounting — tallying up all of your sources of energy income and all of your energy expenditures. Comparing these numbers will enable you to assess your energy account and determine whether you come out even, under or over in the energy equation.

Calculating your caloric intake

Determining how many calories you take in throughout the course of a day can be a little time-consuming but well worth the effort. It's a good idea to do this when you start a fitness program and to reassess your intake every few months. You may be surprised at how fast the calories add up. Or you may discover that you've intuitively moderated your caloric intake so that you're getting just about the right amount. What you learn can help you make changes necessary to accomplish your fitness and nutrition goals.

First, keep an account of everything you eat and drink throughout the day, sort of like a food diary. Record what you eat and drink for each meal and the specific amount. And include all snacks and beverages between meals. Don't be tempted to leave anything out.

Next to the amount of each food item, write down your total number of servings for that item and then multiply it by the number of calories contained in one serving. You can find a comprehensive listing of different foods' caloric contents in the Department of Agriculture's National Nutrient Database on the Web. An easier and less labor-intensive way to keep track of your daily calorie intake is to find a calorie counter online, such as the National Institutes of Health's Interactive Menu Planner. (See "Additional resources" on page 344 for the Web site address.)

At the end of the day, total up your calories to see how much you've consumed. To get an accurate picture of your regular eating habits, keep the diary for four to seven days.

Calculating your caloric expenditure

The next step is to determine how many calories you expend in a day. By determining your BMR and adding in the calories you expend on daily physical activity, you can estimate your daily caloric expenditure.

Basal metabolism

You can have your BMR measured professionally at a hospital or clinic, using a method based on your oxygen consump-

tion. But you can also get an approximate measure of your basal metabolism with the following formula. Unless you're a whiz at doing math in your head, use a calculator.

Formula for women:
655 + (9.6 x weight in kilograms) + (1.8 x height in centimeters) - (4.7 x age) = BMR in kilocalories (kcal)

Formula for men:
66 + (13.7 x weight in kilograms) + (5 x height in centimeters) - (6.8 x age) = BMR in kilocalories (kcal)

To convert pounds to kilograms, divide your weight in pounds by 2.2. To convert inches to centimeters, multiply your height in inches by 2.54.

Example: Rita is a 50-year-old, 5-foot-5-inch woman who weighs 150 pounds. Using the formula for women, her BMR would be 1,372 kcal.
655 + (9.6 x 68.18) + (1.8 x 165.1) - (4.7 x 50) = 655 + 654.53 + 297.18 - 235 = 1,372 kcal

Physical activity

In addition to keeping a food diary, keep a log of physical activity. Record all of your activity including exercise, work-related activity and everyday chores. Even quiet work in the office requires a certain amount of energy.

A unit of measurement that's often used to describe the intensity of physical activity is the metabolic equivalent (MET) level. One MET is equivalent to the

MET values for select activities

Both work-related and recreational activities burn calories. Below are the MET values for various forms of physical activity. The MET values are for a person weighing about 150 pounds.

Work-related		Recreational	
Activity	**MET**	**Activity**	**MET**
Office work	1.5	Ballroom dancing	3.0-5.5
Housecleaning	3.8-4.0	Weightlifting	3.0-6.0
Child care	2.5-3.0	Brisk walking (3.5 mph)	5.6
Assembly work (standing)	3.0	Gardening	4.0
Outside construction	5.5	Jogging	7.0
Chopping wood	6.0	Bicycling	4.2-11.0
Painting	2.2-5.0	Competitive racquetball	11.6
Computer keyboarding	1.8	Canoeing	3.4-8.0
Digging trenches	9.4	Billiards	2.7
		Bowling	6.3
		Golf	5.1
		Softball	5.7
		Soccer	8.0-11.4
		Volleyball	3.4-8.0
		Tennis	7.1-9.5
		Swimming	7.9-11.0
		Yoga	4.0

amount of oxygen used by your body to sit quietly. An activity that measures 5.0 METs requires five times that amount of oxygen. The harder your body has to work to do something, the higher the MET. For example, keyboarding at your desk requires 1.8 METs and brisk walking requires 5.6 METs.

To determine the total energy cost of a physical activity, you can use the following formula (see the chart above for some common MET values):

(MET value of activity) x (weight in kilograms) x (number of hours spent on the activity) = kilocalories (kcal) expended

Take Rita, our previous example. If she walks her dog (a MET value of 3.0) for 30 minutes (0.5 hours), the total amount of calories she spends will be:

3.0 METs x 68.18 kg x 0.5 hr = 102.27 kcal

If you know your BMR, you can approximate the energy cost of an activity by substituting your weight in the above equation with your BMR in kilocalories per hour. We know Rita's BMR is around 1,372 kilocalories a day, so her kilocalories per hour (kcal/hr) would be about 57.2 (1,372 kcal/24 hr). Therefore, a more accurate estimate of the energy cost of walking her dog would be:

3.0 METs x 57.2 kcal/hr x 0.5 hr = 85.8 kcal

Total caloric expenditure

If you've calculated your BMR and the energy costs of your daily physical activities, then you're ready to estimate your total daily caloric expenditure. To see how this works, let's go back to Rita. In addition to being a dog owner, Rita has her own accounting firm where she spends approximately eight hours a day working at her desk or attending meetings. At some point during her workday, she likes to take a 15-minute walk. After work, she takes her dog for his 30-minute walk and then spends about 40 minutes fixing dinner with her husband and children. We already know her BMR is 1,372 kcal/day or 57.2 kcal/hr. Using the MET formula above, her total caloric expenditure on additional work and recreation activities would look something like this:

Working at her firm = 1.5 METs x 57.2 kcal/hr x 8 hr = 686.4 kcal

Brisk walking break = 3.8 METs x 57.2 kcal/hr x 0.25 hr = 54.34 kcal

Walking the dog = 3.0 METs x 57.2 kcal/hr x 0.50 hr = 85.8 kcal

Fixing dinner = 2.0 METs x 57.2 kcal/hr x 0.67 hr = 76.65 kcal

Total physical activity expenditure = 903.19 kcal

Now, let's take a look at the breakdown of Rita's daily caloric expenditure:

Basal metabolism (including kcal expended on digestion) = 1,372 kcal

Physical activity = 903 kcal (rounded)

Total daily expenditure = 2,275 kcal

So, on an average workday, Rita expends 2,271 calories. To meet her caloric needs, she would consume about the

The glycemic index

Currently, a hot topic in the realm of diet and nutrition is the glycemic index. You may have heard about it in connection with diabetes management or low-carb diet plans. Essentially, the glycemic index is a system for classifying carbohydrates according to the effect they have on your blood sugar levels. Carbohydrates that have a high glycemic index are ones that are easily digested by your body and cause an abrupt and often sharp increase in your blood sugar. Conversely, carbohydrates that are low on the glycemic index are digested more slowly and don't have as dramatic an effect on blood sugar.

As you might imagine, some carbohydrates that are easily absorbed — especially those that are highly processed, such as candy, cake, white bread and other products made with refined flour — are high-glycemic foods. Some vegetables, such as potatoes, also are high on the glycemic index, particularly when they've been processed into mashed potatoes or french fries. Some of this has to do with the low-fiber content of the food. Fiber helps to slow down digestion. When foods are highly processed, they're generally stripped of most of their fiber, making them available to your bloodstream soon after they're ingested.

same amount of calories. Most of us don't eat the exact same amount every day. But if you know how many calories you generally expend, it provides a reasonable goal for your average daily intake. If you consume more on one day, you can take in a little less on the next. *Note:* These calculations are somewhat involved. Use them for a day or two to get an idea of your daily total energy expenditure. Then recalculate in a few weeks after you've made changes in your diet and fitness routine, and again every few months thereafter to help you stay on track.

What foods are best to meet energy needs?

Because no single food provides all of the nutrients your body needs, eating a variety of foods ensures that you get all of the necessary nutrients and other substances associated with good health. Eating well doesn't have to be complicated. Unless you're on a special diet for a specific health problem, a good approach is to follow the recommendations contained in the Mayo Clinic Healthy Weight Pyramid (see page 228). If you're very active, you may need more calories and slightly more protein in your diet.

As mentioned previously, carbohydrates, fats and proteins are your sources of energy. How much should you have of each to enhance your well-being and physical activity levels?

Carbohydrates. Carbohydrates are your main source of energy. About 45 percent to 65 percent of your total daily calories — at least 130 grams — should come from carbohydrates. Starches — found primarily in bread, rice, pasta, cereals and vegetables — are complex carbohydrates.

Whole fruits, which consist primarily of simple sugars, still contain some fiber — not to mention plenty of vitamins and minerals — and are lower on the glycemic index than is fruit juice.

Although not everyone reacts in the same way to high- or low-glycemic foods, consuming large quantities of high-glycemic foods can cause fluctuations in blood sugar levels and has been associated with an increased risk of diabetes and cardiovascular disease. Some low-carb diets are based, at least in part, on the idea of lowering your intake of high-glycemic foods (see "Low-fat vs. low-carb diets," page 236).

Keep in mind, though, that carbohydrates are a vital nutrient and provide you with an important source of energy. Fruits, vegetables and whole-grain foods still constitute the basis of a healthy diet. And in some cases, such as an athlete competing for a long period of time, simple sugars can provide a quick energy boost when carbohydrates have been depleted by physical effort.

Sugars — found in fruits, milk and foods made with sugar, such as candy and other sweets — are called simple carbohydrates or simple sugars.

Complex carbohydrates and sugars from fruit are preferred to simple sugars from candy and sweets. Carbohydrates from foods made with whole grains are more desirable than are those found in highly processed foods, such as white bread and cake. Your body requires more time to break down complex carbohydrates — especially when encased in fiber, such as whole grains — than it does simple sugars, thus absorbing them more slowly and providing you with more

energy for a longer period of time. In addition, complex carbohydrates and fruits provide more fiber, vitamins and minerals than do sweets and most highly processed foods.

Right before an intense workout, though, avoid carbohydrates high in fiber, such as beans, lentils and bran cereals. High-fiber foods may give you gas or cause cramping. The pre-exercise meal is one time when simple carbohydrates are acceptable and even preferred.

You can also drink your carbohydrates in sports beverages and fruit juices. Research shows it makes no difference in performance whether you drink your

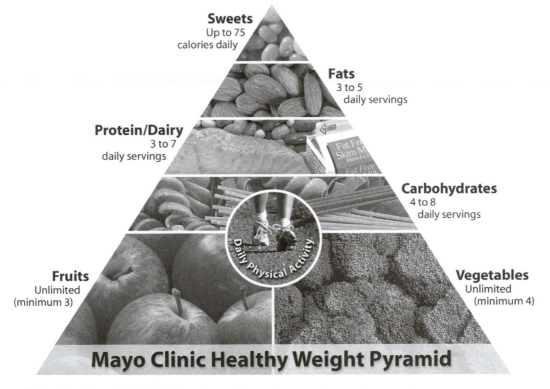

Sweets
Up to 75
calories daily

Fats
3 to 5
daily servings

Protein/Dairy
3 to 7
daily servings

Carbohydrates
4 to 8
daily servings

Daily Physical Activity

Fruits
Unlimited
(minimum 3)

Vegetables
Unlimited
(minimum 4)

Mayo Clinic Healthy Weight Pyramid

© Mayo Foundation for Medical Education and Research.
See your doctor before you begin any healthy weight plan.

Use the Mayo Clinic Healthy Weight Pyramid as a guide to help you get the proper number of servings from each food group.

Carbohydrate-loading

If you're going to be participating in high-intensity exercise for 90 minutes or more, whether for a competition or a long training session, consuming extra carbohydrates before the event might improve your performance. Depending on your level of fitness, after 90 to 120 minutes of exercise, your body may have exhausted most of its immediately available carbohydrate stores and as a result begins to use fat stores for extra fuel. Having extra carbohydrates on board will help your body use these fat stores.

Carbohydrate-loading (carbo-loading) is appropriate for activities like long-distance running and swimming, soccer, and triathlons. But it's not necessary for shorter runs — such as a 5- or 10-kilometer race — weightlifting, recreational biking and swimming. Consult your doctor or a registered dietitian before you start a carbo-loading regimen, especially if you have diabetes, because your blood sugar levels can be affected by increased carbohydrate intake.

How to do it

Carbo-loading is usually done in two steps. The first step actually involves depleting your carbohydrate stores, and the second step involves loading them back.

Step 1. About a week before the high-endurance activity, reduce your carbohydrate intake to about 40 percent to 50 percent of your total diet. Increase protein and fat intake to compensate for the decrease in carbohydrates. Continue training at your normal level. This is designed to deplete your carbohydrate stores and make room for the loading that comes next.

Step 2. Three to four days before the event, increase your carbohydrate intake to about 70 percent of the calories that you eat. Cut back on foods higher in fat to compensate for the extra carbohydrate-rich foods. That means fats should make up about 15 percent to 20 percent of your diet, and protein 10 percent to 15 percent. If you've carbo-loaded properly, expect to put on 2 to 4 pounds that week. Much of this weight is extra water because carbohydrates are stored with water in the body (*hydrate* means "water"). Thus, your lean body weight won't change.

Also gradually reduce the amount of exercise during this time so that you don't deplete your glycogen stores. Plan to rest completely for a day or two before the event. This type of taper will not result in a loss of the conditioning gains.

Cautions

Carbo-loading works best when you've been on a carbohydrate-rich diet throughout your training, because during that time your body learns to more effectively use carbohydrates. If you're unsure about how to carbo-load, talk with a registered dietitian or qualified fitness trainer before trying it.

Watch out for high-fiber foods one or two days before your event because they can sometimes cause gassy cramps, bloating and loose stools.

Even if you've loaded up on carbs for your big event, you still need to replenish them during the event to maintain your blood sugar levels, especially if you've been going for more than 60 minutes. You can replenish carbs with a piece of fruit or a carb-containing drink or gel.

Finally, experiment with carbo-loading as part of your training. That way you'll discover what works and what doesn't. If the weight gained from carbo-loading leads to a decrease in performance, you're probably better off skipping the extra carbs.

carbohydrates or eat them. However, during certain activities, like long-distance running, it's sometimes more convenient to take carbohydrates in liquid form.

Proteins. Although protein isn't your body's food of choice for fueling physical activity, it's important in muscle repair and growth. The amount of protein your body needs varies depending on your weight and the amount of exercise you do. If you perform moderate exercise three times a week, a diet containing 0.8 grams (g) of protein per kilogram (kg) of body weight typically is sufficient. For a person who weighs 150 pounds (remember, to convert pounds to kilograms, divide your weight in pounds by 2.2, which in this case equals 68.2 kg), this comes out to about 55 g of protein a day (68.2 kg x 0.8 g). To give you an idea of the protein content of food, here are some examples:

- 3 ounces lean beef = about 25 g protein
- One bagel = about 11 g protein
- One large egg = about 6 g protein
- 1 cup 2-percent milk = about 8 g protein

If you're a competitive athlete or exercise at high intensity most days of the week, increase your protein intake to 1.0 to 1.2 g/kg of body weight. Most people can easily get the protein they need from such foods as poultry, meat, dairy foods and nuts and don't need protein supplements. The number of grams of protein per serving can be found on the Nutrition Facts label of all packaged foods sold in the United States.

Fats. Fats, along with carbohydrates, provide fuel for your muscles during exercise. But they're a much more concentrated form of energy than are carbohydrates. A little goes a long way.

A good rule of thumb for determining the number of fat grams to consume in a day is to multiply your desired weight in kilograms (pounds/2.2) by 0.45.

Another way to look at it is to keep fat to within 20 percent to 35 percent of your total daily calorie intake. Try to get most of your fat from sources such as nuts, fatty fish and olive oil, which are

What about energy bars?

Energy bars, which are sometimes called nutrition bars, are popular because they're easy to carry, high in carbohydrates, and often contain protein, fat, vitamins, minerals and other supplements, although the benefit of some of these supplements is still unclear.

These bars are often expensive and high in calories, and they typically don't provide much of an advantage over regular snacks, such as fresh fruit or a whole-grain bagel. Many also contain additives that may not agree with your digestive system. Check the nutrition label before you buy any nutrition bar. Anything over 250 calories a serving is probably more than you need.

Sports gels are also high in carbohydrates and are used for energy boosts during endurance events. Unlike energy bars, sports gels come in a semiliquid consistency and are usually consumed without chewing. Some contain caffeine. These products don't contain much fluid, so plan to drink something when you consume them.

Fats aren't all the same

Although all units of fat contain the same amount of calories (1 gram fat = 9 calories), not all fats are created equal. There are several different kinds of fat — including saturated, polyunsaturated, monounsaturated and trans fat — and some types are better for your health than are others. Wisely chosen sources of fat may actually help to improve your health.

Saturated fat. When you think of "bad" fats, think saturated. Most saturated fats can increase your blood cholesterol levels and risk of heart disease. Usually solid or waxy at room temperature, saturated fat is most often found in animal products — red meat, butter, whole milk and other full-fat dairy products. Vegetable products that are high in saturated fat include coconut, palm and other tropical oils.

Trans fat. Along with saturated fat, trans fat may raise your low-density lipoprotein (LDL, or "bad") cholesterol level and lower your high-density lipoprotein (HDL, or "good") cholesterol level, thereby increasing your risk of heart disease. Trans fat — also referred to as trans-fatty acids — comes from adding hydrogen to vegetable oil through a process called hydrogenation. This makes the fat more solid and less likely to turn rancid. Hydrogenated or partially hydrogenated fat is a common ingredient in commercial baked goods, such as crackers, cookies and cakes, and in fried foods, such as doughnuts and french fries. Shortening and some margarines are high in trans fat. The Food and Drug Administration will require in 2006 that nutrition labels list the amount of trans fat contained in a product on a separate line under saturated fat, unless the total fat in the foods is minimal (less than 0.5 grams a serving). You can also look for the words *hydro-genated* or *partially hydrogenated* in the list of ingredients to see if trans fat is included. Some margarine labels state if the product has no trans-fatty acids.

Polyunsaturated fat. Usually in liquid form at room temperature and in the refrigerator, polyunsaturated fats — when used instead of saturated fats — help lower blood cholesterol levels. In addition, they may help reduce the amount of cholesterol deposits in your arteries. Foods high in polyunsaturated fats include vegetable oils such as safflower, corn, sunflower, soy and cottonseed.

One type of polyunsaturated fat — omega-3 fatty acid — may be especially beneficial to your health. Omega-3 fat appears to decrease your risk of sudden cardiac death, protect against irregular heartbeats and help reduce blood pressure levels. It may even protect against some cancers. You'll find omega-3s mainly in fish — particularly in fatty, cold-water fish, such as salmon, mackerel and herring. Additional sources are flaxseeds, soybeans and canola oil. You can get sufficient omega-3 fatty acids by consuming two to three servings of fish a week.

Monounsaturated fat. If used in place of other fats, monounsaturated fat — like polyunsaturated fat — can also lower your risk of heart disease by reducing your blood cholesterol level. In addition, monounsaturated fat, unlike polyunsaturated fat, is more resistant to oxidation — a process that leads to cell and tissue damage in your body. This type of fat is usually liquid at room temperature but may start to solidify in the refrigerator. Foods high in monounsaturated fat include olive, peanut and canola oils. Avocados and most nuts also have high amounts of monounsaturated fat.

high in unsaturated fats (see "Fats aren't all the same" on page 231). Saturated fats are the main culprits in raising your cholesterol and increasing your risk of heart disease. Limit saturated fats to less than 7 percent of your total calories. In addition, avoid eating fatty foods just before exercising. Fats remain in your stomach for a longer period of time, and may cause you to feel uncomfortable during your workout.

Alcohol. Alcohol is essentially empty calories with no nutritional value. It's best to limit alcohol consumption to a moderate amount — no more than one drink a day if you are a woman and two drinks a day if you are a man, and just one drink a day regardless of your sex if you are over age 65. One drink is defined as 12 ounces of beer, 5 ounces of wine, or 1.5 ounces of 80-proof distilled spirits.

Vitamins and minerals

Having the right balance of vitamins and minerals in your body is essential. Prolonged vitamin or mineral deficiencies can cause specific diseases or conditions, such as night blindness (vitamin A deficiency), pernicious anemia (vitamin B-12 deficiency), rickets and osteoporosis (calcium and vitamin D deficiency), and anemia (iron deficiency). But too much of some vitamins and minerals can cause toxic reactions.

You can get your entire daily requirement of vitamin C by just popping a pill. You can get the same amount by eating a large orange. So which is better? In most cases, the orange is. Whole foods — fruits, vegetables, whole grains and lean sources of protein — have three main benefits you can't find in a pill.

- Whole foods contain a variety of the nutrients your body needs — not just one. An orange, for example, provides vitamin C but also beta carotene, calcium and other nutrients. A vitamin C supplement lacks these other nutrients.
- Whole foods often provide dietary fiber, which is important for digestion.

- Whole foods contain other substances that may be important for good health. Fruits and vegetables, for example, contain naturally occurring food substances called phytochemicals, which may help protect you against cancer, heart disease, osteoporosis and diabetes. Although it's not yet known precisely what role phytochemicals play in nutrition, research shows many health benefits from eating more fruits, vegetables and grains. If you depend on supplements rather than eating a variety of whole foods, you miss the potential benefits of phytochemicals. In addition, there are other potential nutrients in whole foods that are still unknown and therefore can't be put into a supplement.

In some cases, a vitamin or mineral supplement may be appropriate to help your body get what it needs, for example, if your body can't absorb nutrients very well, if you're on a special diet or if you're pregnant. Consult your doctor before taking a vitamin or mineral supplement.

HYDRATION

Sometimes the focus of fitness is so much on food and eating that there's a tendency to forget about fluids. But water is one of the most important factors in a healthy body. At least half of your body weight is made up of water. Water makes up more than 75 percent of your brain, about 80 percent of your blood and about 70 percent of your lean muscle. Water also helps to:

- Regulate your body temperature
- Remove wastes
- Carry nutrients and oxygen to cells
- Cushion your joints
- Improve digestion
- Keep your kidney and liver from being overloaded with toxins
- Enhance your body's absorption of vitamins, minerals and other nutrients

Lack of water can lead to dehydration. Even mild dehydration of as little as a 1 percent to 2 percent loss of your body weight can sap your energy and make you lethargic. For example, if you weigh 150 pounds, losing 1.5 to 3 pounds after working out should be a sign that you need to replace lost fluid even if you're not thirsty. Dehydration poses a particular risk for the very young and the very old.

How much should you drink?

Your body loses fluid every day through sweating, exhaling, urinating and bowel movements. Your body can't produce water on its own, so you have to replace what you lose. A panel of advisers from the Institute of Medicine of the National Academies recently advocated allowing thirst to be your guide because most people seem to get adequate hydration by following this rule of thumb and by fluids they consume at mealtimes. While this may be a good general guideline, it may not be adequate to replace fluid after exercise.

Although drinking pure water is often the best way to replace lost fluids, you can also get water from other sources, such as milk, fruit juices, sports drinks, fruit and soup. Some beverages aren't good substitutes for water. Sodas contain sugars that can promote weight gain and tooth decay. Caffeinated beverages increase your excretion of urine and may actually reduce the amount of fluids in your body. Alcohol is also dehydrating and can impair physical performance and mental functioning. If you choose to drink alcohol after exercising, rehydrate with water first.

Hot and humid weather conditions that make you perspire increase your need to replace lost fluids. Cold weather and high altitudes also can increase your fluid requirement because the air you breathe contains less moisture than does warmer air that's closer to sea level. Cold air needs to be warmed and humidified on its way through your respiratory tract, leading to additional fluid loss. Along similar lines, having an illness — particularly if you have a fever or trouble breathing — increases your fluid requirements. Medications, such as diuretics, also may affect your fluid balance.

To help determine if you're getting enough water in your day, a ballpark measure is to look at the color of your urine. If your urine is pale yellow, you're probably drinking enough fluids. If your urine is dark yellow and has a strong odor, or if you urinate less than four times a day, you probably need to increase your fluid intake. Keep in mind, however, that multivitamins and medications can alter the color of your urine, so ask your doctor what to expect.

Another way to measure fluid loss or gain is to weigh yourself at the beginning and end of the day, or before and after exercising. The difference in weight is fluid you've either lost or gained. Older adults often have less of a sense of thirst than do younger people and may not be aware that they need to replace fluids. By weighing yourself, you can tell whether you've lost fluid and whether you need to drink more throughout the day to avoid dehydration. Other signs of inadequate fluid intake may include thirst, dry mouth and constipation. More serious signs and symptoms that you may not be getting enough fluids include fatigue, loss of coordination, mental confusion, irritability, dry skin, elevated body temperature and reduced urine output. For details about recognizing and treating heat-related illness, see Chapter 6.

Energy and sport drinks

These days, there seems to be an endless supply of energy and sports drinks from which to choose, all in a wide array of colors, from delicate blue to violent purple. Take your pick. But are these drinks better for you than water? Not necessarily. Water is a great way to replace lost fluids, and it's inexpensive. Some energy and sports drinks may be useful in certain circumstances, and others may actually be harmful. Here's a brief breakdown from the American College of Sports Medicine.

- **Energy drinks.** These drinks usually contain large amounts of carbohydrates and caffeine. Carbohydrates can boost energy, but too much caffeine, a stimulant, can have adverse side effects, especially if you're also on medications that contain other stimulants. Caffeine can make your heart beat faster, increase your blood pressure, interrupt sleep and cause nervousness and irritability. In addition, caffeine tends to act as a diuretic and can cause fluid loss rather than fluid replacement — not a good choice when you want to replace fluids.
- **Sports drinks.** These usually contain carbohydrates and electrolytes, which can enhance energy and replace minerals lost in sweat. Sports drinks can be useful if you've been exercising for longer than an hour and need to replace carbs and sodium. Some people find sports drinks easier to consume than just water.
- **Fitness water.** This is water enhanced with some vitamins, minerals, carbohydrates, flavoring and sometimes caffeine. The added value of any nutrients contained in these drinks is negligible in the amounts supplied. And the negative effects of caffeine should be considered before choosing a fitness water drink. However, if these drinks help you stay hydrated, then they can be useful.

Staying hydrated while exercising

Exercising or engaging in any physical activity that causes you to perspire increases your water requirement. Be sure to drink at least 1 cup of fluid before and after exercising and every 10 to 15 minutes during your workout. Water is all you need if you're exercising for an hour or less. If you're working out for longer than an hour, have some fruit juice or a sports drink handy to replace carbohydrates and electrolytes. Drinking frequent, small amounts is better than drinking large amounts all at once.

Rarely, endurance athletes consume too much water and dilute their bodies' sodium — a vital electrolyte that helps the body use water to stay hydrated. This can lead to a potentially life-threatening metabolic imbalance (hyponatremia). Signs and symptoms include bloating, nausea, incoherence, confusion, collapse and convulsions. Although this condition is rare, try to drink fluids that contain sodium and potassium — sports drinks, tomato-based drinks, clear broth — in addition to water, if you're running a marathon or performing in a triathlon or other prolonged competition.

WHEN WEIGHT LOSS IS YOUR GOAL

To lose weight, the amount of calories you consume must be less than the amount of calories you burn. This often sounds simpler in theory than in practice, but it's important to grasp this concept mentally so that you can apply it to your daily habits. If you're gaining weight, you're eating too much, exercising too little or both.

When you decide you want to lose weight, it's often tempting to pursue a diet trend that promises rapid weight loss. And why not? Who wouldn't rather shed all their extra pounds at once rather than over months or even years? But the truth is that wide swings in weight over a short time generally reflect changes in body fluids rather than actual gain or loss of body fat. When you discontinue the diet and return to your regular eating habits, you often regain the weight you lost and perhaps even add a few more pounds.

To lose weight and keep it off, it's important to change your daily eating and physical activity patterns in order to create a more healthy lifestyle. This is the difficult part. Humans are creatures of habit, and changing habits requires time and determination. But it's not impossible, and long-term loss of excess weight definitely has its rewards, such as making you feel better, giving you more energy and reducing your risk of disease. It's likely you'll have setbacks — giving up unhealthy eating habits can be almost as hard as stopping smoking. Don't let it get you down. Start each day fresh and remember that you're making lifelong changes — take the time to do it right.

The rate at which you lose weight will depend on your age, height, sex and activity level. A reasonable weight loss goal is an average of 1 to 2 pounds a week or 4 to 8 pounds a month.

Healthy eating habits

Losing weight goes deeper than just deciding to eat less. You also need to identify behaviors or habits that influence the kinds and amounts of foods you eat. This, in turn, can help you determine your motivations for eating and help you change problem eating habits.

Following are some tips to help you establish healthy eating habits. You may also wish to consult a registered dietitian before you start on a weight loss program. A dietitian can help you develop realistic weight loss goals and an eating plan that will help you accomplish those goals. A dietitian can also help you determine what is the best weight for your age, sex and body type.

Low-fat vs. low-carb diets

For a long time, diets low in fat were promoted as the best way to lose weight. But many food products that were touted as being low fat or reduced fat actually contained just as many, or more, calories as the original product did. Even though the calories coming from fat were fewer, calories from carbohydrates and sugar used to enhance flavor were increased. So even though people were consuming less fat, they were still consuming just as many calories. And sometimes they were consuming more calories because they had the idea that you could eat more of a product simply because it was low in fat.

The trend today is toward diets low in carbohydrates. The theory is that carbohydrates raise blood sugar levels, which then trigger insulin production. Insulin drives blood sugar into the cells and prevents fat breakdown in the body, making it harder to burn excess fat and lose weight.

Proponents of low-carbohydrate diets take this one step further. They say that if carbohydrates raise blood sugar and insulin levels and cause weight gain, a decrease in carbs will result in lower blood sugar and insulin levels, leading to weight loss. And because you're not eating the carbs, your body breaks down fat to provide needed energy.

Many people do lose weight on low-carb diets, but the weight loss probably isn't primarily due to increased blood sugar and insulin levels. It's more likely the result of eating fewer total calories, whether they're from carbohydrates, fats or proteins. In addition, much of the initial weight loss with low-carb diets occurs due to loss of water.

The thing about cutting down too much on any particular nutrient is that you may miss out on the benefits of that nutrient. For example, certain fats, such as polyunsaturated and monounsaturated fats, are good for your health when consumed in moderation (see "Fats aren't all the same," page 231). And nutrition experts are finding out more and more about the nature of carbohydrates and how they can affect body weight. Replacing highly processed and refined foods rich in sugar with whole-grain foods rich in complex carbohydrates and fiber is better for your overall health as well.

In terms of weight loss, your body can't violate the laws of thermodynamics. Excess calories, regardless of where they come from, will eventually be stored as fat. Your best bet is to cut calories while maintaining a varied, nutritionally balanced diet. This way you lose the weight but keep the nutrients, vitamins and minerals you need.

Keep a food diary. As mentioned earlier in this chapter, keeping a food diary can be enlightening in terms of showing how many calories you actually consume in a day. Most people tend to underestimate the amount they eat each day. For four to seven days, including a weekend, record what you eat, where you eat it (in front of the television, in bed, and so on), what prompts the eating, how it's prepared and the portion size. Then you'll have a detailed picture of your calorie intake as well as your motivations for eating.

Avoid large portions. By avoiding excessively large portions of certain foods, you're able to eat a wider variety of foods during a meal. Eating a variety of foods will ensure that you get all of the energy, protein, vitamins, minerals and fiber you need. To help reduce food portions:

- Serve food on plates instead of putting serving bowls on the table.
- Serve main dishes on a smaller plate.
- Ask for a take-home container when eating out. Save part of the meal for another time.
- Ignore the urge to clean your plate.

Did you know?

One pound of fat equals 3,500 calories. To lose a pound of fat in a week, you must reduce your calorie intake by 3,500 calories, exercise more to burn 3,500 calories, or do a combination of both to equal 3,5000 calories. Exercising can ensure that the calories you take in help increase your muscle mass rather than your fat reserves.

- Eat larger portions of fresh and frozen fruits and vegetables.

Eat low-energy-dense foods. If it's hard for you to limit yourself to small portions, try to eat foods that contain fewer calories in a given amount, that is, those that are less calorie dense. The higher the energy density of a food, the more likely it is to cause weight gain because even small amounts add up. Low-energy-dense foods, such as most vegetables, fruits and, to a lesser extent, whole grains, contain a small amount of calories in a large volume. This means you can eat a greater amount of low-energy-dense foods than you could of high-energy-dense foods without gaining weight. Examples of high-energy-dense foods include crackers, candy, dried fruit and fruit juices.

Avoid drastic reduction of calories. Drastically reducing your daily calorie intake can cause you to lose weight, but it's difficult to keep up for long periods of time. Nutrition experts recommend reducing your caloric intake by no more than 500 to 1,000 calories a day. This can lead to a weight loss of 1 to 2 pounds a week.

Avoid excessive hunger. Always try to eat three meals a day. Skipping meals — especially breakfast — slows your metabolism and may lead to excessive snacking or overeating at the next meal. To control between-meal hunger, include healthy snacks — such as baby carrots, an apple or an orange — as part of your overall eating plan. Prepare them ahead of time and take them with you so that you won't be tempted by a vending machine.

Supplements and ergogenic aids

Most active people want to be better at what they do, to reach that next level of proficiency and satisfaction. This is especially true when it comes to athletes, and there's no shortage of pills, drinks and powders that promise to provide that boost. These days, even weekend athletes and nonathletes are using supplements and ergogenic aids — substances touted to increase energy output, add muscle mass and decrease fatigue. And adults aren't the only ones interested. Teens involved in school sports are also using ergogenic aids. Studies suggest that 5 percent to 11 percent of high school age boys and 0.5 percent to 2.5 percent of high school age girls have tried anabolic steroids.

Ergogenic aid	What is it?
Creatine	■ Synthetic version of body compound that helps replenish energy (ATP) in your muscles.
Androstenedione (Legal dietary supplement, but banned by many official sports organizations, including the International Olympic Committee.)	■ Synthetic version of hormone produced by the adrenal glands, ovaries and testes; a precursor hormone that's normally converted to testosterone and estradiol in both men and women.
Anabolic steroids (Anadrol, Deca-Durabolin, others) (Illegal to possess or distribute without a prescription.)	■ Synthetic version of testosterone.
Dehydroepiandrosterone (DHEA)	■ Sold as an alternative to anabolic steroids but is still an androgenic steroid and is banned by several sports organizations.

So are these substances effective and safe? Most health and nutrition experts say they're not necessary because you can obtain all of your nutrients from whole foods, unless you're on a special diet. Some substances are illegal or restricted in competition. Most haven't been studied extensively and aren't well-regulated. And even though many are described as natural, this doesn't mean they're safe. Ergogenic aids should be considered with caution and not without the advice of your doctor or a registered dietitian. Following is a list of some of the more common aids in use:

What does it do?	Issues to consider
■ Scientific research indicates creatine can produce small gains in short-term bursts of power and increase muscle mass.	■ The only documented side effect in healthy adults is weight gain; its long-term effects are unknown; effect on performance not consistent. ■ May increase risk of dehydration and related side effects, including cramps. ■ Some studies have shown no benefit. ■ Not effective for endurance performance. ■ Creatine is legal but banned by some sports organizations.
■ Claimed to increase testosterone levels, which proponents say allows athletes to train harder and recover more quickly. ■ Advocates also claim it increases muscle mass.	■ No published safety data. ■ Emerging studies show that supplemental androstenedione doesn't increase testosterone or strengthen muscles. ■ Decreases high-density lipoprotein (HDL, or "good") cholesterol in men and women.
■ Increases muscle mass and strength.	■ In men causes diminished sperm production, male-pattern baldness, shrunken testicles and enlarged breasts. ■ In women causes deepening voice, facial hair, menstrual irregularities and decreased breast tissue. ■ Both men and women may experience increased low-density lipoprotein (LDL, or "bad") cholesterol and decreased HDL cholesterol, liver abnormalities, aggressiveness, hyperactivity, irritability, acne and depression (when use is discontinued).
■ Data are sparse with respect to effectiveness and side effects.	

Ergogenic aid	What is it?
Stimulants	■ Common stimulants include caffeine and amphetamines. ■ Cold remedies often contain the stimulants ephedrine, pseudoephedrine hydrochloride and phenylpropanolamine. ■ Ephedra (ma-huang), an herb that has long been used in Chinese medicine, contains the alkaloids ephedrine and pseudoephedrine. Sale of ephedra-containing products is banned in the United States because of possible lethal side effects.
Chromium	■ Essential dietary mineral that helps break down carbohydrates, proteins and fats.
Glucosamine and chondroitin sulfate	■ Glucosamine is an amino sugar that plays a major role in cartilage maintenance and repair. ■ Chondroitin sulfate, which consists of glucosamine and sugar molecules, is also present in cartilage.
Glutamine	■ The most abundant amino acid in human plasma and muscle. ■ Vital to the production of proteins and urea, and a transporter of nitrogen.
Carnitine	■ A body compound made up of the amino acids lysine and methionine.

What does it do?	Issues to consider
■ Stimulates the central nervous system, increasing your heart rate, blood pressure, body temperature and metabolism. ■ Can reduce fatigue, suppress appetite and increase alertness and aggressiveness. ■ Caffeine can increase free fatty acids and enhance performance in endurance activities. ■ Proponents of ephedra claim it can stimulate weight loss.	■ Although stimulants such as caffeine are relatively safe, they may have side effects that affect performance, including nervousness, irritability and insomnia. ■ Other side effects of high caffeine consumption include nausea, muscle tremors, palpitations and headache. ■ There's no evidence that ephedra improves performance; taking ephedrine may cause heart attack, stroke, seizure or death; combining ephedrine and caffeine can greatly increase side effects.
■ Proponents claim chromium supplements can help burn fat and build muscle.	■ Studies supporting chromium supplement advantages have been criticized for methodology; most studies have found chromium to have little or no beneficial effect. ■ Most people, including athletes, can get the chromium they need from whole foods such as whole grains, nuts, asparagus, cheese and mushrooms.
■ Proponents claim glucosamine and chondroitin sulfate may reduce the pain of osteoarthritis and may help rebuild cartilage.	■ Several studies have reported modest reduction in symptoms in people with osteoarthritis. ■ Long-term effects are unknown. ■ No solid proof of cartilage-building properties.
■ Naturally occurring glutamine increases immune function and is critical during times of metabolic stress and illness. ■ Proponents of glutamine for athletes claim it prevents overtraining syndrome.	■ Preliminary data suggest glutamine supplements may decrease the rate of infections in athletes, but further research is necessary to confirm the results. ■ The benefits of glutamine for athletes during periods of intense training aren't well-established.
■ Proponents claim carnitine supplements promote the use of fatty acids as fuel, decrease body fat and increase endurance.	■ Studies haven't proved these claims as of yet. ■ Carnitine is found in animal foods and isn't typically necessary in supplement form. ■ The L-carnitine version appears to be safe, but D-carnitine may be toxic. There's concern that some L-carnitine supplements may be contaminated with D-carnitine, which can lead to harmful side effects.

Get active

Limiting calories can help you lose weight. But, as you read in Chapters 1 and 3, adding moderately intense exercise most days of the week can increase your rate of weight loss. Even more important, regular exercise helps you keep the weight off.

The goal of exercise for weight loss is to burn more calories. How many calories you burn depends on the frequency, duration and intensity of your activities. For many people it's easier to maintain a routine of longer duration, lower intensity aerobic exercises. The minimum recommendation for weight loss is 30 minutes of moderate activity at least five days a week. If you can do more, that's even better. One of the best ways to lose body fat is through steady aerobic exercise — such as walking — for 30 to 60 minutes most days of the week. (See Chapter 3 for more on aerobic exercise.)

Strength training exercises, such as weight training, also are important because they help counteract muscle loss associated with aging. And because muscle tissue burns more calories, muscle mass is a key factor in helping maintain a healthy weight. The more lean muscle mass you preserve, the bigger "engine" you'll have with which to burn more calories.

Even though regularly scheduled aerobic exercise is best for losing fat, any extra movement helps burn calories. Lifestyle activities may be easier to incorporate into your day. Think about ways you could increase your physical activity throughout the day. For example, use the stairs instead of the elevator, or park at the far end of the lot. Stair climbing, walking, gardening, lawn mowing and even doing housework all burn calories.

WHEN YOUR GOAL IS WEIGHT GAIN

If you would like to bulk up, you need to tip the scales in the other direction by consuming more calories than you burn. But this doesn't mean eating anything and everything. To put on healthy weight and be fit, you need to eat well and exercise so that the extra calories contribute to your muscle mass rather than turn to fat. Changes in weight and body shape take time, whether you're trying to gain or lose. Progress includes more than just pounds.

Eat a well-balanced diet that includes whole grains, vegetables, fruits, low-fat dairy and lean protein sources, such as fish, poultry, meats, beans and legumes. And, although increasing your intake of fats and sweets may help you gain weight, be sure to keep such foods in proportion with healthier foods.

Eating three meals a day plus between-meal snacks on a regular basis helps ensure the balance and variety you need to gain weight. In addition, try to eat high-energy-dense foods, such as dried fruit, nuts, and olive and canola oils. You don't necessarily need sports supplements, such as protein and energy shakes and herbal supplements. While these can sometimes be helpful, wholesome food is the preferred fuel for building muscle.

Strength training will help increase lean muscle mass, and increased lean muscle will add weight. Develop a program of exercises that includes all of the major muscle groups in your upper and lower body and trunk. Proper technique is key. Select a weight that tires your muscles at about 15 to 20 repetitions when first starting. As you progress, your goal should be 8 to 12 repetitions. One set two or three times a week may be all you need, although if muscle mass gain is your goal, you may want to progress to multiple sets. Avoid working the same muscle group on consecutive days. (For more on strength training, see Chapter 3.)

FROM FOOD TO FITNESS

Just as you select exercises to help you reach your fitness goals, you also choose foods that help you achieve fitness. Whether your goal is to lose a few pounds and be able to take a brisk walk, or to run a 10-kilometer race, what you eat will play a key role in the outcome. Try to get a good mix of healthy foods in your diet — complex carbohydrates such as whole-grain pastas and breads, lean sources of protein, and plenty of fresh fruits and vegetables. As with exercise, planning a healthy diet may take extra time in the beginning. But once you've established good eating habits, the dividends will last a lifetime.

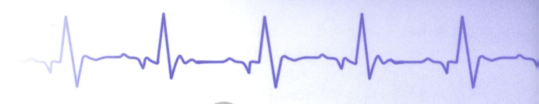

Exercise & medical conditions

CHAPTER 8

It used to be that if you had a medical condition or were pregnant, you were told to take it easy and rest as much as possible. Adequate rest does play an important part in managing ongoing medical conditions, but sometimes too much rest can be detrimental. In fact, research shows that physical activity actually improves the health of many people with medical conditions.

Chronic conditions such as cardiovascular disease, arthritis and diabetes usually can't be cured. But often they can be managed with medications and healthy lifestyle choices, including physical activity. For many people with such medical conditions, regular attention to health is required to maintain quality of life. An appropriate level of physical activity combined with proper nutrition can go a long way toward helping you feel and perform your best, in spite of a medical condition.

If you have a chronic medical condition, you may feel that increasing your physical activity is the last item on your list of things to do. But you might be surprised at the tangible benefits that such activity can bring you. For one thing, physical activity offers many of the same benefits to people with chronic illnesses as it does to people without them. But for a person with added aches and pains, physical

Measuring the intensity of your activity

Physical activity is typically described as light, moderate or vigorous.

Recommendations for activity intensity are often made in terms of how much energy must be expended, such as 50 percent to 80 percent of your maximum heart rate, or 3 to 6 metabolic equivalents (METs). For most people, these methods provide a good indication of effort. But measurements are based on healthy adults and may not be appropriate for someone who has a physical limitation.

Ratings of perceived exertion

Another way of measuring the intensity of your exercise is by rating the total amount of effort, physical stress and fatigue you perceive during an activity. This may be done by using the Borg ratings of perceived exertion (RPE) scale and reflects your individual fitness level. For more information on the Borg scale, see page 71.

The Borg method is appropriate for measuring activity intensity in people who have an irregular heart rhythm or whose heart rate is affected by medication and for whom heart rate measurements may not be reliable. If you have significant cardiovascular or pulmonary concerns, ask your doctor about using this method. He or she may have you take an exercise test that will help you adjust your efforts and use the scale more effectively. This typically applies to aerobic activity, but may also be applied to strength training (anaerobic activity).

Talk test

Another easy way to help you regulate your exercise intensity is to carry on a conversation — but not sing a song — while exercising. If you're too winded to talk, you're probably pushing too hard and should slow your pace.

activity may actually offer even more value. Here are a few examples:

- Improved heart and lung function
- Decreased blood pressure and cholesterol levels
- Increased energy, muscular strength and endurance
- Increased independence and ability to perform activities of daily living
- Better body composition and weight control
- Increased disease-fighting immune cell activity
- Improved pain control
- Fewer medical complications
- Reduced anxiety and depression
- Improved self-esteem
- Greater sense of control
- Better general quality of life

The activities you pursue may depend on your particular physical limitations, but many options are available. Regardless of your condition, you'll likely be able to engage in some form of physical activity. It's just a matter of modifying the activity to meet your individual needs. In this chapter, you'll find out what can work for you.

THE IMPORTANCE OF SEEING YOUR DOCTOR

If you have a medical condition, it's essential that you talk with your doctor before increasing your level of physical activity, whether through a formal exercise program or on your own. Your doctor can help you

determine the level of intensity, frequency and duration with which you should perform specific physical activities. He or she may recommend a graded exercise test to determine your current level of fitness and help you determine your training heart rate and intensity goal using the Borg scale, or by using other methods. Your doctor may also be able to tell you what benefits you can expect from a specific activity based on your condition. Such a consultation with your doctor and perhaps other health care professionals will result in an individualized fitness program that's right for you.

If you're taking medications, ask your doctor how they may affect your exercise plan. Drugs for diabetes, high blood pressure and heart disease, as well as sedatives, antihistamines and cold medications, can cause side effects such as dehydration, impaired balance and blurred vision. In addition, some medications can affect the way your body reacts to exercise. Your doctor may be able to adjust your medications in order to minimize problems during exercise.

A doctor who specializes in physical medicine and rehabilitation physiatry may be especially suited to address your needs. Certain situations — such as following a heart attack or a stroke, or if you have severe osteoporosis — may require that you exercise under medical supervision. This might entail participation in physical therapy or a supervised rehabilitation program.

After you begin exercising, continue to have your doctor evaluate your physical fitness program or activity on a regular basis. This can help ensure that you don't make your condition worse by pushing yourself too hard or by doing specific exercises improperly.

Finally, remember to tailor your routine toward your specific physical needs at any given time. Sometimes you can be more active, but other times you may need to take it easy. For example, if you're being treated for cancer, you may need to focus on resting and recuperating immediately after a chemotherapy session. As you rebuild your energy, you'll be able to tolerate more strenuous activity.

In addition, if you're a smoker, take steps to stop. Smoking complicates any medical condition and makes exercising more difficult. If you smoke, talk with your doctor about starting a smoking cessation plan.

TIPS AND PRECAUTIONS

Physical activity is almost always an option, no matter what medical condition you face. But a condition may affect two people differently. One person may benefit from aerobic exercise, another from strength training. In addition, different conditions impose different limitations.

This chapter has tips and precautions for various chronic illnesses. Under each condition, different types of activity and training are mentioned. (To find out more about a specific exercise, go to the "Exercise guide," beginning on page 134.) If you don't see your particular condition here, talk to your doctor. He or she will be able to point you in the right direction to find out more about how to integrate physical activity into your life.

Key points to remember

As you increase your physical activity, remember these key points:

- **Start out slowly.** Begin at a comfortable pace and gradually increase the duration of your activity, for example, by adding a couple of minutes each week. Don't go for dramatic increases in strength or endurance over a short time. This can increase the risk of burnout or injury.
- **Warm up.** If you have a chronic illness, warming up before you begin an activity is especially important. Warm up slowly by starting your activity at a very low intensity. Gradually increase the intensity until you're at your target level for the day.
- **Cool down.** At the end of your activity, take the time to cool down. This can consist of light activity and some flexibility exercises. Cooling down will help prevent your muscles from becoming too sore and give you time to get your heart rate back to normal.
- **Have fun.** Choose an activity that you enjoy. If you like what you're doing, you're much more likely to continue doing it than if you consider it a chore.

Medications and their potential effect on exercise

Some medications may have an effect on your exercise capacity. This effect can be beneficial and help to increase your ability to move. However, some medications may have a negative effect. Be sure to tell the person who's helping to develop your exercise plan what medications you're taking so that your plan can be tailored accordingly.

Medication	Effect on exercise
Beta blockers, nitrates and calcium channel blockers	Increase exercise capacity if you have received a diagnosis of chest pain (angina) or congestive heart failure. Calcium channel blockers may cause low blood pressure after exercise. To avoid this, make sure you include an extended cool-down period in your exercise program. *Note:* Beta blockers and some calcium channel blockers decrease your heart rate, so the standard formula for calculating target heart rate (see page 42) doesn't apply. In such cases, an exercise stress test is needed to determine your target heart rate.
Diuretics	Generally leave exercise capacity unchanged, but may improve it if you have congestive heart failure because these drugs can decrease fluid in the lungs and around the heart. Carefully monitor fluid and electrolyte replacement to avoid dehydration.
Vasodilators	Generally leave exercise capacity unchanged, but may improve it if you have congestive heart failure. Vasodilators may cause low blood pressure following exercise. This effect can be prevented with an extended cool-down period.
Anti-arrhythmic drugs	Generally leave exercise capacity unchanged. Anti-arrhythmics in general may cause new or worsened arrhythmias during vigorous exercise. If you're taking an anti-arrhythmic drug, exercise only under the guidance of your doctor.
Bronchodilators	Increase exercise capacity if you have asthma and have difficulty breathing (bronchospasm). Some bronchodilators may improve performance in people with chronic obstructive pulmonary disease.

Medication	Effect on exercise
Cholesterol-lowering drugs	Some of these drugs, for example, HMG-CoA reductase inhibitors, may contribute to muscle damage during exertion. If you develop severe muscle pain during or after exercise, see your doctor.
Drugs to prevent blood clots (anti-thrombosis drugs)	May improve walking performance in people with claudication due to peripheral arterial disease. May increase risk of bruising or bleeding with trauma.
Drugs for diabetes	May alter your blood sugar levels (glycemic response) during exercise. Be sure to check your blood sugar levels before and after exercising (see page 266).
Drugs for osteoporosis	Allow you to place more stress on your bones while reducing risk of fracture. Exercise combined with bisphosphonates may help increase bone density more than just exercise or bisphosphonates alone. When taking bisphosphonates orally, be sure to drink plenty of water and avoid exercise for one hour afterward.
Anti-cancer drugs	Drugs used in chemotherapy can cause excessive fatigue, anemia or gout, decreasing exercise capacity. Some anti-cancer drugs, such as anthracyclines and mitoxantrone, can damage or enlarge the heart muscle, a condition called cardiomyopathy.
Antidepressant drugs	Tricyclic antidepressants may cause an elevated heart rate and an increased risk of dehydration. Tranylcypromine, a monoamine oxidase inhibitor (MAOI), can cause increased blood pressure. Anti-anxiety medications and sedatives, such as phenobarbital and diazepam, should be used with extreme caution when exercising due to the risk of serious, potentially lethal, side effects.
Stimulants	Stimulants such as amphetamines and methylphenidate (Ritalin) should be used with extreme caution while exercising, and only under a doctor's supervision. Ephedra is a dietary supplement that has also been used as a stimulant. Its sale is banned in the United States. Don't assume that products marketed as substitutes for ephedra are safe.

Danger signs during exercise

If you develop any of the following warning signs or symptoms, stop whatever physical activity you're doing. If any of these signs or symptoms persist or become worse, seek medical attention immediately. Even if they go away, tell your doctor or the supervisor of your exercise program before resuming any physical activity. Danger signs and symptoms include:

- Severe shortness of breath, that is, you can't talk or carry on a conversation
- Pain, pressure or aching in the chest, arms, jaw, neck, shoulders or back
- Extreme fatigue more than an hour after exercising
- Lightheadedness or dizziness
- Very rapid or very slow heart rate
- Distinct joint or muscle pain

Cardiovascular disease

If you have cardiovascular disease, regular exercise can help prevent a heart attack by reducing pressure on damaged arteries and reducing buildup of cholesterol-containing deposits (plaques). Daily physical activity can reduce your low-density lipoprotein (LDL) cholesterol level, or "bad" cholesterol, and increase your high-density lipoprotein (HDL) cholesterol level, or "good" cholesterol. Physical activity also helps combat other risk factors for coronary artery disease, such as obesity and high blood pressure.

If you've had a heart attack, regular physical activity can help reduce the risk of a second heart attack. Studies show that participation in an exercise program after a heart attack results in a 20 percent to 25 percent reduction in total and cardiovascular-related deaths. Some people worry that they'll have a heart attack during exercise. The chances of that happening during light to moderate physical activity are very small. If you participate in a cardiac rehabilitation program — you

may be enrolled in one by your doctor if you've had a heart attack or other cardiovascular problem — you'll be monitored for signs of danger. In the rare case that something does happen, you'll receive immediate attention.

Any aerobic activity is likely to be of benefit if you have a heart condition. Your goal is to maintain or gradually increase the strength and endurance of your heart and other muscles. By following a consistent schedule of aerobic activity, you can recondition your heart and circulatory system so that they'll work more efficiently. To minimize your health risks and maximize your benefits, consider the following tips:

- Moderate walking on a level surface or riding a stationary bicycle with low resistance may be the only exercise you need at first. This will improve your fitness level without significant danger to your heart. Your doctor may suggest other activities.
- Start and finish your workouts slowly, with warm-up and cool-down periods

of at least 10 minutes each. Abruptly starting or stopping a workout may lead to heart irritability and arrhythmia.

- Remember to keep your exercise light to moderate in intensity, especially at first. Never exercise to the point of chest pain, labored breathing or extreme fatigue.
- At least initially, avoid competing in athletics, where you may be tempted to go all out in order to win a game or a match.
- If your doctor has prescribed nitroglycerin for you, take it with you during workouts in case of an emergency.
- For an added measure of safety, exercise with a partner. If you do exercise alone, carry a cell phone or pager with you in case of an emergency.

Peripheral vascular disease

Peripheral vascular disease (PVD) is a disorder in which blood vessels in the lower extremities become blocked by cholesterol-containing plaques, thus reducing blood flow. This condition typically causes pain in the calves, thighs or buttocks while walking — a symptom called claudication — that sometimes can be relieved by a few minutes of rest. In severe cases, people with PVD may have pain even at rest, at which point PVD is called critical ischemia (is-KE-me-uh). Claudication and critical ischemia can impair your ability to walk and affect your daily physical activities. Moreover, these conditions are associated with an increased risk of cardiovascular disease, heart attack and stroke.

If you have PVD, you'll want a thorough medical exam before beginning an exercise program. Aerobic exercise can help control risk factors and may increase the distance that you can walk without pain. As with cardiovascular disease, many aerobic activities may be of benefit. People with PVD may begin with low-intensity walking on a treadmill.

Use pain as your guide when exercising with PVD. You may continue walking after initial mild discomfort. However, if the discomfort continues to increase, you should stop. If the pain remains stable and you can tolerate it, you may continue walking. In some people, the pain subsides as they continue walking.

Exercising at least three times a week has been shown to increase the distance that people with PVD can walk without pain, leading to overall improvement in physical conditioning and quality of life.

People with PVD are prone to skin problems, including foot ulcers. For this reason, appropriate foot care and good walking shoes are essential. For more information, see "Anatomy of an athletic shoe" on page 127 and "What shoes are best for walking" on page 129.

High blood pressure

High blood pressure (hypertension), defined as a systolic pressure of 140 millimeters of mercury (mm Hg) or higher, or a diastolic pressure of 90 mm Hg or higher, is a major risk factor for cardiovascular disease and stroke. But you can lower your blood pressure through regular moderately intense exercise. Blood pressure classifications are detailed on page 7.

If you're at risk of developing high blood pressure — for example, you have a family history of the condition — being physically active can have a protective effect. If you already have high blood pressure, regular exercise may be enough to prevent you from having to take medication. If you're taking medication, exercising may help make your medication work more effectively, and may also reduce the dose that you need.

To lower your blood pressure, you don't need to engage in high-intensity activity. Moderate-intensity activity appears to lower blood pressure just as much as, and perhaps more than, high-intensity activity. In general, consistency is more important than intensity. Your goal should be to get 30 to 60 minutes of moderately intense activity most if not all days of the week. You might start out with 10 to 15 minutes and gradually increase the duration of your activity over four to eight weeks to reach your goal. It takes approximately one to three months for regular exercise to have a stabilizing effect on blood pressure, and the benefits last only as long as you continue to exercise.

Although strength training can be beneficial when it's incorporated into an overall fitness program that includes plenty of aerobic activity, it's generally not very effective in lowering blood pressure and may temporarily raise your blood pressure if you exert yourself too much. This doesn't necessarily exclude you from

obtaining the many benefits of strength training, but you need to take appropriate precautions. For example, when performing strength training exercises, don't hold your breath because doing so can cause your blood pressure to fluctuate dramatically and increase your risk of fainting. Exhaling during the lifting, or exertion portion, of the strength training exercise and inhaling during the relaxation portion can help prevent this. Focus on completing a higher number of repetitions with light to moderate weights rather than doing short sets with heavy weights.

Avoid exercise if your resting systolic blood pressure is greater than 200 mm Hg or if your resting diastolic blood pressure is greater than 115 mm Hg. An exercise program can be implemented after your blood pressure is controlled through medications.

Stroke

A stroke occurs when the blood supply to your brain is interrupted and brain tissue is deprived of oxygen and nutrients. As with cardiovascular disease, high blood pressure and abnormal blood cholesterol levels are major risk factors for stroke. Physical activity as part of a healthy lifestyle can help prevent stroke, but it can also be beneficial during recovery from stroke, whether you do it on your own or within a formal exercise program.

After a stroke, flexibility exercises can increase the range of motion of limbs on the side of your body that has been affected and help prevent tightening of your tendons (contractures). Strength training can maximize your muscle mass and help increase your independence in performing daily tasks. It can also help prevent shrinkage (atrophy) of your muscles. If balance is a concern, most flexibility and strength training exercises can be done from a chair or on the floor. Coordination and balance activities can help you get back on your feet and improve your safety when moving around. Strength training can be performed two to three times a week. In most cases, your doctor or therapist will ask that you perform flexibility and balance exercises daily.

Aerobic exercise can help increase your independence, as well as your walking speed and endurance. Plus, it helps decrease your risk factors for a second stroke. Your physical therapist might start you out on a treadmill or, if you have difficulty with movement while standing, a recumbent stationary bicycle. Aerobic exercises can be performed daily.

Your posture may also be affected by loss of muscle tone and balance. Posture retraining — involving extension of your head, neck, trunk, hips and knees — can help restore normal movement. In addition, core exercises for your trunk muscles can improve your posture, breathing and overall muscle tone. See the chest stretches and core exercises in the "Exercise guide" beginning on page 134.

Congestive heart failure

At one time, people with congestive heart failure (CHF) were told not to exercise. CHF is a condition in which the heart is weakened through coronary artery disease, high blood pressure or other illness and has trouble pumping enough blood to meet the body's needs. Studies have shown that moderate exercise helps your heart pump more efficiently, reducing the demands on your heart muscle, and that it can be beneficial for people with stable CHF.

If you have CHF, you likely have a lower tolerance for exercise intensity, but this doesn't mean you can't exercise. To obtain the maximum benefit from exercise, you may wish to join a supervised exercise program that assists you in carefully monitoring your activity.

Aerobic activity can help increase your endurance and your heart's functional capacity. Someone with heart failure will probably obtain the most benefit from exercising five to seven days a week. Ideally, you should have an exercise test to determine your exercise capacity and help your doctor in providing specific exercise guidelines. As you implement your exercise program, you'll want to gradually increase the duration of your activity session until you can exercise for at least 20 to 30 minutes.

If you can't exercise for more than a few minutes at a time, that's OK. Several shorter exercise sessions of two to four minutes each day may be preferable. Sessions shouldn't cause excessive fatigue or discomfort. If you have enough endurance, working toward a goal of 30 to 60 minutes of low to moderately intense activity a day can further improve your fitness.

Safe aerobic exercises for someone with CHF include walking on a treadmill and using a stationary bicycle. Using an exercise machine allows you the advantage of controlling your pace and thus the intensity of your exercise. Outdoor walking or bicycling can be hard to pace and may be difficult to finish if you become fatigued some distance from your house or car. Swimming can be problematic because the water pressure increases blood flow return to the heart, which may overstress the heart. If you would like to swim, ask your doctor about it before starting.

If you're considering a strength training program, be sure to discuss it with your doctor before beginning. Some people with CHF may benefit from strength training, but only with medical supervision.

Asthma

Exercise is a common trigger of asthmatic signs and symptoms, a condition called exercise-induced asthma. You're more prone to exercise-induced asthma if you have asthma due to allergies. Signs and symptoms of exercise-induced asthma include coughing, wheezing, chest tightness, shortness of breath and fatigue.

Having asthma doesn't preclude you from engaging in physical activity. In fact, it's best if you're active. There are many professional athletes who have asthma. Here are some tips for exercising with asthma:

- To help prevent signs and symptoms, inhale a fast-acting bronchodilator medication 15 to 30 minutes before exercising. This type of medication typically requires a doctor's evaluation and prescription.
- Before beginning vigorous activity, warm up for five to 10 minutes with light activity and stretching, to help open your airways.
- Consider activities that involve short or intermittent periods of exercise and are less likely to trigger asthma signs and symptoms. Examples include golf, volleyball and softball. Sports that involve a lot of continuous running, such as soccer or basketball, are more likely to trigger signs and symptoms. In general, strength training with rest periods between sets is unlikely to trigger asthma signs and symptoms.
- Cold-weather activities, such as skiing or hockey, are more likely to cause wheezing in people with asthma. If you do exercise in cold weather, wear a face mask to warm the air you breathe. Avoid exercising in extremely cold conditions.
- Try to exercise in an environment that doesn't aggravate your condition. For instance, if there's a high pollen count or air quality alert, exercise indoors.

Cancer

For many people, cancer is a chronic illness. According to the National Cancer Institute, approximately 9.6 million cancer survivors live in the United States. Side effects from cancer treatment can be

Exercising with cancer

Condition	Precaution
Low hemoglobin levels, which may indicate anemia	Avoid high-intensity activities.
Low neutrophil (white blood cell) count, which may indicate a problem with your immune system	Avoid activities that might increase your risk of infection, such as swimming, or exercising to exhaustion.
Low level of blood platelets, which may be associated with a bleeding problem	Avoid activities that increase your risk of bleeding, such as contact sports or high-impact aerobics. Avoid lifting heavy weights and holding your breath during physical activity.
A fever greater than 100.4 F, which may indicate infection	Tell your doctor. Avoid high-intensity activities and exercising outside in warm weather.
Difficulty coordinating movement, numbness in your extremities, such as your feet, which may indicate peripheral neuropathy	Avoid activities that require significant balance and coordination, such as walking or jogging. Instead choose swimming, a treadmill with handholds or a stationary bicycle.
Severe weight loss	Loss of muscle mass tends to limit exercise intensity, but you can still perform short bouts of low-intensity activities.
Difficulty breathing	Tell your doctor. Ease up on the intensity and duration of your activity.
Bone pain	Avoid impact activities such as running, walking and contact sports. Also avoid heavy weight training. Talk to your doctor before resuming physical activity.
Severe nausea	Tell your doctor. Ease up on your activity. Drink plenty of fluids to avoid dehydration, especially if you're vomiting.
Extreme fatigue and weakness	Don't overdo it. Instead consider multiple, short bursts of low-intensity exercise.

Source: Adapted from "Coping With Cancer: Can Exercise Help?" The Physician and Sportsmedicine, May 2000

significant and long term, typically including fatigue, weakness, abnormal blood counts, anxiety, depression and a general decline in well-being. Although no studies show a relationship between physical activity and cancer recurrence or overall survival, exercise has been shown to reduce cancer's negative side effects. Even if you're living with advanced cancer, some degree of physical activity may be helpful in increasing appetite, relieving constipation and counteracting fatigue.

If you're currently receiving treatment, the goal of exercise may be to preserve and perhaps even improve function. If you're finished with treatment and are cancer-free, your goal may be to return to or initiate a healthy and active lifestyle where exercise is a daily part of life. If you're dealing with recurrent or metastatic cancer, exercise can help you maintain mobility and independence and provide relief from stress and anxiety.

Because cancer treatment often affects your whole body (that is, it's systemic), activities that work your entire body, such as walking or swimming, are especially recommended. Certain types of exercises can be helpful for different side effects of treatment. For example, flexibility exercises that emphasize range of motion can be helpful for lymphedema, a condition characterized by swelling in your arms and hands that may result from breast cancer treatment. In addition, men and women — usually those with prostate or breast cancer — who are treated with hormones, may be at a higher risk of osteoporosis and may benefit from strength training, which increases bone strength.

Although most people with a history of cancer can be physically active to some degree, in some cases exercise may not be immediately appropriate or may need to be modified or more closely monitored. A group of researchers conducted a review of the scientific literature and clinical trials regarding the effects of exercise on people with cancer and cancer survivors from 1980 to 2000. The researchers derived a number of precautions from their study (see "Exercising with cancer" on page 255).

Osteoporosis

Osteoporosis is a condition that causes your bones to slowly lose their mineral content and internal support structure.

Keep up the good work!

With most forms of exercise, several months of regular physical activity are required to see changes in your health. For example, it generally takes one to three months of consistent aerobic activity to produce cardiovascular benefits. If you have osteoporosis, you may begin to see the benefits of exercise in a few months, but it typically takes nine months to a year to see a significant change in your bone density. In addition, the health benefits you gain from exercise tend to stick around only as long as you keep exercising.

Eventually, your bones can become so weak that they break easily. The bones in your spine and hips are most commonly affected by osteoporosis. When bones in your spine fracture, it's called compression fracture because they compress together. Hip fractures are often a result of falls in people with osteoporosis.

Regular exercise can help maintain, and perhaps even increase, the density of your bones, making them stronger and less prone to fracture. Exercise also strengthens your muscles and improves your overall fitness. Together, strong bones and muscles will improve your posture and balance, which can reduce your risk of falls.

Three types of activities are often recommended for people with osteoporosis: strength training exercises — especially those for the back — weight-bearing aerobic activities and flexibility exercises. Because of the varying degrees of osteoporosis and the risk of fracture, ask your doctor or physical therapist whether you're at risk of osteoporosis-related problems and what exercises are appropriate for you.

- **Strength training** may include use of free weights, weight machines, resistance bands or water exercises to strengthen the muscles and bones in your arms and upper spine. Strength training can also work directly on your bones to slow mineral loss.

  Compression fractures resulting from osteoporosis often lead to a stooped posture and increased pressure along your spine, resulting in even more compression fractures. Exercises that gently arch your back and ones that focus on the muscles between your shoulder blades can strengthen back muscles while reducing stress on your bones. Rows, prone cobras and other core exercises are some examples.

- **Weight-bearing aerobic activities** involve doing aerobic exercises on your feet, with your bones supporting your weight. A seated activity is a non-weight-bearing activity. Examples of recommended weight-bearing activities include walking, dancing, low-impact aerobics and gardening. These types of activities work directly on the bones in your legs, hips and lower spine to slow mineral loss. They can also provide aerobic benefits, such as reducing your risk of cardiovascular disease.

  Swimming and water aerobics have many benefits but don't provide the impact on bones needed to slow mineral loss. However, these activities can be useful in cases of extreme osteoporosis or during rehabilitation following a fracture when impact exercise isn't possible.

- **Flexibility exercises** help increase your flexibility, another key component of overall fitness. Having full range of motion around a joint helps prevent muscle injury. Increased flexibility can also help improve your posture — tight abdominal and chest muscles tend to pull you forward and make you more stooped. Chest and shoulder stretches, and prone push-ups, may be helpful. Stretches are best performed after your muscles are warmed up, such as at the end of your exercise session. They should be done gently and slowly, without bouncing. Relax and breathe deeply while you stretch. Avoid stretches that flex your spine or cause you to bend at the waist. Ask your doctor which stretching exercises would be best for you.

If you have osteoporosis, avoid the following types of exercises:

- **High-impact exercises** such as jumping, running or jogging. These produce added compression in your spine and lower extremities and can lead to fractures in weakened bones. Avoid jerky, rapid movements in general. Try to move in a slow and controlled manner.
- **Bending and twisting forward at the waist,** including touching your toes, doing sit-ups and using a rowing machine. These also have a high compressive effect on the bones in your spine and shouldn't be done. Other activities that may require you to bend or twist forcefully at the waist are golf, tennis and bowling. Don't do these activities if you have severe osteoporosis.

Note: If you have only mild bone deterioration and don't have osteoporosis, the above exercises may be beneficial.

Arthritis

If you have arthritis, the pain and stiffness that accompany this disease may make exercise and physical activity in general seem unappealing. But an important way to keep your joints func-

tioning at their best is to move them and strengthen the muscles that support them.

Arthritis takes many different forms. The two most common are osteoarthritis and rheumatoid arthritis. Osteoarthritis results from wear and tear on your joints and usually affects people later in life. It typically involves the knee, hip and spine. Rheumatoid arthritis is an inflammatory condition believed to be an autoimmune disease — caused by an attack from your body's immune system on the tissue that lines your joints. It tends to involve joints such as the hands, wrist, feet and ankles, but it may also involve larger joints, such as the knees, hips and shoulders. People with rheumatoid arthritis may experience flare-ups of the disease, when joints become acutely inflamed and painful. At other times, signs and symptoms may decrease or disappear.

Exercises generally recommended for people with arthritis include flexibility and range-of-motion exercises, strength training and aerobic conditioning.

- **Flexibility and range-of-motion exercises** can help reduce pain and stiffness and increase your mobility. Gentle forms of yoga and tai chi are examples of flexibility exercises that can help arthritic joints stay mobile. If you've had joint replacement surgery, discuss specific stretching recommendations and precautions with your surgeon.
- **Strength training** strengthens the muscles around your joints, helping to take pressure off your cartilage and bones. The resistance you use to improve your

strength can be tailored according to your abilities. It may include using free weights, weight machines, elastic tubing or bands, and even household items such as unopened soup cans.

- **Aerobic exercise** can strengthen your muscles, as well as improve joint stability and increase your endurance and overall fitness. In addition, by increasing endurance, you can ensure that your muscles are working to control joint motion and stress.

The main precaution to take during exercise is to protect your joints from further damage. Your doctor or physical therapist can help you design a program suited to your needs. Low-impact activities such as cycling, swimming and cross-country skiing are desirable because they place less stress on your joints than do high-impact activities, such as those that involve jumping or running. Even walking can sometimes increase pain in arthritic joints.

Be careful not to overdo it. If you experience a flare-up, you may need to rest or reduce your activities in order to minimize joint damage. In general, avoid overstretching affected joints. If you feel pain, don't force a motion. If your muscles ache for more than an hour or two after your workout, or you notice an increase in swelling in a joint, cut back on the intensity of your exercises. Cross-training — alternating between a variety of exercises throughout the week — helps prevent overworking a particular set of muscles or joints.

If stiffness is an issue, it may be helpful to employ the "heat before, ice after" principle. Apply heat to the affected joint before exercising it, then begin your exercise with an appropriate warm-up activity. Follow the exercise with the application of ice to reduce inflammation. Avoid heat on swollen joints.

Experts often recommend that people with arthritis do water exercises such as swimming, water walking and water aerobics because water's buoyancy reduces stress on the joints. Water also offers resistance as you move about, providing a form of strength training. If possible, try to exercise in warm water (83 to 88 F), which helps relax your muscles and allows for increased blood circulation. The Arthritis Foundation has developed an aquatic exercise program. Your local gym or community health club may offer a similar program under the guidance of a trained instructor.

Chronic pain

People often think that exercise aggravates chronic pain, but this is a misconception. It's true that acute injury requires rest in order to heal, but inactivity isn't be... active, you b... strength and... can contribut...

When you'... body releases... enkephalins)... reaching your... help alleviate...

Exercising after joint replacement surgery

The most common reason for joint replacement surgery is severe pain and disability caused by arthritis. Other reasons include a severe fracture involving a joint or other trauma-induced injuries. Although it's important not to place too much wear and tear on your prosthesis after joint replacement surgery, this doesn't mean you should be inactive. In fact, low-impact activity after joint replacement surgery may be important for increasing bone density and improving fixation of your prosthesis. In addition, improved muscle strength, balance and coordination resulting from regular exercise can help prevent falls and injuries.

Recommended regular activities after joint replacement surgery include those that don't place too much stress on your joints, such as walking, swimming, golfing and bicycling. But if you're used to doing certain higher impact activities for pleasure, such as dancing, playing tennis, hiking or cross-country skiing, you may be able to continue doing them, as long as you do them only occasionally and not regularly. To reduce the load on your hips and knees, use a walking stick or ski poles while hiking. Ski on flatter surfaces using long, wide turns, and avoid moguls.

In general, avoid high-impact activities such as contact sports, high-impact aerobics, running, racquetball, squash and other activities that involve lots of running and jumping. If you've had total shoulder replacement surgery, your doctor may recommend avoiding sports that require you to throw with the affected arm. Also avoid positions that may place your new joint at risk of dislocation, such as some extreme stretches and yoga positions. Discuss these with your doctor before attempting them.

Physical activity after joint replacement surgery

	Recommended	OK if you have experience	Not recommended
After hip replacement	Stationary bicycling Croquet Ballroom dancing Golf Horseshoes Shooting Shuffleboard Swimming Doubles tennis Walking	Low-impact aerobics Road bicycling Bowling Canoeing Hiking Horseback riding Cross-country skiing	High-impact aerobics Baseball or softball Basketball Football Gymnastics Handball Hockey Jogging Lacrosse Racquetball Squash Rock climbing Soccer Singles tennis Volleyball

	Recommended	OK if you have experience	Not recommended
After knee replacement	Low-impact aerobics Stationary bicycling Bowling Golf Dancing Horseback riding Croquet Walking Swimming Shooting Shuffleboard Horseshoes	Road bicycling Canoeing Hiking Rowing Cross-country skiing Stationary skiing Speed walking Doubles tennis Weight machines Ice-skating	Racquetball Squash Rock climbing Soccer Singles tennis Volleyball Football Gymnastics Lacrosse Hockey Basketball Jogging Handball
After shoulder replacement	Cross-country skiing Stationary skiing Speed walking and jogging Swimming using the breast stroke Doubles tennis Low-impact aerobics Road and stationary bicycling Bowling Canoeing Croquet Shuffleboard Horseshoes Dancing	Golf Ice-skating Shooting Downhill skiing	Football Gymnastics Hockey Rock climbing

Source: *"Athletic Activity After Joint Replacement," American Journal of Sports Medicine, May-June 2001*

conditions that can make your pain more difficult to control.

Musculoskeletal problems, such as lower back pain, shoulder problems and foot problems, are a common source of chronic pain. A regular exercise program that includes flexibility, aerobic exercises and strength training can improve your overall fitness and help control your pain. Exercise also improves sleep and promotes weight loss, thus reducing stress on your joints, and it increases muscle and bone mass, reducing your risk of injury.

Following are some general exercise suggestions if you have low back pain, shoulder problems and foot problems. Your doctor or physical therapist can help you create a more specific fitness program with the most benefit and least risk for your particular condition.

Lower back pain

Improper lifting and sudden twisting movements are common causes of lower back pain. Although most experts agree that physical activity in general is good for people with low back pain, exercises that specifically target the deep abdominal muscles and core may provide additional benefit. Exercise can also reduce stress and anxiety about your condition, improve your mood and make you more confident in your body.

If you've been inactive for a while, start out slowly. Generally, swimming, cycling and other non-weight-bearing exercises are safest because they place minimal strain on your lower back. Warm up before starting your exercise to avoid strain and injury. Strength and flexibility training and core exercises, which aim to strengthen your trunk muscles, are also crucial to keeping your back strong and limber (see the "Exercise guide" on page 134 for more on these types of exercises). Lack of flexibility in your hips can lead to overstressing your back muscles during movement.

Comprehensive spine fitness also includes endurance and aerobic training. Poor endurance has been cited as a risk factor for back pain, whereas increased aerobic fitness has been associated with reduced back pain. But choose your activities wisely. Your back is at greatest risk when you're doing high-impact activities and activities that involve forceful twist-

Choosing a stationary bicycle — Upright or recumbent?

For low back pain, a semireclining (recumbent) stationary bicycle may provide more comfort and support for your back than does an upright one. Recumbent bikes allow you to sit with your legs and feet in front of you, rather than under you, which places less strain on your back.

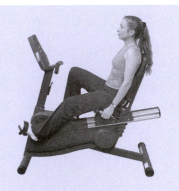

Don't push through pain

Some exertion and muscle soreness is to be expected with exercise, but if you experience pain while doing an exercise, stop the exercise immediately and relax. If the pain goes away, repeat the exercise slowly and less forcefully. If the pain persists after you've stopped exercising, talk to your doctor or physical therapist before resuming the exercise.

ing or bending at the waist and quick stops and starts.

Shoulder problems

Shoulder problems can be caused by sports injuries, excessive overhead motion or diseases such as arthritis. Some shoulder problems include:

Rotator cuff injury. Your rotator cuff is made up of four muscles and their attached tendons. The muscles connect your upper arm bone (humerus) with your shoulder blade. They also help hold the ball of your upper arm bone firmly in your shoulder socket, as if holding a golf ball on a tee. These muscles travel through a bony and ligamentous tunnel on their way to the arm and therefore are at risk of getting pinched during repetitive motion. This is called impingement and can lead to pain, inflammation and, potentially, tears in the rotator cuff.

Frozen shoulder. When frozen shoulder (adhesive capsulitis) occurs, the shoulder socket becomes inflamed and stiff. The inflammation may cause the tissue to become "sticky." As a result, pain and subsequent loss of movement may occur.

Doctors aren't sure what causes it, but it may occur after an injury or prolonged immobilization of your shoulder.

People with certain health conditions, such as diabetes or heart disease, may have an increased risk of developing frozen shoulder.

Shoulder osteoarthritis. This condition is less common than are the preceding two. It may be associated with a previous injury that has led to abnormal wear and tear of the cartilage in your shoulder.

A daily shoulder fitness program will help you improve your motion, strength and function, as well as reduce pain. Applying heat to your shoulder muscles before exercising promotes muscle relaxation and may help prevent further injury. Avoid overhead reaching and lifting, including overhead weightlifting techniques such as the military press. In general, during exercise keep your arm close to your body to decrease stress on your shoulder.

Depending on the type of shoulder problem, your doctor or physical therapist may prescribe a variety of exercises. Basic rotator cuff exercises include internal and external rotation exercises, punches and rows (see exercises on pages 150-151 and 154-156). Shoulder exercises should be done with light weights and higher repetitions. It's desirable to have full range of motion in your shoulder before beginning strengthening exercises. This is particularly important if you have frozen shoulder, but it may not be possible if you have severe osteoarthritis.

Endurance, not brute strength, is the goal for rotator cuff strengthening. In addition, exercises to improve your posture and stabilize your back and shoulder blade muscles can help to avoid further impingement of your rotator cuff.

Foot problems

One of the most common causes of chronic foot pain is plantar fasciitis, an inflammation of the fibrous tissue that runs along the bottom of your foot (plantar fascia). A flattening of your arch or overuse of your feet can cause this tissue to stretch and pull on your heel bone. This can result in microscopic tears in tissue, inflammation, a piercing pain, ache or burning sensation.

Achilles tendinitis is another cause of foot pain, characterized by strain and inflammation of the tendon just above your heel (Achilles tendon). Achilles tendinitis often results from sports such as basketball and high jumping, which place exceptional stress on the calf muscles and Achilles tendon.

Daily stretches of your plantar fascia and calf muscles can increase their flexibility and reduce stress on the plantar fascia and Achilles tendon (for more, see foot exercises on pages 148-149 and 171-172). Tightness in these areas is a major risk factor for plantar fasciitis. It's also important to strengthen the muscles that support your arch to further reduce stress on the plantar fascia. This can be done with toe curls and ankle strengthening exercis-

Bunions and hammertoes

A bunion is a painful enlargement of the joint at the base of your big toe. A hammertoe is a toe that's curled due to an abnormal bend in its middle joint. These common foot problems are often associated with ill-fitting shoes and can be helped by switching footwear. For example, shoes with a wide toe box can better accommodate a bunion, whereas extra depth in your shoe's toe box can alleviate the pain of a hammertoe. Removable metatarsal pads placed just behind the ball of the foot can relieve pain (metatarsalgia) associated with a hammertoe.

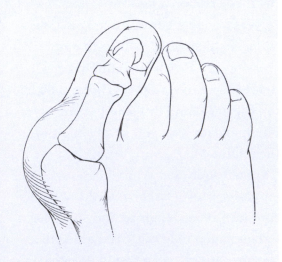

es including heel raises and ankle inversion and eversion (see page 149). Achilles tendinitis is generally treated with rest, ice, compression and elevation. Stretching and strengthening of your calf muscles can also reduce your risk of straining your Achilles tendon.

Stretch your calf and foot muscles several times a day, especially before going to bed at night and getting up in the morning — the plantar fascia can get particularly tight overnight. Your doctor may recommend wearing a night splint to keep the plantar fascia and Achilles tendon stretched while you sleep.

While your foot is healing, temporarily reduce walking or jogging. Instead, try exercises such as swimming, water aerobics and bicycling, which put less weight on your heel. You might also try wearing heel pads or cups in your shoes to cushion and support your heel.

Diabetes

Regular physical activity can be a useful tool in managing your diabetes. It can help you control your blood sugar levels, manage your weight and improve your cardiovascular health.

If you have type 2 diabetes — formerly called noninsulin-dependent diabetes or adult-onset diabetes — your body becomes resistant to insulin and your pancreas can't make enough insulin to overcome the resistance. As a result, your blood sugar levels become abnormally high because insulin helps to regulate your blood sugar. Regular exercise can help you lower your blood sugar levels by tapping into your blood's sugar supplies for energy and increasing efficient use of insulin. Some people who exercise regularly are able to manage their type 2 diabetes with diet and exercise alone.

If you have type 1 diabetes, your body is unable to produce enough insulin to ensure proper metabolism. This means you have an absolute need for insulin, which must be supplied to your body every day, usually in the form of injections. Although exercise alone can't normalize your blood sugar levels if you have type 1 diabetes, it can increase your sensitivity to insulin and may reduce the amount of medication that you need.

Physical activity contributes to weight loss, which also increases your body's sensitivity to insulin, regardless of what type of diabetes you have. In addition, regular exercise can help prevent some of the cardiovascular complications of diabetes, such as high blood pressure and cardiovascular disease.

Long-term regular physical activity can help in a number of ways. Depending on the status of your condition and diabetes-related complications you may have, you might have to take some extra precautions while exercising. Following are some general tips on exercising with diabetes. Before you begin, talk to your doctor about your individual abilities and limitations, especially if you have long-standing diabetes, which is a risk factor for cardiovascular disease.

■ Try to exercise at least 30 minutes a day

most days of the week. Most experts recommend low- to moderate-intensity aerobic activities, such as walking, bicycling, swimming and rowing. In addition, maintain a fairly steady intensity throughout each session. Varying intensity significantly may alter your blood sugar levels.

- Follow a general strength training program to increase muscle mass and insulin sensitivity, thus decreasing required dosages of medication.

- Check your blood sugar before, during and after exercising. If it's below 100 milligrams per deciliter (mg/dL), eat a snack before you exercise to avoid low blood sugar. You may wish to have a snack or fruit drink handy while you're exercising, in case you need a carbohydrate boost. Don't exercise if your blood sugar is above 250 mg/dL and ketones are present in your urine or if your blood sugar is above 300 mg/dL. Wait until your blood sugar level drops before increasing your physical activity. Exercising with very high blood sugar levels can lead to the overproduction of toxic acids in the blood (ketones) or to ketoacidosis, a serious condition that can lead to coma or death if untreated.

- Take good care of your feet. With diabetes, the skin of your feet is predisposed to ulcers and other problems because of reduced blood flow. Proper foot care is especially important if you have reduced sensation in your feet (peripheral neuropathy). Consider using silica gel or air midsoles in your shoes plus polyester or polyester-blend socks to help prevent blisters and keep your feet dry. After exercising, check your feet for blisters.

- Wear a medical identification bracelet that lets others know you have diabetes.

- Drink plenty of fluids before, during and after activity, especially when it's hot. Dehydration can affect blood sugar levels and heart function.

- If you have eye problems related to diabetes, such as abnormal growth of blood vessels on your retina, avoid strenuous activities, including weightlifting, boxing and other contact sports. These can increase the risk of bleeding in your eyes.

Metabolic syndrome

Metabolic syndrome isn't a disease. Rather, it's a cluster of disorders, including high blood pressure, high insulin levels, excess body weight and abnormal cholesterol levels that increase your risk of diabetes, cardiovascular disease and stroke. This condition has become increasingly common in the United States. As many as one in four American adults and 40 percent of adults age 40 and older have metabolic syndrome, an increase of 61 percent over the last decade. You may be at risk if you're overweight and don't exercise regularly. In fact, if you have three or more of the following — abdominal obesity, high triglycerides and low high-density lipoprotein (HDL) cholesterol, a blood pressure measurement greater than 130/85 millimeters of mercury and blood sugar levels greater than 110 milligrams per deciliter — you may have metabolic syndrome. Weight loss and increased participation in regular physical activity are essential to prevent and treat this condition. A healthy diet that includes plenty of fruits and vegetables and that's low in sodium is important in managing or delaying the onset of metabolic syndrome. A regular exercise program that emphasizes aerobic activity is also important. See Chapter 4 for a sample aerobic workout plan and Chapter 7 for tips on nutrition and exercise.

Obesity

Physical activity and dietary modifications are your best allies in the fight against obesity. But answering the call to action may not be easy if you're obese. Even simple movements such as bending over may be difficult, and you may not be able to stay on your feet for very long. Many overweight people avoid exercise because it hurts, they're out of shape, they're embarrassed or they aren't athletically inclined. Overcoming obstacles may be challenging but, in the long run, well worth the effort.

At first, your main goal will be to simply increase your daily activity. Anything that gets you moving — even if only for a few minutes a day — is a good start. This can be as simple as:

- Walking around your living room a few times each day
- Taking two- to three-minute walking breaks at work a few times each day
- Parking farther away from your destination and walking the rest of the way
- Storing the TV remote control and getting up to change the channel
- Marching in place during TV commercials or while talking on the phone
- Walking the dog
- Walking around the house while you talk on a cordless phone
- Climbing stairs
- Gardening
- Housecleaning

It's important to start out slowly. This will help you avoid burnout and injury. Focus on taking small steps, not giant ones. Spend a few minutes warming up for any activity — even walking. Shrug your shoulders, tap your toes, swing your arms or march in place. Don't forget to cool down. Slow down gradually. Stretch for a few minutes.

Set realistic goals for yourself. And find an activity you like doing so that you're more likely to stick with your plan. As you consistently perform small amounts of activity, you'll find you can keep going longer each time. In the short term, you may try to walk five minutes at least three days a week. In the long term, in six months for example, you might aim to walk 30 minutes most days of the week. Generally, when weight loss is your goal, working up to 60 minutes a day will bring you even more benefits. If you can't set aside a big block of time for physical activity, do shorter sessions of 10 or 15 minutes each. Several short sessions of activity produce health benefits similar to those of a single long session, although weight loss may occur more slowly.

Strength training can help you develop and retain lean muscle mass. But aerobic exercise may be more effective at helping you lose weight because you can maintain the activity for a longer time and thus burn more calories. Therefore, you may want to incorporate both strength training and aerobic activity into your workout.

Because excess weight can increase the amount of stress placed on your joints, go for low-impact aerobic activities such as walking, cycling and using an elliptical trainer. If your feet or joints hurt when you stand, try non-weight-bearing activities, where you're not required to support the weight of your body on your feet. Examples include swimming, cycling and water exercises.

People who are obese are also more prone to heat intolerance. For this reason, wear loosefitting clothing, drink an adequate amount of fluids and avoid working out in very hot or humid weather. For more on staying properly hydrated, see Chapter 7.

For some people, body image and self-esteem issues can present significant barriers to being physically active. If you're self-conscious about exercise, find a place where you're comfortable being active. This might include participating in an exercise class for obese people or using exercise equipment set up in your own home. Psychological counseling can also be of great benefit. And don't forget to enlist support. Get a family member or friend to be active with you. You'll be doing your companion a health favor, and the whole experience may be more fun as you cheer each other on.

Exercise and pregnancy

If you're pregnant and have no known medical conditions that may call for a particularly cautious approach to physical activity, moderate aerobic exercise can help you feel healthy and boost your spirits. Even if you've never exercised, pregnancy is a good incentive to get started. Just be sure to get your doctor's approval before you begin any activity. After pregnancy, physical activity can help you return to your normal weight and maintain your overall health.

During pregnancy

Throughout your pregnancy, the conditioning that results from exercise can help prevent back pain, muscle cramps, swelling and constipation. It can also reduce fatigue and help you sleep. In addition, exercise during pregnancy can help prepare you for labor and childbirth. Increased stamina and muscle strength can decrease stress on your ligaments and joints and allow you to push for longer periods during labor without fatigue.

Many sports and exercises are suitable for pregnant women. One of the best is swimming. It provides a good cardiovascular workout with minimal risk of injury because of the water's buoyancy. Walking and low-impact aerobics also are excellent forms of exercise. If you were practicing a sport regularly before you became pregnant, you'll likely be able to continue doing so into your pregnancy, although you may need to decrease your intensity if you find yourself becoming more fatigued than usual.

Each sport that you participate in should be reviewed with your doctor. Scuba diving in particular should be avoided because it places the fetus at an increased risk of decompression sickness. In addition, avoid prolonged exposure to high temperatures, such as in a hot tub or sauna, especially during the first trimester. Excessive heat may cause injury to the fetus.

Keep in mind the following guidelines:

- Always warm up before exercising.
- After your 20th week of pregnancy, don't do any exercises that require you to lie flat on your back. This position makes it more difficult for your blood to circulate to your baby.
- Avoid activities that require you to jump or change directions quickly, particularly during the third trimester. The cartilage and ligaments that support your joints soften during pregnancy and are more easily strained.
- Don't let yourself get overheated. This can lead to fluid loss and dehydration.
- Don't exercise in hot, humid weather or if you're sick.
- Don't continue to exercise to the point of exhaustion.
- Start slowly if you haven't exercised for a while. Begin with as little as five minutes a day and add five minutes a

week until you're active for 30 minutes a day.

Stop exercising if you experience:

- Vaginal bleeding
- Difficulty breathing
- Dizziness
- Headache
- Chest pain
- Muscle weakness
- Calf pain or swelling — have your doctor check for signs of a blood clot in your legs
- Preterm labor
- Decreased fetal movement
- Leakage of amniotic fluid

After pregnancy

After your baby arrives, you may be eager to start exercising to regain your pre-pregnancy shape and fitness. But it's important to start out gradually, perhaps with some Kegel exercises and brief walks. Kegel exercises are done to repair and strengthen your pelvic floor. To do them, you tighten and hold the muscles in your vaginal wall and opening — the ones you'd use to stop the flow of urine — and hold for up to 10 seconds, then release. You can increase the length of your walks as time goes by. After about six weeks, you'll likely be able to get back into a full-fledged aerobic routine.

Flexibility and core stability exercises are also important in the postpartum period. Now that your uterus isn't pressing against your abdomen anymore, the abdominal wall is loose and unable to adequately support your lower back.

Making exercise work for you

Exercise can benefit nearly everyone, including individuals who are pregnant or facing a medical condition. Just be sure to check with your doctor before beginning your program.

Condition	Risks of not exercising	Benefits of exercising
Cardiovascular disease	Low levels of high-density lipoprotein (HDL) cholesterol, narrowed arteries, risk of heart attack or other cardiovascular event	Aerobic exercise reduces buildup of cholesterol-containing plaques and pressure on damaged arteries. It helps to increase HDL cholesterol and decrease low-density lipoprotein (LDL) cholesterol and to reduce risk of a second heart attack.
High blood pressure	Development of cardiovascular disease or stroke	Aerobic exercise helps to lower blood pressure and maintain its control.
Stroke	Uncontrolled high blood pressure, abnormal levels of blood cholesterol	Aerobic exercise can help prevent stroke. After a stroke, flexibility exercise can restore range of motion, aerobic exercise can increase mobility, and balance exercise can improve posture.
Congestive heart failure (stable)	Weakened heart	Aerobic exercise increases the heart's working capacity, reducing the heart muscle's workload and increasing its endurance.
Asthma	Weak heart and lungs, being overweight with all its complications	Aerobic exercise strengthens heart and lungs and promotes weight control, facilitating breathing.
Cancer	Potentially increased difficulty dealing with treatment's side effects	Aerobic exercise helps counteract fatigue, weakness, anxiety, depression, loss of appetite and constipation. Other kinds of exercise may help with different side effects, such as flexibility exercise for swelling (lymphedema) of the arm.

Condition	Risks of not exercising	Benefits of exercising
Osteoporosis	Loss of bone density and increased risk of fracture	Weight-bearing exercise can strengthen bones. Strength and balance training can build muscles and improve joint stability, posture and balance.
Arthritis	Pain and joint stiffness	Flexibility exercise can increase mobility and reduce pain and stiffness. Strength training strengthens muscles and stabilizes joints. Low-impact aerobic exercise increases endurance and overall fitness.
Diabetes	Uncontrolled blood sugar levels, increased need for medication	Regular exercise increases the body's sensitivity to insulin, which helps to control blood sugar. It also reduces the need for medication.
Disability	Underuse or overuse of certain muscles, decreased independence, being overweight	Regular exercise helps to balance and develop muscle groups. It increases independence and helps to counteract infections, weakness and fatigue. It also promotes weight control.
Obesity	Excess weight and increased risk of cardiovascular disease, diabetes and other illnesses	Regular exercise promotes weight loss and long-term weight control.
Chronic pain	Loss of muscle tone, strength and flexibility, which can contribute to pain	Regular exercise promotes release of pain-blocking chemicals, strengthens muscles, and improves balance, posture, overall fitness, and ability to function.
Pregnancy (Some coexisting conditions may prohibit you from exercising. Check with your doctor.)	Excessive weight gain, increased fatigue and weakness	Regular exercise helps prevent back pain, muscle cramps, swelling and constipation. It reduces fatigue and stress, promotes weight control, and helps you prepare for labor and delivery.

Exercises that strengthen abdominal, back and trunk muscles can be especially helpful. Don't overdo it on abdominal exercises — start out slow, such as with pelvic tilts or abdominal hollowing exercises.

Most women lose 18 to 20 pounds within the first month after delivery. The last few pounds are usually the hardest to get rid of, but with patience and consistent activity, you'll get there.

General disability

Don't be fooled into thinking that if you use a wheelchair, physical fitness isn't for you. Again, it's mostly a matter of adapting exercise techniques to your particular situation. Many people mistakenly equate disability with disease and forget that most people with disabilities can achieve physical fitness. Some of the benefits of physical activity that are particularly important for people with disabilities include:

- **Managing secondary conditions.** If you have a disability, you're more likely to develop additional physical or mental conditions because of your disability. These secondary conditions can include obesity, pressure sores, infections, osteoporosis, fatigue and depression. These secondary conditions can lead to further disability and possible loss of physical independence, but they can be controlled or avoided through good physical health.
- **Balanced muscles.** Many people with disabilities are prone to underuse, overuse or misuse of various muscle groups. For instance, a person who uses a

wheelchair may have very developed anterior chest and shoulder muscles — those toward the front — from pushing his or her chair, but might need to develop his or her upper back muscles to avoid a slouched posture. Structured physical activity can help to balance these differences.

- **Independence.** Developing the physical capacity and strength to move around and manage daily tasks, such as showering or getting dressed, can help people with disabilities to achieve or maintain independence.
- **Enjoyment.** If you're doing an activity that you enjoy, it can be a great time. And many activities provide an opportunity for you to meet new people and make friends.

A moderate amount of physical activity most days of the week can improve your health. This can be achieved through longer periods of less intense activity, such as wheeling yourself in your wheelchair for 30 to 40 minutes, or in shorter amounts of more strenuous activity, such as playing wheelchair basketball for 20 minutes.

If you're currently inactive, begin with short amounts — five to 10 minutes — of physical activity and gradually increase the time as you progress. By increasing the amount of physical activity — increasing duration, intensity or frequency — you can achieve greater health benefits.

Machines called ergometers, which measure the amount of work or exercise you do, can be used for aerobic exercise. Various types are wheelchair-accessible, including upper and lower extremity ergometers and dual extremity ergometers. These often offer motorized movement that allows for passive, active and active-assisted forms of exercise.

Strength training helps develop your muscles and can be particularly helpful in counterbalancing muscle development in your upper extremities acquired through daily moving about. Your physical deficit, coordination, strength and muscle control determine the type you use. For example, if you have a hand dysfunction, you may use specially designed gloves that improve your grip or wrist cuffs that secure your hands to free weights. Cuff weights or weight machines or both may also be a good choice if you have cerebral palsy and also have athetosis — a condition that causes involuntary movements in one or more of your limbs. If you have a condition that directly affects your muscles — such as muscular dystrophy, multiple sclerosis or polio — use caution when deciding to pursue strength training and be sure to consult your doctor before attempting it.

Flexibility exercises are critical to keeping you moving independently. Improved flexibility increases your range of motion, reduces muscle soreness, improves your posture, reduces injuries, increases muscle relaxation and controls muscle rigidity (spasticity). Flexibility exercises can be done several times a day and are particularly helpful if you're sedentary. You can do these while seated by stretching your upper body forward with one leg extend-

ed straight out and the other bent. You might start out by reaching to your knee. Make it your goal to gradually lengthen your stretch until you can reach your toes. Discontinue your stretching exercises if they produce spasms or abnormal reflexes, and have your doctor or therapist re-evaluate them to make sure they're appropriate for you. There are a number of seated exercises in the "Exercise guide," which begins on page 134.

SUMMARY

It can be a challenge to follow an exercise plan when you're pregnant or dealing with a chronic illness or another medical condition. But as you've read, having a medical condition doesn't mean you can't be physically active. By working closely with your doctor, physical therapist, trainer or fitness counselor, you can develop a plan that keeps you fit and better able to manage your medical condition.

Remember that the warm-up period is an important part of any program, but especially so when you're exercising with a health problem. Take your time and ease into your workout, and be sure to cool down and stretch afterward. Be patient with yourself and avoid activities that are painful. Be aware that medications you're taking may have an effect on how your body reacts during exercise. Periodically discuss your progress with your doctor.

Training
for your sport

CHAPTER 9

If you're a sports fan, you know that college and professional athletes follow specifically designed training regimens to enhance their performance. A baseball team's spring training looks quite different from a basketball team's practices. What works for a golf pro won't take a top swimmer very far.

But you don't have to be a professional athlete to benefit from working out in a way that's tailored to the sports or activities you enjoy. Training isn't just for Olympic hopefuls. If you're physically active, you can condition yourself to perform at a higher level.

Training for a particular physical activity means getting in shape to play your sport, not just playing your sport to be in shape. A sport-specific training program can help you avoid injury and do better in your activity, whether you're in a weekly volleyball league, are a dedicated mall walker, want to run a 5-kilometer (3.1-mile) race or play golf twice a week.

All physical activities require some degree and combination of strength, endurance,

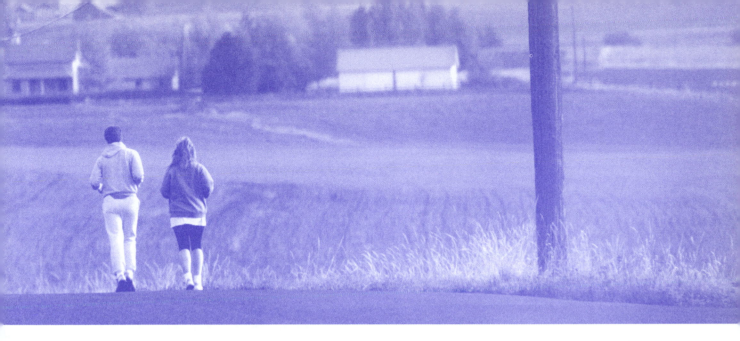

flexibility, coordination, speed, agility, balance and skill. A good overall fitness program will include activities designed to improve strength, aerobic capacity (endurance), flexibility and balance.

But each sport or activity requires a specific set of skills and energy output. For example, sprinting and jumping are high-energy activities that require a relatively large production of energy for a short time. Long-distance running and swimming are longer duration activities that require steady, more moderate energy output. Different sports also use different muscle groups, with varying requirements for strength, flexibility and balance.

Because of these differences, a training program that's effective for one sport may not be well suited for another. One of the key principles of sports training is to specifically develop the muscles and energy systems involved in a given activity.

This chapter presents specific ways to train for a variety of sports and activities. It will help you recognize the major muscle groups used for each activity and will

give you suggestions on how to avoid injury. You'll also find tips on how to kick up your performance to a higher level.

Although everyone can benefit from learning a few secrets of the pros, you'll want to tailor your training program to meet your unique needs and goals. Whether your goal is to participate in a race, prime yourself for the ski or golf season, maintain your fitness, or improve some aspect of your sports performance, this chapter will help you plan an appropriate training program.

TRAINING FUNDAMENTALS

Understanding how your body responds to training (physical conditioning) can help you design a program that's geared to your individual needs and capacities as well as your particular sport or activity. Several basic principles of training apply to any type of exercise and can help you determine what to do to maximize your participation and performance.

Specificity

The best way to train for any sport or activity is to do it. But a good training program goes beyond just doing your sport or activity and nothing else. Most people don't have all the physical attributes they need for optimal participation or performance in a given sport or activity and can benefit from developing them.

One of the basic principles of physical training is specificity — the effects of training depend on the type of sport or activity you do. In other words, specific exercises result in specific adaptations in your body. If you want to swim better, you have to swim. But you also need to train your aerobic system and strengthen the muscles you use in swimming.

One reason activity-specific training is important is because your brain remembers patterns of muscle use. That's why, as the old saying goes, "You never forget how to ride a bike." If you practice a skill such as a tennis serve or golf swing, you become better at it as the nerve pathways between your brain and muscles are reinforced. In other words, the brain stores memories of how you're using your muscles. Even if you can't or don't participate in an activity throughout the year, you can help maintain this muscle memory by choosing other exercises that mimic the components of movements you use in your activity and involve the same neuromotor skills. The closer the exercise is to your activity, the more it will help you maintain your abilities.

In keeping with the specificity principle, your training program should develop the muscles, energy systems and skills you need to perform your sport or activity. For example, you may swim several times a week, but you haven't done anything to strengthen the core muscles of your trunk. A weak core can slow you down in the pool and make you more susceptible to injury. Or your golf swing

Training for everyday activities

You don't have to be a member of a sports team or a hard-core athlete to benefit from physical training. Even if your everyday activity is simply gardening, walking the dog, snow shoveling, raking leaves or another routine task, you'll be able to perform more efficiently, with more stamina and less soreness and injury, if you prepare with some training.

Many everyday activities, just as with sports, require varying amounts of flexibility, strength, endurance and balance. Doing exercises that train these components will improve your everyday work capacity and ability to recover from physical effort.

A good aerobic base is helpful for any physical activity. Beyond this, figure out what muscles your activity uses, and strengthen and stretch those areas. For example, before the snow flies, you can get in shape for shoveling by doing resistance exercises or lifting weights to strengthen your back muscles, abdomen, shoulders and arms.

With the right preparation, your annual window-cleaning spree doesn't have to leave you feeling sore for days.

may be hampered by a lack of flexibility in your hips and back.

The repetitive use of specific muscles can also increase your risk of injury. A soccer player who lacks a balanced exercise program that includes flexibility training is likely to have tight hip flexors from repetitive kicking. Tight hip flexors increase the likelihood of pulled groin muscles or low back pain.

Overload

When you engage in a physical activity at a level above your normal daily activity, or load, you overload the muscles and their energy support systems. When you do an exercise regularly, your body begins to adapt to the overload. The exercise induces a variety of adaptations that enable your body to function more efficiently. This is known as the overload principle.

If you want to improve your fitness and your performance in a particular activity, your body must work harder than it's used to working. The overload should increase with time, a concept known as progressive overload. You can increase the load by changing the frequency, intensity or duration of your workouts.

Energy demands

As explained in Chapter 2, your body relies on three different sources of energy to fuel its activities. Different physical activities draw on different energy sources, depending on the duration and intensity of your activity. The three major energy systems are:

- The immediate system (anaerobic), which relies on adenosine triphosphate (ATP) and phosphocreatine (PC) for power energy
- The short-term system (both anaerobic and aerobic), which relies on stored glycogen for speed energy
- The long-term system (aerobic), which relies on aerobic metabolism of carbohydrates, fats and proteins for endurance energy

As you're working out, the three energy systems don't simply switch on and off. Rather, they blend together smoothly on a continuum, with one energy source overlapping another. The three systems work together to support short, intense bursts of activity and more sustained periods of less intense activity.

Most sports use a combination of aerobic and anaerobic metabolism. For example, in baseball or softball, long periods of low activity are interspersed with short bursts of high-intensity sprinting, throwing or batting. Some physical activities, such as long-distance running, cycling and hiking, rely almost exclusively on the aerobic system, while others, such as hockey, are mostly anaerobic. In some activities, including soccer and basketball, the predominant energy system is constantly changing.

ASSESSING YOUR TRAINING NEEDS

To get started on crafting a tailored training program, do a needs analysis of your sport or activity. What motions does it require, and what muscle groups are working? What are the demands for endurance, flexibility, strength and balance?

Next, figure out where you stand with respect to the needs you identified. Do you lack flexibility in certain muscle groups? Do you have room to improve in strength or endurance? Do you have bal-ance trouble? Then prioritize where you'd like to focus your efforts.

As a general guideline, the following key areas can serve as focus points for training:

- **Energy systems (aerobic and anaerobic).** The total duration of your activity will guide you in determining how much aerobic conditioning you need. The

Energy systems used in different sports

Different physical activities use the three energy systems to varying degrees. This table shows a number of sports and activities and the approximate percentage of each system that supplies energy for them. (See Chapter 2 for detailed information about the body's energy systems.)

Sport or activity	Immediate (ATP-PC) anaerobic	Short-term (glycogen) anaerobic and aerobic	Long-term (oxygen) aerobic
Baseball, softball	80%	15%	5%
Basketball	60%	20%	20%
Bicycling (long-distance)	Negligible	10%	90%
Bowling	90%	10%	Negligible
Golf (with cart*)	95%	5%	Negligible
In-line skating (under 10 kilometers)	5%	25%	70%
Kayaking, canoeing (long-distance)	20%	40%	40%
Running (long-distance)	Negligible	5%	95%
Skiing (downhill)	50%	30%	20%
Skiing (cross-country)	5%	10%	85%
Soccer (goalie, wings, striker)	60%	30%	10%
Soccer (halfbacks, sweeper)	60%	20%	20%
Swimming (short-distance)	20%	40%	40%
Swimming (long-distance)	10%	20%	70%
Tennis	70%	20%	10%
Volleyball	80%	5%	15%
Walking and hiking	Negligible	5%	95%

*The aerobic demands of golf increase if you carry your own bag and walk the entire course.

Source: Adapted from Merle L. Foss, Steven J. Keteyian and Edward L. Fox, *Fox's Physiological Basis for Exercise and Sport*, Sixth Edition (New York: McGraw-Hill College, 1998)

longer your activity lasts — whether it's a 45-minute soccer game, four-hour golf round or five-hour marathon — the more important aerobic conditioning is.

- **Strength and power.** Following the specificity principle, choose exercises that develop the specific muscle groups used in your sport and that work your muscles in patterns similar to those used while performing your activity. The intensity of strength training is determined by your goals, as outlined in Chapter 4. Think about the length of time you use your muscles during your sport (muscle endurance) to figure out how long each set of weight-training or other resistance exercises should be. For example, if you're training for skiing or snowboarding and your average run is three to six minutes, then focus on working your muscles for several minutes per set. To achieve this duration, you'll need to use lighter weights or less resistance.

Training tips for the weekend warrior

You know the type — and you may even be one yourself. The guy who rouses himself from the couch once a year to play softball at the company picnic. The gal who hasn't golfed in six months but starts hitting 200 balls a day as soon as the driving range opens in the spring. The every-once-in-a-while basketball or volleyball player. The weekend warrior participates in sports infrequently, but sometimes with great enthusiasm.

People who play in a seasonal league or sport, such as bowling, softball, skiing or snowboarding, may also fall into the weekend warrior syndrome when they start the season cold, with no preparation or conditioning in the months beforehand.

Being physically inactive or active on a sporadic, infrequent basis increases your risk of injury. Many significant injuries also occur as a result of lack of conditioning in the offseason. For example, you're more likely to get a tiny crack in a bone (stress fracture) if you do too much too soon, which is common among weekend warriors.

Here are some tips for avoiding getting hurt when you start your sports season or a new physical activity:

- Get fit before you play. If you're in a league or participate in a seasonal sport such as skiing, start training well before the start of the season. Ideally, you'll stay conditioned throughout the year. Your preparation should include some activity-specific skills as well as strength and flexibility training.
- Make sure to warm up before your activity and cool down afterward.
- Start slow and progress slowly. If you haven't pitched in years, don't start out throwing 50 balls at a time.
- Avoid sudden changes in intensity or type of exercise.
- Be steady and consistent with your workouts.
- Listen to your body — it will tell you when to slow down. Stop your activity if you feel pain, especially in joints.

In addition, follow the suggestions for preventing injuries listed in Chapter 6.

For power training useful in sports such as basketball and volleyball, plyometric activities are one of the best choices. Plyometric exercises use the body's natural stretch reflex. They involve rapid muscle stretches followed immediately by contractions of the same muscles. The goal is to produce a stronger, faster muscle response and forceful, explosive movement. Plyometrics include hopping, bounding, jumping quickly from one height to another and tossing a medicine ball or other heavy object. (For examples of plyometrics, see pages 185-187.)

Plyometrics (plyos) are hard on your body and can be dangerous if done incorrectly. It's best to get some training from a fitness specialist about how to do them. It's also a good idea to do plyos on a mat or other softer surface.

- **Flexibility.** Good flexibility is essential to successful performance and injury prevention in any sport or physical activity. After determining which muscles and motions are involved in your activity, choose a few exercises that stretch those muscles and move the joints through a full range of motion.
- **Balance.** Balance training is most important for sports and activities that are performed on unstable surfaces, such as wet grass, hills, snow or slippery roads, or activities that reduce your base of support, as when you stand on one leg. Almost any strength training exercise can be modified to simultaneously add a balance challenge,

which builds your strength in a more activity-specific manner. (For balance exercises, see pages 181-184.)

SPORTS TO CONSIDER

Whether you're new to a sport or have been doing it for years, you can tailor your workouts to your activity. When designing your training program, consider the sport's specific energy demands, muscular action, sport-specific movements and common injuries.

In the wide world of sports, your choices are endless. This section offers tips on training for a variety of common sports. These are starting points for improving your performance and minimizing your chance of injury.

Basketball

Basketball requires speed, agility and power. Players must be able to run the court, change direction quickly and jump repeatedly. And because the game moves in a continuous flow, players need an endurance base.

Basketball uses all three energy systems — immediate, short-term and long-term. The quick bursts of power for fast breaks, steals and jumps are fueled by the immediate and short-term systems. Slower-paced play, longer sustained actions and brief recovery periods draw fuel from the long-term aerobic system. The aerobic system helps prevent fatigue.

How to train. Throughout a basketball game, periods of high-intensity work are followed by quick recovery periods. To play well, you need both a strength base and an aerobic base.

Aerobic and anaerobic training are both important, but success in basketball depends more on anaerobic power and muscle endurance. That's why many professional basketball players look more like football players than marathoners. Strength training is a key component of a basketball program. Try to develop a base of strength through total-body weight training, with emphasis on legs and hips. For example, squats are a good way to build leg strength. You can make the squats even more effective for basketball by placing your feet in the same position as for a jump shot, and by alternating the speed, depth of squat and weight used. Other leg-strength exercises include lunges, step-ups, leg extensions, heel raises and leg curls. Multidirectional lunges will help improve your ability to rapidly change directions.

Anaerobic training for basketball may also include sprints and jumping plyometrics. Plyometrics help you develop explosive force — the strength you need to jump fast and high. These exercises,

Protect your eyes

According to Prevent Blindness America, many eye injuries are sports- or play-related. Sports-related eye injuries usually result from a blow to the eye and can include scratches on the cornea, retinal detachment, inflamed iris, fracture of the eye socket and bleeding inside the eye.

Prevent Blindness America recommends that people wear eye guards when participating in sports. For many sports, prescription glasses, sunglasses and occupational safety glasses don't provide adequate protection. People who wear glasses with plastic or case-hardened lenses have some protection against eye injury, but it's safer to wear prescription eye guards.

Sports eye guards come in a variety of shapes and sizes. Choose the eye protection that's appropriate for your sport. Eye guards designed for use in racket sports are also commonly used for basketball, baseball and soccer. Baseball and softball players should also wear batting helmets.

Follow these tips for buying eye guards:

- Shop at sports specialty or optical stores. Ask a sales representative to help you find an appropriate protector and adjust the fit.
- Make sure the eye guards have lenses that either stay in place or pop outward in case of an accident. Avoid eye guards without lenses or with lenses that pop in against your eyes.
- Choose eye guards that fit securely and comfortably and, if necessary, can be worn with a helmet.
- Some eye guards have an anti-fog coating or side vents to help prevent fogging of the lenses, which can occur when you're sweating.
- Eye protectors made of polycarbonate material are the most impact resistant.

including hops and jumps from different heights, use your body weight and the force of gravity for resistance.

Focus the aerobic component of your basketball training program more on maintaining an aerobic base than on improving your aerobic capacity. If you're playing basketball frequently — a couple of times a week or more — the practice and games may be enough to maintain aerobic fitness without having to do anything else. At times when you're not playing, do aerobic activities such as running, cycling and swimming at least three days a week for 30 minutes at a time.

How to prevent injury. Ankle sprains are the most common basketball injury. In addition, the repetitive jumping, pivoting, and rapid acceleration and deceleration in basketball put players at risk of overuse injuries such as jumper's knee, which is inflammation of the tendons of the kneecap (patella). Tears of the knee's anterior cruciate ligament (ACL) are also common. To reduce your risk of injuries, follow these precautions:

- Maintain appropriate flexibility, especially in the hamstring muscles. Tightness in this area is associated with the development of jumper's knee.
- Use balance and plyometric exercises to help prevent knee injuries such as tears of the ACL. Use strength and balance training to reduce the risk of initial or recurrent ankle sprains. Build core strength to help prevent back pain, another common complaint among basketball players.
- Choose basketball shoes that fit snugly,

offer good support and are nonskid. For people who've sprained their ankle before, ankle braces can reduce the likelihood of re-injury, although their role in preventing a first sprain is less clear.
- Wear protective knee and elbow pads to help prevent bruises and scrapes.
- Wear a mouth guard.
- Use safety glasses or eye guards to protect your eyes. (See "Protect your eyes," page 281.)

Biking

Bicycling is one of the most popular activities in the United States. Almost 60 million people ride at least once a year, and more than 15 million enthusiasts average at least one ride a week.

The right training program for cycling depends on whether you do road biking or mountain biking. As the name implies, road biking takes place on paved roads. For this type of cycling, you can ride a cruiser (comfort) bike, a recumbent bike, a fitness (hybrid) bike, or a road (touring, racing) bike. Mountain biking, one of the world's fastest growing sports, takes you off-road to hills, trails and rough roads. Mountain bikes are sturdier than the average road or hybrid bicycle (see "The right bike for you," on page 283).

Road biking and cross-country mountain biking require mainly aerobic metabolism. Downhill mountain biking is a power sport that relies more on the anaerobic energy systems. Road cyclists also use anaerobic energy sources when they climb hills or sprint.

The right bike for you

What type of bike should you get? That depends on how you want to use your bicycle. Think about where you'll ride and what type of riding you'll do. Are you planning on an occasional ride for pleasure, or will you be commuting by bike to work every day?

  To help choose the right bike for your needs, here are some guidelines.

Type of bike	Features	Uses	Advantages and disadvantages
Mountain	• A sturdy frame • Wide tires with extra tread • A semiupright riding position • Straight handlebars	Biking in off-road areas, such as dirt roads, trails, rough terrain and steep, rocky slopes	Not suited for long-distance or high-speed road riding
Road (also referred to as touring or racing)	• Lightweight • Drop handlebars • Narrow, smooth tires • 24 to 30 speeds	Riding long distances or in races	Best choice for dedicated cyclists who regularly go for long rides; may be uncomfortable for people with back problems because of bent-over riding position
Fitness (hybrid)	• A blend of mountain and road bike • A semiupright riding position	Commuting, doing fitness riding, riding on smooth off-road paths	Heavier than a road bike, with a less aerodynamic riding position
Recumbent	• A lightweight frame • A large seat with full back support • Pedals in front, not below • Lower to ground	Riding on flat roads and downhill	Comfortable riding position, especially for people with back, neck and shoulder problems; less pressure on arms and wrists; knees may get sore, especially when biking uphill; limited visibility in traffic
Cruiser (comfort)	• An upright riding position • A wide saddle • 1 to 3 or more speeds • A heavier frame	Taking short, leisurely rides	Not well suited for hills, longer distances

Helmet savvy

When you're biking, in-line skating, skiing or snowboarding, you're at increased risk of falling. Even a low-speed fall can change your life forever if your head hits the street, sidewalk, curb, a car, tree or other hard object. A head injury can cause brain damage or even death.

The best way to reduce your chance of head injuries is to wear a helmet whenever you engage in an activity that leaves your head vulnerable. In many states, bike helmets are required for riders under age 16.

If you don't own a helmet or have one that's several years old, invest in a new one. Newer helmets are better ventilated and offer more features than older styles do. Still, any helmet is better than none.

When shopping for and using a helmet, consider these tips:

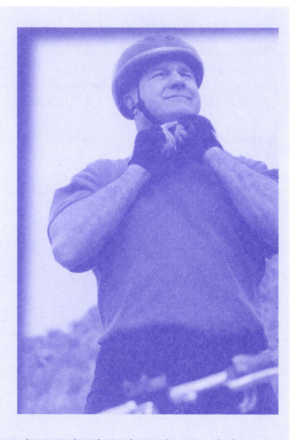

- All bike helmets are suitable for in-line skating, but helmets for skateboarding, snowboarding, skiing and other sports have different designs. If you're going to be snowboarding or skateboarding, choose a helmet designed for that sport.
- Look for a bike helmet with a label that indicates it meets the standards of the American National Standards Institute or Snell Memorial Foundation. All bike helmets must meet the Consumer Product Safety Commission standard for impact absorption.
- To be effective, your helmet should be the right size, with a proper fit. It should sit flat on your head about an inch above your eyebrows and have snug straps. It should stay in place when pushed upward from the front and shouldn't tilt in any direction or slide from side to side. In general, choose the smallest helmet that fits without feeling too tight. Try it on before you buy it.
- Look for a helmet that breathes. Effective ventilation helps keep you from overheating.
- Ease of use is also important. If you have trouble adjusting the helmet to fit your head or find it uncomfortable to wear, you're less likely to use it.
- Replace your helmet if it has been in an accident. Helmets lose the ability to cushion a blow after they've been damaged.
- Replace your helmet at least every five years or if its impact-absorbing foam is dented or cracked due to an accident or dropping. Replace the chin strap if any part of the buckle breaks so that the helmet doesn't come off in an accident.

How to train. A good aerobic foundation is essential for all types of cycling. Even if you're mainly climbing hills or sprinting, aerobic training allows you to recover more easily from hard exercise. To build your aerobic capacity, bike or do another aerobic activity for 30 minutes or more three to six times a week. Cyclists who ride in long-distance road races use a technique called overdistance training, which involves biking for a longer time than the race time at a slower pace than usual.

For anaerobic training, consider interval training two or three times a week. For example, alternate two to five minutes of hill climbing or sprinting with periods of biking at a lower intensity. For strength training, concentrate on resistance exercises that develop muscle strength and balance on both sides of the body, particularly the legs. Squats, lunges, leg extensions, leg curls, step-ups and heel raises are all useful exercises for biking.

How to prevent injury. The most common bicycling injury is abrasion, also known as road rash, caused by a crash or fall from the bike. With an abrasion or scrape, the wound can be deep.

Falls account for about half of all bicycle mishaps, while collisions with cars, other bikes or objects also cause accidents. Collisions and falls can result in a variety of injuries, from minor bruises and cuts to concussions, other head injuries and broken bones, particularly in the upper extremities. Head injuries are the most serious bicycle injuries and are responsible for most of the approximately 1,000 bicycling deaths in the United States each year.

Overuse injuries are also common in cycling. They're often the result of biking for too long or at too high an intensity, such as overdoing hills or higher gears. The knee is the most common site of overuse injuries in cyclists. Low back pain, sunburn, and saddle sores or chafing are other common complaints.

Spinning

Spinning classes are the biggest thing to hit the fitness industry since step aerobics. In these indoor cycling classes, an enthusiastic instructor guides you through a varied workout, complete with exciting visual imagery and music. But even though these classes are often promoted as being suitable for beginners, the workouts can be very intense, lasting 40 minutes or more. The intensity may be far beyond what most novices can maintain.

If you're considering a spinning class, it's worthwhile to get into shape for it by doing some cycling-specific training beforehand. Work on cardiovascular conditioning by riding a stationary bike or doing another aerobic activity. You can increase your endurance by interspersing periods of high-intensity cycling with more relaxed pedaling.

The training suggestions for bicycling also work for an indoor cycling class. When you do get to class, make sure to exercise at the right pace for you. It's easy to be intimidated by the high speeds and furious intensities of the people around you. Listen to your body and adjust the bike's tension and your pedaling speed accordingly. Don't be afraid to sit back and take a break when necessary.

Most cycling injuries can be avoided with proper training, bike maintenance, sizing and fitting of your bike, and protective equipment. Using a helmet reduces head-injury rates by as much as 85 percent to 95 percent. To help prevent cycling injuries, follow these guidelines:

- Wear a helmet. (See "Helmet savvy," page 284.)

- Check the size and fit of your bicycle. Be sure it's not too large or small for your frame. While seated on the bicycle, you should be able to put a foot on the ground to steady yourself. In addition, when you pedal, your knee should be nearly — but not quite fully — extended. To ensure a proper fit, have your bike fitted at a bike shop.

- Keep your bike equipment well maintained and in good working order.

- Aim for a pedaling rate of around 80 revolutions a minute. Setting the gears to make pedaling too hard can strain your knees.

- When pedaling up a hill, use a low gear. Climbing hills in too high a gear is hard on the knees. If the hill is too much for you, get off and walk.

- Bicycle gloves can protect against scrapes from falls, blisters and other injuries. If you're mountain biking, wear knee and elbow pads as well.

- If you develop low back pain when biking, try tilting the saddle slightly forward or changing the handlebars to a more upright position.

- To prevent knee pain, maintain flexibility in your leg and knee muscles with stretching. Pay particular attention to stretching your leg muscles and your Achilles tendon before and after you ride. Strength training with knee extensions, hamstring curls and hip work also can help.

- To prevent or reduce wrist pain, which is relatively common in long-distance riders, periodically change your grip and hand position.

Bowling

Bowling isn't the most physically demanding sport, but it does require strength, balance, flexibility and good eye-hand coordination. Bowling mainly draws on the immediate and short-term energy sources. Aerobic endurance plays only a minor role in bowling.

How to train. Strong muscles help you maximize power and control in your bowling game. A strength training program for bowling should focus on the areas you use in the sport as well as areas in which you're weak or injury prone. Train your leg muscles to improve balance, your torso to improve stability, and your upper body muscles to improve strength, power and accuracy. Aim for two to three strength training sessions a week.

To improve your balance, consider exercises such as weight shifts and ball tosses while standing on one leg.

How to prevent injury. Bowlers are susceptible to back, shoulder, knee, hip, elbow, wrist, hand and finger injuries. Hand injuries are common. The finger joints may become somewhat stiff, and compression of a nerve in the thumb can result in numbness, a condition known as bowler's thumb. Back injuries are also common, often due to imbalances in the strength of different trunk muscles.

To bowl safely and reduce your risk of injury, consider these tips:

- Warm up before bowling. Start with a few minutes of light aerobic exercise, followed by stretches that work the muscles you use in bowling — including your low back, hamstrings and trunk muscles.
- Use protective bowling gloves to help prevent skin disorders and injury to the hands.
- Pay attention to the grip and fit of your bowling ball. Have your hands and fingers measured to determine the proper grip. Balls with large holes, rounded smooth holes or rubber inserts can help prevent hand problems.
- When strength training, make sure to work areas that are prone to injury, including your shoulders, hips, low back, elbows and wrists. Strengthening your core muscles will help prevent back pain.

Golfing

For millions of people, golf isn't just a sport, it's a passion. And with the success of Tiger Woods — who spends time training in the gym as well as on the course —

more golfers are realizing the importance of overall fitness. A golf-specific training program can improve your game.

Golf requires strength, flexibility, endurance, agility, balance, coordination and skill. Your muscles, particularly those of your legs and torso, must be both strong and flexible to generate club speed and brace against injuries.

The quick burst of energy and power needed to swing a golf club comes from the immediate and short-term energy systems. Golf relies almost exclusively on these anaerobic energy sources. Even if you don't use a cart, golf isn't considered an aerobic sport because of its stop-and-go nature.

How to train. A thorough golf training program focuses on all the major areas of fitness — strength, flexibility, balance and aerobic endurance. Such a program can reduce the risk of injury and improve your performance on the course. Strength and flexibility training also help limit or delay the decline in spine strength and flexibility that happens as you age.

Most of the power for a golf swing comes from the lower body and trunk. Your training should focus on these areas. Low back pain is one of the most common complaints among golfers at all levels. This isn't surprising because tremendous forces are generated in the spine as the trunk coils during the backswing to unwind during the downswing.

Strengthening the lower body builds a base of support, and strengthening the trunk, including the low back, hips and core, helps generate power and protect the spine. One set of eight to 12 repetitions lifting lighter weights three days a week works well.

Flexibility exercises are also critical for developing a fluid, full golf swing and preventing injury. A golf swing requires a considerable range of motion of many joints. Stretching exercises help you maintain or increase your range of motion in your shoulders, trunk, hip flexors, low back and hamstrings. Your stretching exercises should include these areas as well as the elbows and wrists. It's best to do stretching exercises every day. Always warm up your muscles before you stretch them.

Although golf isn't an aerobic sport, cardiovascular conditioning helps keep you from getting tired during a long round of golf. Aim to fit in at least 30 minutes of walking, cycling or other aerobic activity at least three times a week.

Some golfers use plyometric exercises to increase their swing velocity. These exercises train your muscles to swing faster and more explosively. One such exercise involves tossing a medicine ball very quickly. Balance exercises are also useful because golf takes place on unstable, uneven surfaces, such as sand traps and hills. Some golfers find yoga useful for improving balance, flexibility, posture and mind-body awareness.

How to prevent injury. Although golf is often regarded as a safe sport, injuries are common in golfers of all levels. Among recreational golfers, the most common injuries are to the lower back, elbow, shoulder and wrist. The frequency of low back injuries is attributed to the high forces and repetitive nature of golf swings and the twisting motion of the swing. These actions place stress on the lower back and can lead to overuse injury and nonfluid body mechanics when swinging.

Poor swing mechanics can contribute to shoulder and elbow injuries. Golfer's elbow is pain on the inside of the elbow where the tendons of your forearm muscles attach to the bony prominence (epicondyle). The pain may spread into the forearm and wrist.

Wrist injuries are common in golfers. Because of the large number of tendons crossing the wrist, many forms of tendinitis can occur.

Other injuries happen when players are hit with golf clubs or balls or when they're exposed to lightning, high heat and humidity, and sun.

To reduce your risk of injury on the golf course, follow these guidelines:

- Warm up properly before a round of golf. After five minutes of walking, do some simple stretches to loosen your back, shoulders, elbows, wrists, forearms and legs. Some gentle swings of one or two clubs will also help limber you up. A few minutes of chipping and putting can get you in the rhythm.
- To prevent back injury, tailor your strength training for a combination of stronger abdominal muscles and

more flexible back muscles. Modifying your swing may also help prevent back injury.

- To avoid overuse injuries, give your body time to adapt to repetitive loads. If you haven't golfed since last September, don't go out in May and start hitting 200 balls a day.

In-line skating

In-line skating, also known as rollerblading, is one of the fastest growing recreational sports in the world. More than 30 million people in the United States skate for fun and exercise. In-line skating is a highly aerobic, low-impact sport that's easy to learn.

In-line skating is also a favorite cross-training activity for people who participate in winter sports such as skiing, skating and hockey. It's a good cross-training choice for runners who want to add a low-impact activity to their programs.

The push-and-glide action of in-line skating uses both the anaerobic and aerobic energy systems. Pushing off requires power and strength, as does balancing on a set of narrow, rolling wheels. The sustained, large-muscle work of in-line skating taps the aerobic system. Skating burns as many calories as running does and provides a better aerobic workout than cycling does. It strengthens the muscles of your legs, buttocks and lower back.

How to train. A training program for in-line skating should focus on cardiovascular conditioning, but strength, flexibility and balance are also important. Strength-

ening exercises can make skating easier, flexibility exercises can help you avoid muscle injury and strain, and balance training can help reduce your risk of falls.

Build your aerobic endurance by skating or doing other aerobic activities for at least 30 minutes five or six times a week. Options for anaerobic training include skating up hills, lifting weights, hiking in the mountains, bicycling up hills and doing strength exercises such as lunges, squats, toe raises, ab crunches, hip abductor strengthening and lateral jumps. A training tool called a slide board can help you develop lateral strength as well as balance and agility. The slide board has a slick top surface. Wearing special booties, you glide from side to side over the board in a skating motion. Modified strength training exercises that challenge your balance can also be useful (see the "Exercise guide," pages 181-184).

Two or three sessions of these strength-building activities each week are adequate. Focus on working the muscles you use in skating — those of the legs (quadriceps, hamstrings, calves, shins), groin (abductor, adductor), buttocks (gluteus minimus, gluteus maximus), hips, low back and abdomen.

Add flexibility exercises to your workout before and after you skate. After warming up with a five-minute walk or jog, stretch your calves, hamstrings, quadriceps, upper and lower back, torso and neck. Other important areas for flexibility include the adductors and hip flexors. Trunk rotation exercises are also useful.

How to prevent injury. Along with the surge in popularity of in-line skating has come a dramatic increase in skating-related accidents and injuries. Fortunately, most of them are minor and don't require treatment, but serious injuries and even deaths have occurred. Because skaters can reach high speeds and braking is tricky, falls and collisions are common and account for almost all injuries among recreational skaters. Typically, falls occur when a skater loses his or her balance, runs into an uneven surface or has trouble stopping when going downhill. Beginning skaters are at greatest risk of falling.

Wrist, forearm and elbow injuries are the most common skating injuries. Falling onto an outstretched hand with your wrist and elbow extended can cause a fracture of the wrist or elbow. Scrapes and bruises from falling are also common. Other injuries associated with in-line skating are head injuries, knee pain, stress fractures to the foot, lower leg or ankle, and other problems with the lower leg and ankle, such as tendinitis, bursitis and sprains.

Take these precautions to reduce your risk of falling and getting hurt:

- Always wear protective gear, including wrist guards, knee and elbow pads, and a helmet. A bike helmet works fine. (See "Helmet savvy," page 284.) Although safety gear doesn't provide 100 percent protection, it reduces the frequency and severity of injuries. In one study, skaters who didn't wear wrist guards were 10 times more likely to injure their wrists than were those who wore the guards. (For more information about wrist guards, see "Wrist-ready," page 301.)
- Warm up before your workout. Muscles that are warmed up are more pliable and relaxed, which helps them better absorb a fall.
- Learn safe-skating techniques and the basic skills of the sport, especially how to stop properly. Learn from a qualified instructor or watch an instructional video.
- Keep your body loose at all times, with your knees bent, arms to your sides and center of gravity low. This puts you in a better position to absorb a fall.
- Make sure your skates fit properly. They should be snug — your feet shouldn't have a lot of room to move around. But don't buy skates that put too much pressure on any part of your foot because this can cause blisters.
- Keep your equipment in good working order. Skate wheels should be rotated every 40 to 50 miles and replaced when damaged or worn out.
- Skate in safe areas and under good conditions. Anticipate hazards such as hills,

potholes, water and sand. Avoid public roads, if possible, and obey traffic regulations and signals if you have to use public roadways. Don't skate at night not only because it's difficult for others to see you but also because it's harder for you to see obstacles.

Kayaking and canoeing

Kayaks and canoes have been used for centuries as a means of transportation. They'll still get you from point to point, but these watercraft have moved beyond function to fun and fitness. Kayaking and canoeing are popular for casual recreation and serious training.

Kayaks are generally smaller than canoes. You sit in the craft with your feet in front of you and use a double-bladed paddle. You can kayak on lakes, rivers or oceans. Some kayaks are designed for white-water paddling or surfing.

When canoeing, you sit or kneel and generally use a single-bladed paddle. Canoes range from all-purpose types such as the ones at summer camps to solo touring canoes to white-water craft.

Kayaking and canoeing rely on both anaerobic and aerobic energy pathways. Upper body strength is important for paddling, and aerobic fitness provides the endurance needed for long outings.

How to train. The aerobic component of your training program can be kayaking,

canoeing or another aerobic activity such as walking or jogging. Do these activities 30 minutes a day three to six times a week. Vary the intensity of your training to simulate low- and high-intensity aspects of rowing and paddling.

In addition, incorporate strength exercises about three times a week. Focus on the muscles you use to power your stroke, which are the chest, abdomen, upper and lower back, shoulders, arms, wrists and hands. In particular, it's important to strengthen the rotator cuff and the shoulder blade (scapula) muscles. Useful strengthening exercises include a variety of rows, lat pull-downs, back extensions, core work including rotation exercises, biceps curls, wrist curls, reverse wrist curls and triceps extensions. Doing upper body strength training in the seated position can simulate how muscles will be used in kayaking and canoeing. Performing these exercises seated on a stability ball can simulate an unstable surface similar to being seated in a kayak or canoe on the water. (For more information about stability balls, see Chapter 5.)

Flexibility exercises are also important for preventing injury. Pay special attention to your low back, hamstrings, shoulders, forearms and wrists.

How to prevent injury. Paddle sports carry a risk of hypothermia, which is dangerously low body temperature. It can happen when you're wet and cold, from either falling in the water or doing activities in inclement weather. Your risk of hypothermia increases in cold water and in cold, windy, damp weather.

Shoulder injuries are also prevalent among paddlers. Chronic shoulder pain caused by damage to the rotator cuff (impingement syndrome) is the most common shoulder injury that paddlers experience. Back strain and elbow and wrist injuries are frequently seen in kayakers and canoeists.

Here are some guidelines to help avoid injury:

- Wear a personal flotation device (PFD).
- Dress appropriately for the weather and water conditions. If the water is cold, wear a wet suit or dry suit and dress in layers. In hot, sunny weather, wear lightweight clothing, waterproof sunscreen and a wide-brimmed hat. If you're going to be venturing onto white water or into the surf, wear a helmet.
- Get some training in basic paddling strokes and techniques and rescue skills. Take a class.
- To protect your shoulders, keep your hands in front of your body when paddling. During the part of the stroke when the paddle blade is behind you, turn to look at it by rotating your upper body, including your shoulders. This helps you to maintain better alignment between your trunk and shoulders. Also follow a shoulder-exercise routine designed to strengthen your rotator cuffs.

- Make sure your craft is in good repair, with the appropriate safety equipment.
- Grip the paddle loosely.
- Develop good swimming skills.

Running

Ever since the running boom of the 1970s, the sport has been part of the American scene. About 40 million to 50 million people in the United States run at least two or three days a week. Many people find running is the fastest way to reach and maintain a desired fitness level. Others enjoy the challenge of running in races, from 5-kilometer (5K, or 3.1-mile) events to marathons (26 miles, 385 yards).

Running draws primarily on the aerobic energy system. Sprinting short distances, by contrast, relies almost exclusively on the anaerobic systems. Which energy source is used depends on the intensity and duration of the run. A long-distance run at a slow-to-moderate pace will produce constant energy with little or no buildup of lactic acid, a byproduct of anaerobic energy production. This type of training is referred to as pure endurance.

If you increase your speed, continuing at a steady pace, there will be a minor increase in lactic acid, and a mixture of anaerobic and aerobic energy will be used. Higher running speeds result in a buildup of lactic acid and other metabolic byproducts that eventually forces you to stop or slow down.

How to train. A training program for running will stem from your specific goals. Do you want to simply maintain

Getting started on a running program

If you're new to running or getting back to it after an extended break, take it easy. To avoid injuries, plan a progressive program that takes you from walking to jogging. Progressing slowly allows your muscles to adapt to the rigors of running.

The American Council on Exercise suggests the following training plan to ease into jogging and running. Exercise according to this plan three days a week, with days off in between. Begin jogging when you can easily tolerate brisk walking for at least 22 minutes. Don't forget to warm up before, and cool down after, exercising.

Week	Time (in minutes)	Intensity
1	20	Walk
2	22	Walk
3	22	Jog 30 to 60 seconds, walk 5 minutes and repeat
4	24	Same as week 3
5	24	Jog 30 to 60 seconds, walk 4 minutes and repeat
6	26	Same as week 5
7	26	Jog 30 to 60 seconds, walk 3 minutes and repeat
8	28	Same as week 7
9	28	Jog 30 to 60 seconds, walk 2 minutes and repeat
10	30	Same as week 9
11	30	Jog 2 minutes, walk 1 minute and repeat
12+	30	Gradually progress to continuous jogging

Running after injury

If you're returning to running after an injury, take precautions to avoid re-injury. First, talk to your doctor about when and how to get back to running and whether you need to observe any limitations. Here are some general guidelines:

- Make sure to warm up before running.
- Start with a slower pace, perhaps jogging or brisk walking, and gradually work up to a faster running pace.
- At first, run only on alternate days. Build up your frequency gradually.
- At first, you may need to avoid running on hills.
- Make sure your shoes aren't contributing to your risk of injury. (See "The ideal running shoe," page 294.)
- Listen to your body. Stop if you have pain.

aerobic fitness? Are you training for a 10K (6.2-mile) or longer race? Are you running primarily to lose weight? Whatever your goals, the basis of any training program will be runs of fairly long duration (30 to 40 minutes or longer) at a steady pace.

If you're just starting out, ease into a training program by first walking the distance you want to run. Over time, move up to relaxed runs broken into segments interspersed with walking for a total exercise session of 30 to 40 minutes.

Once you've become proficient at running, your usual run should be 30 to 40 minutes or longer at an intensity of about 75 percent of your maximum heart rate

The ideal running shoe

Shoes are a runner's most important piece of equipment. Properly fitting running shoes can help prevent injuries, blisters and sore muscles. Worn or ill-fitting shoes can lead to hip and low back problems as well as foot and leg injuries.

If you're a runner, you'll want to select your shoes carefully. But with hundreds of models to choose from, how do you find the ideal running shoe? Start by evaluating your feet. Do you have high, low or neutral arches? Do your feet tend to tilt inward (pronation) or outward (supination)? (See "Shopping tips" on page 128 for information on determining what type of foot you have and how to buy a shoe that's right for you.)

The three most important features of a running shoe are shock absorption (cushion), motion control and stability. The best combination of these depends on the characteristics of your feet. For all running shoes, flexibility in the forefoot is important to allow easy flexing motion of the foot as you push off the toe.

The shoe's midsole is probably the most important part because it provides cushioning, supports the foot and absorbs shock. A running shoe's midsole shouldn't be too hard or too soft. Midsoles are typically made of ethyl vinyl acetate (EVA), a spongy, cushy material that's a good shock absorber. Often the EVA is molded and compressed, a process that makes the

If your feet have:	Look for these features:
Low arches, inward tilt (pronation)	• Good motion control and stability • Firm, stable heel counter • Forefoot flexibility • Hard midsole • Good arch support • Straight or slightly curved last • High rear-foot stability (heel stabilizer)
High arches, excessive outward tilt (supination)	• Good cushioning • Firm, stable heel counter • Forefoot flexibility • Soft midsoles • Curved or slightly curved last • Lower rear-foot stability
Neutral features	• Firm, stable heel counter • Forefoot flexibility • Firm midsoles • Semicurved or slightly curved last • Moderate rear-foot stability

(MHR) — a pace at which you could pass the talk test and carry on a conversation. (To calculate your MHR, see page 49, and for more on the talk test, see page 79.)

If you're training for competition, you might also include longer runs and harder sessions in your routine. These might be:

material more resistant to flattening. A flattened midsole loses its shock-absorbing capability. The chart at the bottom of page 294 shows shoe features that are appropriate for different foot types. (See also "Anatomy of an athletic shoe" on page 127.)

A good fit is essential. Buy shoes to fit your larger foot if your feet aren't the same size. There should be at least a thumbnail's width between the end of your longest toe and the end of the shoe. A properly fitted shoe will bend where your foot bends.

The shoes should be of quality construction. Shoes with synthetic fabric uppers, such as nylon or mesh, are lightweight, washable and breathable, so your feet don't overheat. Running shoes should have a padded tongue to cushion against pressure and a padded ankle collar to cushion the ankle.

Keep in mind that your shoes may still feel comfortable but might not be providing you with enough shock absorption or support. Running shoe midsoles might be worn down to the point of causing chronic wear-type injuries, but you may not actually be able to see the wear and tear. Sixty percent of a shoe's shock absorption is lost after 250 to 500 miles of use. Running shoes should be replaced about every 300 to 400 miles. If you run up to 10 miles a week, that means getting new shoes every seven to 10 months.

- Tempo or speed endurance runs, in which you run at a fast pace that you can maintain for only 15 to 20 minutes
- Hill runs
- Interval training, in which you alternate intensive and more relaxed exercise segments within a single session
- Fartlek (speed play) training, a form of interval training in which you vary your pace from slow to fast.

To minimize the risk of injury and muscle and joint discomfort, run on alternate days, no more than three or four times a week. Although you may gain some additional benefit by training five to six days a week, the risk of injury also increases. On alternate days you can cross-train with other aerobic activities, such as biking, swimming and in-line skating.

Anaerobic training such as weightlifting and hill running will improve your muscular endurance. In addition, strength and stretching exercises will help provide a balanced and varied workload for your body, increase your overall strength and preserve a full range of motion in all your joints. In these exercises, focus especially on your lower body muscles, including the quadriceps, hamstrings, gluteals, hip abductors, groin, lower back and abdomen.

Runners often believe that their hips and lower bodies are strong because running uses the legs, but that's not necessarily true. Exercises that strengthen the lower body are important for all runners. These include lunges, squats and hip abductor exercises. Adequate core strength is also important.

How to prevent injury. Running can be hard on your joints. The impact from repetitive pounding can lead to overuse injuries to the knees, lower legs, feet and ankles. Studies suggest that 40 percent to 60 percent of runners sustain an injury each year.

One of the primary causes of overuse injuries in runners is poor shock absorption. Your muscles are your body's primary shock absorbers. Without strong muscles, bones and ligaments are subjected to too much stress, which can lead to injury. That's another reason strengthening exercises are so important. Proper shoes also play a role in shock absorption. (See "The ideal running shoe," on page 294.)

Another common cause of running injuries is overdoing it — running too much or too intensely without adequate recovery time. Runners who consistently log more than 40 miles a week or run seven days a week without rest days are injured more than are those who run less.

Runner's knee (patellofemoral stress syndrome) is the most common running injury. It encompasses a variety of conditions characterized by pain around the front of the knee. Pain at the side of the knee (iliotibial band syndrome), shin pain, stress fractures to the shinbone (tibia) or forefoot, Achilles tendon injuries, heel pain, and pain along the bottom of the foot (plantar fasciitis) are other common problems in runners.

Blisters on the feet and chafing of the skin in the groin area are also common problems, especially for long-distance runners. Blisters may occur when you run long distances in new shoes before they're broken in. Wearing dry, comfortable running socks can also help prevent blisters. Use of over-the-counter powders may help reduce chafing. Wearing clothing that fits firmly and doesn't rub against your skin with every stride may also help protect against chafing.

Many running injuries can be prevented by following these guidelines:

- Warm up before running. Start with a five-minute walk or jog, followed by stretching exercises. Stretching is even more important after running. Make sure your stretching and flexibility exercises include your calf muscles, hamstrings, quadriceps, hip abductors, hip flexors, lower back and trunk.

- Don't overdo it. Run on alternate days, no more than three or four days a week. Cross-training with low-impact activities allows you to maintain your cardiovascular conditioning with less risk of injury. Limit speed training, interval training and other hard workouts to twice a week.

- Use good form. Keep your head level and your shoulders down and relaxed. Avoid bouncing, and lean forward slightly from the ankles, not the waist. Strike the ground relatively flat-footed, then push off from the toes.

- Wear the right shoe for your foot. Shoes are the most important piece of equipment for runners. (See "The ideal running shoe," page 294.)

- Dress appropriately for the weather conditions. (See "Clothing," page 131, and "Weather and climate" on page 203.) Start your run feeling a little cool because your body temperature will increase as you run.

- When possible, run on a clear, smooth, flat and reasonably soft surface.

- Avoid always running in the same direction on an angled or sloped circular track in order to reduce stress on the same leg.

- Avoid running when you're overly fatigued — at the point where your muscles aren't working well. When your muscles are tired, they're less able to absorb shock.

Skiing

Downhill (Alpine) skiing and cross-country (Nordic) skiing are very different sports, though both give participants a chance to get out and enjoy the winter. Millions of people worldwide take to the slopes and trails to stay fit, compete in races and appreciate nature.

Embodying the timeless sensations of speed and rhythm, downhill skiing requires strength, balance, coordination, agility, endurance and flexibility to maintain control as you work against the forces of gravity, friction, wind and centrifugal force. Downhill skiing relies primarily on the anaerobic immediate and short-term energy systems, which are used when you turn and change position. The aerobic long-term energy pathway also contributes, making it easier to work out at high altitude and protecting against fatigue.

Cross-country skiing is an endurance sport that takes the skier across various types of terrain. You can ski in your own backyard, on a local golf course, up and down hiking trails or along groomed cross-country ski trails. Skiers may use the traditional (classic) style, with skis placed parallel to each other, or the more recent ski-skating style, which involves diagonal movements that are similar to those used in ice-skating and in-line skating.

Both traditional cross-country skiing and ski skating rely much more on the aerobic energy system than on the anaerobic systems. However, the latter can come into play during sprints or uphill climbs.

How to train. Start a conditioning program specifically for skiing at least eight to 10 weeks before the beginning of the ski season. For Alpine skiing, use a program that emphasizes strength training, jumping and plyometric exercises, and flexibility exercises. For strengthening, focus on exercises that work your quadriceps, hamstrings, low back, hip abduc-

tors, triceps and core muscles. Examples include squats or leg presses, lunges, hip abductor strengthening, back extensions and core work on a stability ball. When you're doing resistance training, set your number of repetitions to allow you to work for the duration of your typical Alpine ski run, which may be several minutes. Because cross-country skiing requires more upper body work than does Alpine skiing, upper back and shoulder strengthening is helpful.

Jumping and plyometric exercises, such as hopping from side to side or jumping off a box or over a line, help prepare you for the weight transfer and shifting essential to skiing. Other ways of building anaerobic power include sprint or interval training with running or biking, or use of a slide board.

Flexibility exercises are important for both downhill and cross-country skiing. Focus on stretching the quadriceps, hamstrings, groin, hip flexors, low back (especially with rotation) and abdomen.

Because balance is crucial in skiing, try training on unstable surfaces. For example, you could do strength exercises on a stability ball or while standing on a pillow or on one leg. See the "Exercise guide" beginning on page 182 for examples of how to increase the balance challenge in your strength training workouts.

Low-intensity, long-duration activities such as running and biking can help establish a good base of aerobic fitness for skiing. In-line skating and roller skiing are aerobic activities that imitate the movements of skiing. Roller skis are like short cross-country skis on wheels, and the action of roller skiing mimics cross-country skiing (skating or classic style). To use them, you mount ski boots on the roller skis.

For cross-country ski training, a wide range of activities can help you maintain and improve aerobic capacity. These include in-line skating, roller skiing, running, cycling, swimming and hiking.

How to prevent injury. Different types of injuries prevail in downhill skiers and cross-country skiers. Of the two sports, downhill skiing carries more risk because of the high speeds involved. In the 1960s, the most common downhill ski injuries were broken shinbones and ankle sprains. Thanks to modern ski boots and bindings, those types of injuries have declined. Unfortunately, knee injuries have increased sharply since 1980 because rigid ski boots transmit force to the knee.

Knee injuries include sprains and rupture of the anterior cruciate ligament (ACL), one of the crossing ligaments in the center of the knee. Other injuries frequently seen in downhill skiers include thumb sprain or fracture (skier's thumb), shoulder injuries and fractures of the upper leg or hipbone. Head injuries and spinal cord injuries, though not common, can be devastating. About 20 to 30 people die in skiing accidents each year in the United States. Most deaths occur when the skier goes out of control and hits a tree or other object.

Factors that may contribute to injury include fatigue, poor visibility, crowded slopes and equipment failure. Beginners are at much higher risk of injury than are more experienced skiers. Older skiers may also be at increased risk because of decreases in flexibility, ability to balance and degeneration of joint tissue.

In cross-country skiing, overuse injuries are more common than are acute injuries. As with downhill skiing, the knee is the most common site of injury in cross-country skiing. Low back pain is also common.

To reduce your risk of a ski-related injury, observe these guidelines:

- Before you put on your skis, make sure you're in good overall shape, including strength, flexibility, endurance and balance. Include the exercises described in the "How to train" section. Preseason conditioning is one of the most important elements of injury prevention.
- Pace yourself and rest when you're tired. Most ski injuries occur in the afternoon or at the end of the day.
- Give yourself time to get acclimated to higher altitude. If possible, slowly ascend to your high-altitude destination. Drink plenty of water and other fluids, but avoid alcohol, especially for the first several days you're acclimating. If you're concerned about altitude sickness, talk to your doctor about possible preventive measures.
- Dress appropriately for the weather.
- Wear a helmet to protect against head injuries. Most helmets designed for winter sports can be used for both skiing and snowboarding. Various types of helmets are available. Some are designed for com-

petition, and others are more suitable for recreational use. Many skiers prefer an open-face helmet. Some helmets have a built-in visor or can fit a visor attachment, which can cut overhead glare and help protect your face in wet or windy weather. Some helmets include venting to help prevent overheating.

- At the start of the day, take a couple of slow ski runs to warm up. Stretch major muscle groups before and after skiing.
- Watch out for rocks and patches of ice on ski trails. Stay on marked trails.
- Check the binding of each ski before skiing. Your bindings must be properly adjusted to your height and weight. Have your bindings set, adjusted, maintained and tested by a ski shop that follows standard practices.
- When downhill skiing, avoid using the safety strap on your ski poles. If you're falling, let go of your poles.

Snowboarding

Snowboarding is the new kid on the block of winter sports, but its popularity has exploded since the 1980s. It's the fastest growing winter sport in the United States, and snowboarders make up about 20 percent to 30 percent of all slope users at U.S. ski resorts.

Snowboarding differs from downhill skiing in many respects. Snowboarders ride with both feet affixed to a single board, standing sideways on the board. Unlike skiers, snowboarders don't use ski poles. The two sports also require some different skills.

Both sports, however, work some of the same muscle groups and have similar energy requirements. Like downhill skiing, snowboarding uses all three energy systems — immediate, short-term and long-term. The anaerobic energy sources contribute most to the demands of snowboarding, which include the power to carve turns by digging the edge of the board into the snow. Some snowboarders also take on the more extreme challenges of jumps and aerial or acrobatic maneuvers.

How to train. Year-round fitness is the ideal preparation for the snowboarding season. At a minimum, start training for snowboarding six to eight weeks before you hit the slopes for the first time of the season. With proper preparation, you can board more, feel better, and avoid injury and soreness.

A good base of aerobic fitness will help keep you from running out of steam halfway through a day on the slopes. To maintain aerobic endurance, participate in aerobic activities for 30 minutes four to six times a week. Anything that provides a good aerobic workout, including running, cycling, hiking and swimming, will work. In-line skating and mountain biking are great because they work your body in a way similar to that of snowboarding.

To maintain your snowboarding skills during the off-season, cross-train in activities that involve similar actions, such as surfing and skateboarding.

Incorporate the same strength exercises used for downhill skiing into your training program three days a week. However, because snowboarders tend to have one leg that's stronger than the other, exercise both legs independently. For example instead of doing squats on two legs, do them on one leg.

Don't neglect stretching, flexibility and balance exercises. Make sure to regularly stretch your legs, ankles, buttocks, hips, back and trunk rotator muscles. Balance challenges are also crucial. Many top snowboarders practice yoga for flexibility and balance. Exercising on an unstable surface such as a stability ball or while standing on a pillow or on one foot can be useful in strengthening balance.

How to prevent injury. Falling is an inevitable part of learning to snowboard. It's also the leading cause of snowboarding injuries, followed by jumps. Snowboarders usually fall backward, landing on their buttocks and head, or forward, landing on outstretched arms. Muscle strains and overuse injuries, including hip and back pain, are also common.

Compared with downhill skiers, snowboarders have a lower risk of knee injuries but a much higher risk of wrist and ankle injuries. Broken wrists are the most common snowboarding injury. The second most common injury is ankle injuries, including sprained ankles and snowboard-

Wrist-ready

Wrist injuries are common among snowboarders and in-line skaters because participants in these sports often use their arms and hands to break a fall. Wrist guards can help prevent injury by absorbing the impact of a fall and keeping the wrist from overextending. In addition to keeping your wrists relatively rigid, the guards may prevent your hands from getting scraped.

Several studies have shown that wrist guards are effective in preventing wrist injuries among snowboarders and in-line skaters. For example, a 10-year study published in 2002 and conducted by the Colorado Snowboard Injury Survey found that of the more than 7,400 snowboarders whose injuries were studied, those who wore wrist guards were half as likely to injure their wrists as were those not wearing the protection.

A variety of styles of wrist guards are available for both snowboarders and in-line skaters. Some snowboarders wear wrist guards similar to those worn by in-line skaters. Most of these guards are made of two plastic splints that hold the wrist in a relatively rigid position. Wrist guards designed specifically for snowboarders are also available. Some styles are worn over your gloves, and others fit inside the glove or are integrated into the glove itself.

A small 2004 study published in the *Journal of Sports Science and Medicine* suggested that wrist guards could be improved with the addition of padding. In a test of a prototype guard with padding on the palm side of wrist guards, the researchers found that splints and padding were substantially better than wrist guards without splints and padding.

er's ankle, which is a fracture of part of the ankle. Knee injuries are also frequent, but they tend to be less severe than knee injuries that occur in downhill skiing.

Beginning snowboarders often hit the back of the head in a fall, which may cause concussion. Most head injuries aren't serious, but head injury is the leading cause of death among snowboarders.

Reduce your risk of injury by following these guidelines:

- If you're new to the sport, take lessons from an instructor. Beginners have the highest injury rate. Indeed, almost one-fourth of all snowboarding injuries happen during a person's first experience. Most beginners need more training than a book or video can provide.
- Get in shape before the season, and prepare with sport-specific training. Without adequate preparation to specific muscles, even experienced boarders can suffer muscle strains at the start of the season.
- Strength training, flexibility and balance exercises can help reduce injury risk. Make these exercises part of your year-round routine.
- Wear wrist guards designed for snowboarding or in-line skating. (See "Wrist-ready," page 301.) Try to avoid breaking a fall with open hands. Hold your hands in closed fists while you ride. If possible, tuck and roll when you fall.
- Protect your head by wearing a helmet. Hard-packed snow or ice can be especially unyielding. Choose a helmet designed for snowboarding or skiing. Most snowboard helmets have a poly-

carbonate shell that's both strong and lightweight. For serious snowboarders who do a lot of tricks or faster snowboarding, a full-face, full-shell helmet or one designed for competition is appropriate. A helmet with good ventilation is the best choice for most conditions.

- Protect your knees, hips and elbows with pads. These can soften the blow when you fall.
- Consider hybrid boots. Snowboarding boots come in three styles — hard, soft and hybrid. Soft boots provide less ankle support, so wearing them makes you vulnerable to ankle injuries, but hard boots increase the risk of knee injury. A hybrid boot with moderate support may provide the best protection.

Soccer

Soccer is one of the most widely played sports in the world. Participation is steadily increasing in the United States as more men, women and children join recreational leagues.

Soccer is a physically demanding sport involving bursts of intense activity interspersed with periods of low-to-moderate-intensity activity and occasional rest periods. Although a college soccer game lasts 90 minutes, the ball is typically only in play for about 60 minutes.

A soccer player has to sprint, jog, stride, walk and move sideways and backward. To handle the game's jumping and rapid changes in speed and direction, a soccer player needs to be coordinated, agile and able to react quickly.

Because of the varied demands of the game, soccer taps both the anaerobic and aerobic energy systems. The many sprints, jumps, tackles, and quick starts and stops use the immediate and short-term energy sources of adenosine triphosphate-phosphocreatine (ATP-PC) and glycogen. These are interspersed with periods of slow jogging that use the long-term energy system.

How to train. Build your aerobic capacity with moderate-intensity aerobic activities, such as jogging, cycling and swimming, four or five times a week throughout the year. A generalized strength training program that works all the major muscle groups can help prevent injuries.

As you get closer to the season, you may want to add some specific soccer drills to your routine. These might include doing sprints and practicing overhead throws. Hip abductor, hip flexor and core exercises are also helpful.

Flexibility is also important. Stretching exercises for the hamstrings, quadriceps, low back, hip flexors, groin muscles (adductors) and trunk rotators are all useful for reducing the risk of injury.

How to prevent injury. Soccer is unique in the use of the head and feet to advance the ball. Not surprisingly, most soccer injuries occur in the lower extremities. The most common injuries are bruises, scrapes, sprains — especially ankle sprains — and muscle strains. Stress fractures and over-

use injuries also occur frequently. ACL tears are common, especially in female soccer players. Injuries of the hands, wrists and fingers are far more common in goalkeepers than in other players.

Fortunately, serious injuries in soccer are rare. Although injuries to the head, face and neck make up 5 percent to 15 percent of soccer injuries, most of these are minor cuts, scrapes and bruises.

Take these steps to reduce your risk:

- Always take time to warm up and stretch before a game. Pay close attention to the muscle groups mentioned earlier for the flexibility exercises.

- Wear shinguards. Studies show that these guards help prevent lower leg injuries. Many leagues now require use of shinguards.

- Wear shoes with molded cleats or ribbed soles rather than screw-in cleats. But if you're playing on a wet field with high grass, screw-in cleats may be a better choice.

- Use synthetic, nonabsorbent balls on wet playing fields. Leather balls can become waterlogged and heavy.

- Strength training and balance exercises can help prevent injuries. Balance exercises on one leg or an unstable surface — such as a stability ball — are useful. Balance programs have been shown to reduce the risk of recurrent ankle sprains in soccer players, and combined balance and strength programs may reduce the risk of ACL injuries.

- Jumping and plyometric movements, such as hopping from side to side or jumping on and off a box, can also help keep you in good form for soccer.

Softball and baseball

Players of all ages enjoy America's pastime of baseball and its companion sport, softball. With more than 40 million league players, softball is the largest team sport in the United States.

Baseball and softball use similar skills and have similar energy requirements. Most elements of the games, including pitching, batting, base running and throwing, require anaerobic fitness. Baseball and softball don't involve continuous activity, but players need to be skilled, coordinated and able to react quickly.

How to train. A base of cardiovascular endurance will help prevent fatigue during a longer game. To build such a base, do moderate-intensity aerobic activities for 20 to 30 minutes several days a week.

A strength training program using light weights and high repetitions is useful for strengthening the muscles worked in baseball and softball. Strength training helps prepare your arm for the rigors of throwing and keeps your arm from getting tired and injured. When training, emphasize the shoulder muscles, including the rotator cuff and the muscles of the wrists, elbows, arms, legs and core. Specific exercises include rows, lat pull-downs or chin-ups, external and internal shoulder rotation, push-ups, lateral raises, bent-over lateral raises, core work including rotations, squats, lunges and wrist curls. See details for these in the "Exercise guide" beginning on page 134.

Flexibility is also important. Stretching exercises should include the same muscles as those you focus on in strength training. Because throwing involves all the muscles in your body, stretch all the muscle groups before throwing. Start with your legs and include your trunk, back, neck and arms. Stretching the inferior and posterior shoulder muscles are particularly important.

The ability to balance on one leg is especially important for pitchers. Leg balancing exercises are found in the "Exercise guide" on pages 181-185.

How to prevent injury. Baseball and softball are fairly safe sports. Most serious injuries happen when a player slides into a base. Other injuries occur when a player falls, runs into another player or is hit by the ball or bat.

Overuse injuries can result from overhead throwing, a complex motion that puts great stress on the shoulder joint. Shoulder injuries are the most common injury in adult baseball players. Elbow, head, neck and eye injuries are also common.

One of the most common causes of shoulder injury is going back to throwing a softball or baseball after a long interval away from the game. For example, a man who hasn't played since his days as a high-school pitcher takes up softball again in middle age and immediately begins throwing dozens of balls. Before long he develops shoulder pain and has to stop playing.

Sports medicine specialists have developed a return-to-throw program for pitchers and other throwers who return to the game after an injury, surgery or a long break from play. The program is designed to gradually restore motion, strength in the throwing arm and minimize the chance of re-injury. It emphasizes pre-throwing warm-up and stretching.

The basic premise of a return-to-throwing program is a gradual progression of throwing interspersed with rest periods. For example, at the beginning of the program, you might start with some warm-up throws, followed by 10 to 25 regular throws, followed by 15 minutes of rest before repeating the cycle. Begin by throwing from a short distance, then gradually increase distance and intensity in a pain-free manner. Proper warm-up and throwing mechanics are essential. After completing your throwing session, you can do weight training. Do such a program every other day at the most. Use the day in between for flexibility exercises and recovery.

To play safely, follow these precautions:

- Use breakaway bases rather than traditional stationary bases, which become a rigid obstacle to sliding. A breakaway base is stable during normal base running, but dislodges when a runner slides into it.
- Follow your league's guidelines about the number of innings that should be pitched during a week. Many injuries occur from excessive pitching. When considering the work you do with your shoulder, include your practice throws in addition to game throws.
- If you're returning to throwing after an injury or time away, start gradually, as described earlier. If you experience numbness in your arm, or sharp or increased pain, especially in your shoulder joint, stop throwing. If the pain persists, consult a doctor.
- Wear a batting helmet at the plate, while waiting to bat and when running bases. If your league has batting helmets with face guards, use them. They help prevent injuries to the face and eyes.
- Wear the appropriate glove for your position. Catchers should always use a catcher's mitt and wear full protective gear.
- Men and boys — wear a plastic athletic cup, especially when catching, to protect against testicular injury.
- Wear molded, cleated baseball shoes that fit properly.
- When pitching, throw the ball in a natural way. If you're new to the sport, take at least one lesson with a pitching coach.
- Include flexibility and strength exercises that work the legs, hips, trunk, wrist and forearms.

Swimming and water workouts

According to the National Sporting Goods Association, swimming is America's second most popular fitness activity after walking. About 100 million people in the United States swim for fun and fitness. People young and old compete in swim meets, and the increasing popularity of masters swimming and triathlons has contributed to the sport's continued growth.

In addition to swimming — in pools, lakes and oceans — other popular water workouts include water aerobics, walking, jogging or running in water, and games such as water polo. All types of water sports provide low-impact exercise that's easy on the joints.

Swimming uses both anaerobic and aerobic energy sources, depending on the intensity with which you swim and how far you swim. Because water provides about 12 times the resistance of air, working out in water requires a certain amount of power to overcome the resistance. But even in a swimming sprint, which relies heavily on anaerobic energy systems, aerobic training is needed.

How to train. Swimming and water aerobics require a solid base of aerobic fitness for endurance. You can achieve this by swimming for 30 minutes several times a week and by cross-training with other aerobic activities. To become a faster swimmer, however, you have to swim. Elite competitive swimmers spend two to four hours a day in the pool.

Strength training is also important, both because of the anaerobic demands of faster sprint swimming and to lessen the risk of overuse injuries. A properly developed core is essential because when you're in the water your body doesn't have a hard surface against which to generate

force. A firm midsection serves as the foundation from which your shoulders and hips can generate the power for your stroke. Without a strong midsection, injury risk increases and performance decreases.

Working out in water helps to strengthen your muscles because the water provides resistance. You can add more resistance by using hand-held paddles, weighted boots, webbed gloves and swim fins. Most competitive swimmers also participate in a strength training program using free weights, machines, and resistance tubing or bands.

Strength training for swimming includes the exercises used for baseball plus core work on a stability ball to increase your ability to generate force in an unstable water environment. Shoulder pain is common among swimmers, so it's important to include rotator cuff exercises. And while balance isn't very important in swimming, flexibility is essential. Full-body stretching, with emphasis on the shoulder area, is important.

How to prevent injury. Because swimming and other water exercises are low-impact activities, most injuries are a result of repetitive motions rather than trauma. In general, swimming is a safe sport with a low injury rate.

Shoulder injuries are the most common problem in swimmers, due to the repeated demands on the shoulder joint, which is the least stable joint in the body. A variety of shoulder injuries can occur, including swimmer's shoulder (rotator cuff tendinitis), impingement and instability.

Swimmers who primarily do the breast stroke are vulnerable to knee injuries. People who spend a lot of time in the water are also prone to swimmer's ear, an infection of the outer ear canal.

To keep your swimming or water workout safe:

- Be sure to warm up before and cool down after exercise. Stretch your front and back shoulder muscles, forearms, arms, legs and trunk.
- Increase the intensity and duration of your workouts gradually. Include the most vigorous activities at the beginning of your workout.
- Use proper stroke mechanics — get instruction if you're unsure of your technique.
- Don't swim if you're too tired, too cold or overheated.
- To prevent swimmer's ear, consider using an astringent solution of aluminum acetate and water (Burow's solution) after swimming.
- Don't swim alone. Swim in areas supervised by lifeguards.
- Don't dive into shallow water.
- If you're swimming outdoors, be aware of water and weather conditions. High surf, undercurrents, thunderstorms, flooding, fog and high winds all present hazards.

Tennis

Tennis is the most popular American racket sport with 20 million people playing at least once a year. It's similar to other racket sports, including squash, racquetball and badminton.

Tennis requires speed, agility, coordination, strength and endurance. It's an intermittent activity, with alternating bursts of intense, quick effort and periods of rest. Approximately 60 percent to 90 percent of the energy for tennis comes from the anaerobic sources — primarily ATP-PC — and the rest from the aerobic system. The metabolic requirements of the sport depend on what the player is doing at any given moment. Serving and hitting the ball draw on the immediate and short-term energy sources, but the aerobic system allows for recovery between points.

How to train. To build aerobic endurance, you can cross-train with aerobic activities, such as brisk walking, swimming, jogging and dancing. Interval training is effective for tennis. For example, alternate short periods of fast running or sprinting with jogging or walking for a total workout of 30 minutes or so. This conditions both your aerobic and anaerobic systems and is more specific to the way your body works in tennis.

A strength training program can help prevent overuse injuries. Improving your strength can also increase your power, which will help to improve your serve and forehand and backhand strokes. Because much of the hitting in tennis is done while you're barely in contact with the ground, it's important to have excellent core strength and stability.

Ground reaction forces are transmitted up to the shoulder and arm through your core. The stronger it is, the more power you'll generate.

Exercises suggested for baseball and swimming will also help you prepare and stay in shape for tennis. In addition, because of the heavy lateral legwork associated with tennis, include hip abductor exercises and multiangle lunges in your routine. Plyometric exercise will help you with the rapid front-to-back and side-to-side movements required in tennis.

Stretching of all major muscles — every day, if possible, after you play — is a key component of training for tennis.

Balance is important if you play on a clay court, an unstable surface. To improve your balance, include exercises that are performed on an unstable surface (pillow) or from a reduced base of support (on one leg).

How to prevent injury. Tennis and other racket sports place participants at high risk of overuse injuries. Playing tennis for too long or without adequate preparation can increase the risk. Overload injuries are more common in older and more sedentary tennis players, who tend to be less flexible, and in beginners, who often have poor stroke mechanics.

The impact between a tennis ball and a racket produces a significant amount of force. When the ball hits the sweet spot — the area where the initial impact is at a minimum — the shot feels good. If the ball doesn't hit that spot, more force is transmitted to your hand, wrist and elbow. This can cause such injuries as tennis elbow (lateral epicondylitis), pain on the outside of your elbow.

Tennis injuries occur in the upper body and lower body. Common injury sites include the back, knee, ankle, foot, elbow and shoulder. Most injuries are mild. Common problems include rotator cuff tendinitis, tennis elbow, low back pain, leg muscle strains and cramps, ankle sprains and heel pain, including plantar fasciitis. Hand and wrist problems are also common. In addition, tennis players are subject to heat-related illness and sunburn.

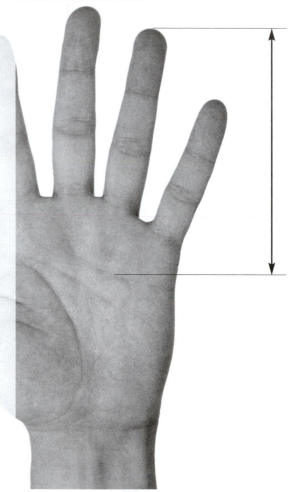

To chose the proper tennis racket grip size, measure the distance between the tip of your ring finger and the nearest crease in the palm of your hand. Select the racket with a grip size as close as possible to that length.

To minimize your risk of injury, take these precautions:

- To reduce risk of tennis elbow, incorporate wrist flexor and extensor stretches and wrist curls and reverse wrist curls into your program. In addition, start backhand swings from your shoulder. Bend your arm slightly for forehand shots and when you serve. If you're not sure about your technique, take a lesson with a tennis instructor.

- Choose the largest comfortable grip size on your racket, and avoid gripping too tightly. Don't try to get more support for your backhand by placing your thumb behind the racket's grip. Choosing the right grip size is important, because a grip that's too small or too large can contribute to tennis elbow. To determine grip size, measure the distance between the tip of your ring finger and the nearest crease in your palm (see page 308). Cushioned grips can reduce the shock of the ball's impact and force of contact into the arm.

- A lighter weight, stiffer tennis racket, such as one made of titanium or graphite, allows you to hit power strokes with less fatigue. Players who are recovering from an injury of the shoulder, arm or wrist may want to use a lightweight racket.

- Most new tennis rackets have an oversize or large frame. This increases the area that you can use to hit the ball, as well as the size of the sweet spot. Using an oversize racket can reduce your number of off-center hits and decrease the amount of impact force your arm has to absorb.

- To prevent ankle injuries, wear tennis shoes with good support. If you have foot pain from plantar fasciitis, a shoe with extra arch support or a heel cup may help.

- When serving or hitting an overhead shot, don't arch your back unnecessarily. Instead, bend your knees and raise your heels.

- Avoid landing on the ball of your foot, which could result in an Achilles tendon injury.

As with pitching in baseball, sports medicine specialists have developed a return-to-tennis program (see page 339) for people who return to the game after an injury, surgery or a long break. As with the return-to-throw program for baseball, the return-to-tennis program is designed to gradually restore motion, strength and confidence in the racket arm and to minimize the risk of re-injury.

Volleyball

Volleyball is a fast-paced game of explosive power, speed, strength, precision and agility. Volleyball players start and stop quickly, jump, dive and change directions frequently. They rely most heavily on the anaerobic energy system for fuel. The immediate ATP-PC system supplies energy for the strength, power and speed they need for serves, spikes, blocks and digs. Glycogen fuels short-term actions such as a 30-second rally, and the aerobic system provides energy for rallies lasting more than two minutes, as well as recovery periods.

How to train. Training is aimed at improving agility and power. Power is important to be able to accelerate quickly, a crucial skill in volleyball. Several types of exercises can build power and strength. These include strength training and plyometric exercises.

Strength training for volleyball is similar to that used for baseball with the following variations. Most core work should be done on an unstable surface because in volleyball, you're often airborne while hitting the ball. Plyometrics are important and should emphasize vertical jumping onto, off and over boxes. Aim to do some kind of strength training three times a week, and plyometrics at least once a week. Before and after the playing season, emphasize fewer repetitions with heavier weights in your strength training. During the season, include more repetitions with lighter weights at a faster pace.

Interval training is useful for volleyball. This might involve alternating sprinting or running with jogging or brisk walking. A base of aerobic fitness is also important. This can be achieved with 20 to 30 minutes of running, biking, swimming or other aerobic activity several times a week.

Balance training is also useful because many times, hits are made while you're off balance.

Make flexibility training with stretching exercises part of your daily routine. Stretch your legs, hips, low back, groin, arms, trunk, shoulders and forearms.

How to prevent injury. An array of injuries affect volleyball players. Some injuries that happen close to the net when a player is blocking, hitting or setting might include jammed or broken fingers and injuries to the face. More persistent, long-term injuries may result from poor technique and overuse syndromes. Diving or falling onto a hard surface can cause injuries in the upper extremities, and playing in sand or grass may lead to lower extremity injuries.

Different volleyball maneuvers can cause different injuries. For example, the jumping required for blocking, attacking and jump serving can lead to jumper's knee — inflammation of the tendons of the patella — or Achilles tendon problems. Blocks can cause finger and shoulder problems, and awkward landings at the net after blocking can result in ankle, foot and knee injuries. The high-velocity overhead movements of serving and hitting can lead to shoulder and back injuries. Rotator cuff tendinitis and shoulder instability may occur. Overall, most volleyball injuries occur at the net while players are blocking and spiking.

Ankle sprains are the most common injury in volleyball players. ACL knee injuries are also frequent, particularly in women. Other common injuries include elbow and shoulder problems, wrist injuries, carpal tunnel syndrome, sprained or dislocated fingers, and low back pain.

To prevent volleyball injuries, follow these tips:

- Follow a combined program of strength, plyometric and balance exercises. Such a routine has been demonstrated to reduce the risk of serious knee injuries in female volleyball players.
- Use kneepads to protect yourself from injury when you fall or dive onto the court.
- To prevent floor burns and bruises, consider defensive pants, which are padded from hip to knee.
- Wear lightweight shoes that provide strong ankle and arch support and good shock absorption.

Walking and hiking

Walking is the No. 1 fitness activity in the United States. It's not hard to see why. Walking is an instinctive, natural activity that our bodies are engineered to do. It's simple, inexpensive and requires no lessons or other participants. The only piece of equipment you really need is a pair of sturdy, comfortable shoes. Hiking draws on the same basic skills, but takes place off-road over variable terrain.

Walking relies almost exclusively on the aerobic energy system. Hiking also uses this system, though trekking up steep hills requires anaerobic energy as well.

How to train. To condition your body for walking and hiking, your primary activity will be endurance training. This makes your heart work harder and increases the fitness of your cardiorespiratory system. This might involve walking and cross-training with other aerobic activities, such as swimming, cycling, pool walking or running, or water aerobics. Add a different activity once a week or so to give your body a break from walking. Ideally, your cross-training activities will use different muscles or the same muscles in different movement patterns. For example, swimming uses more upper body muscles, while biking uses your quadriceps more.

Start out slowly and gradually increase the duration and pace of your walks or hikes. Aim to walk 30 to 60 minutes a

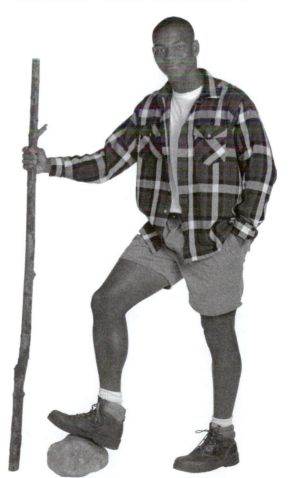

day. If you work on making your walking more efficient, you can walk longer and farther yet feel less tired. (For tips on walking efficiently, see "Walk this way," below. For a sample walking program, see "A 12-week walking schedule," page 86.)

Adding to the intensity of your walking or hiking workout can build both your aerobic and anaerobic fitness. Options include hill walking, interval training and walking with poles. Using poles gives your upper body a workout, too. For interval training, alternate fast speed walking with moderate speed walking. For example, walk fast for two minutes and walk at a moderate pace for three minutes. Repeat this multiple times for a total of 30 to 60 minutes.

Strength training and flexibility exercises

Walk this way

Almost everyone picks up some bad walking habits in a lifetime of walking. To walk more efficiently, consider these tips:

- Hold your head high, with your chin parallel to the ground. Keep your back straight and gently tighten your stomach muscles. To begin, position your feet parallel, about shoulder-width apart, with toes pointing straight ahead. Allow your arms to swing loosely at your sides, or bend your elbows and keep your arms close to your body.
- As you step, land on the heel of your foot and roll forward to drive off the ball of the foot. Take long, easy strides.
- Breathe! When you're trying to walk fast, you may "forget" to breathe, or your breathing pattern may be disrupted.

are also important for your overall fitness and to lessen the chance of injury. Walking may tighten the muscles in your back and the backs of your legs, and stretching helps keep them from becoming stiff and inflexible. Use a weight training program or other resistance program to work your whole body. Pay particular attention to strengthening and stretching the muscles of your legs (quadriceps, hamstrings and calves), low back and hips.

How to prevent injury. Walking isn't a dangerous activity, but it can lead to overuse problems, particularly in the feet. Most foot injuries come on slowly and are caused by abnormal foot structure or poorly fitted shoes.

Walking shoes should cushion your feet, flex easily at the ball of the foot and keep your feet from rolling excessively side to side. (See "What shoes are best for walking?" on page 129.) For hiking, shoes that offer good traction, stability, protection against water, and thick, rugged soles are a must. Some shoes are specifically designed for trail walking.

To keep your feet happy and prevent injuries, follow these guidelines:

- Don't forget to warm up and cool down. Warm up with slow walking followed by stretching. Stretch your calves, hamstrings, quadriceps, knees, low back and trunk. These areas are also important for strength training.
- Wear the right shoe. Walking and hiking shoes are usually made with stiffer soles than are running shoes, for more support. Some shoes are designed for both

running and walking. Hiking boots are made specifically for hiking. These often have an upper that comes above your ankle. Some people feel more comfortable wearing running shoes for walking, and that's fine.

- Make sure your shoes fit well. A comfortable fit is the most important consideration in a walking or hiking shoe. If your foot rolls excessively inward as you walk, a condition called overpronation, look for shoes that provide extra arch support and firm inner foot midsoles. If your feet tend to roll outward (a condition called supination), the appropriate shoe may be more cushioned, with a curved or semicurved last. (The parts of an athletic shoe are described on page 127.) Orthotics and shoe inserts such as heel cups can also help.

- Blisters can occur when your shoes don't fit properly, if your socks are wrinkled or lumpy, or in hot weather. To help prevent blisters, consider wearing a thin undersock and a heavier oversock.

- When heading out for a hike, bring some water and a snack. Whether you're walking or hiking, stay hydrated.

- Dress appropriately for the conditions. Dress in layers, and as you warm up, remove layers. Use sunscreen and insect repellent as needed.

- Don't wear ankle or wrist weights when you walk. These are intended to add a strength training component to your walk, but they can change your normal gait and lead to loss of balance and injury.

- When hiking, stick to trails. Avoid foliage to reduce risk of poison ivy, and don't go hiking after dark.

TRAINING TO IMPROVE PERFORMANCE

When you first start a sport-specific training program, you'll soon notice improvements in your performance. You'll become stronger and able to work out for longer or harder sessions more easily. Over time, your body adapts to the increased demands you've placed on it, and you'll find that your fitness and performance level off. If you keep working out at the same intensity, duration and frequency, you'll stay fit, but your performance won't improve.

If you want to move up to a higher level of performance — go faster or farther, play better, faster, harder or longer — you have to continually increase your training challenges. This goes back to one of the fundamental concepts of training — the overload principle. When you apply a certain overload to your muscles and energy systems, they adapt to the stress by making repairs that increase their ability to perform and endure. The result is higher levels of strength, speed and endurance.

The goal of a training program is to progressively stress muscles to produce the right amount of overload. You can increase the workload by changing your workout frequency, duration or intensity.

But trying to bring about continual improvements in performance can sometimes place excessive strain on your body and lead to injuries or the burnout of overtraining. (For more information on overtraining, see Chapter 6.) Your body needs a certain amount of rest after long-duration or high-intensity workouts in order to rebuild and repair itself in ways that lead to positive adaptations rather than muscle breakdown or damage. For this reason, it's important to plan your training regimen carefully, especially if you want to work up to a challenging event such as a marathon or triathlon.

As you work toward the next level of performance, your training program should give you the right amount of overload and enough rest. It should keep you from doing too much all at once or the same workout week after week.

As you did when you first started training, set a realistic, specific goal for your next step. "Improve my performance" is not specific. Does this mean you want to be able to walk for 60 minutes instead of your current 30 minutes? Or that you want a stronger volleyball serve? Or that you want to drive the ball farther in golf?

To formulate your plan, start by assessing where you are now. In a training log, note the extent (duration) of your activity (for example, running six miles a week), training frequency (for example, running three times a week) and the intensity of your workout (for example, running a mile in 11 minutes). Then figure out what the next step up or goal might be. Per-haps you want to compete in an event, to improve a particular aspect of your performance, or to exercise for longer periods or more often. (For more details on goal setting, see Chapter 4.)

Is your goal realistic — specific and achievable? If you're a beginning runner, for example, running a marathon two months from now is probably too much of a stretch. Start with a goal of running a 5- or 10-kilometer (3.1- or 6.2-mile) race.

The goal you set will determine how you blend the frequency, duration and intensity of your activity into a comprehensive training plan.

Working out a training schedule

Many people who are trying to improve their performance or prepare for an event don't follow any particular training system other than making sure their workouts progress over time. This method works just fine for most recreational athletes. If your goal is to improve your tennis serve, run farther or finish a triathlon, you probably don't need an elaborate, complicated training scheme.

Serious athletes use a system called periodization to structure their training. Its purpose is to produce fitness peaks at the right times while avoiding overtraining. Periodization breaks a training plan into short, medium and long time periods. These periods, called microcycles, mesocycles and macrocycles, allow you to break your training into more manageable units and peak at particular times. Coaches and athletes in a wide variety of sports rely on this system to take players through preparation for the playing season or event, the season or competition itself, and major championships.

If you want to try structuring your training program based on the concept of periodization, find resources that are specific to your sport. Books, Web sites, trainers and coaches can offer ideas.

Tips for training up

To achieve a higher level of performance, gradually increase the intensity of your workouts. You can also increase the duration and frequency, but you don't want to train hard every day of the week. Working out too long or too often can lead to injuries, fatigue, and burnout or overtraining.

You can also achieve a higher level of performance by decreasing the length of the rest periods between exercises, or by changing the order in which you do your exercises without changing the intensity, frequency and duration of each exercise.

To reach a new goal, consider these tips:

- Build up gradually. A weekly increase of no more than 10 percent to 20 percent in total exercise time, distance or intensity is best. Don't try to be faster every time you train. For cardiovascular activities, it takes the body about four to six weeks to adapt to a new level of performance.
- Alternate hard and easy workouts. After an intense workout one day, rest the next day or do an easy workout or cross-training activity. Keep track of your target heart rate through one of the methods discussed on page 42.

- Watch your technique. Maintain good technique whether you're doing a hard or easy workout, warming up or cooling down.
- Avoid increasing more than one variable at a time. For example, if you're increasing your distance, don't up the intensity of your workout at the same time.
- Pay more attention to the intensity of your exercise than to the quantity. Working out for hours a day every day can be counterproductive. Studies have shown that training three to five times a week produces the greatest benefits for the time invested, and additional workouts have diminishing returns.
- Review your progress each month. Are you following your intended plan and making progress toward your short-term and long-term goals? Use this time to reinforce your progress.
- Get to know your own strengths and weaknesses. Adapt your program to fit your individual needs. Work on weak areas as well as strengths for all-around improvement.
- Remember that rest is a key component of your training program. Make sure you're not overtraining (see page 216).

Working up to marathons and triathlons

For increasing numbers of fitness enthusiasts, the ultimate challenge and dream is to run a marathon or take part in a triathlon. These heavy-duty events are not just for elite athletes. But they do require commitment and intensive training. The rewards include a deep sense of accomplishment and the fun and camaraderie of taking part in a community event. For some people, an endurance event is the carrot on the stick that keeps them training.

Are you ready for a marathon or triathlon? If you're just getting started on a physical activity program, you're better off starting with less ambitious goals. Most beginning runners and walkers choose a 5K as their first race. This race is the perfect length to aim for as a beginner. From there you can work up to a 10K. Triathlons often include 1.5 kilometers (0.9 miles) of swimming, 40 kilometers (25 miles) of biking and 10 kilometers (6.2 miles) of running. These distances are daunting even for fit exercisers, but many communities and organizations sponsor minitriathlons of shorter distances.

If you start slowly and commit to a training program over the course of several months, you can build up to a major event. Gradual training is the key to long-term success. Adequate rest is critical. To avoid burnout or injury, don't push your limits and overtrain. For your first major event, your main goal should be to finish — and to have fun and enjoy the experience.

Marathons. Running a marathon takes a lot of preparation, whether you are a beginner or run several races every year. The better shape you're in before you start training, the easier it'll be. Some coaches suggest that you should be running for about a year and be able to cover 15 to 20 miles a week comfortably before you start training for a marathon. It also helps if you've run one or two 5K races and enjoyed the experience.

Finishing a marathon takes courage, perseverance and commitment. The more prepared you are through training, the better your chances of finishing. Begin training for a marathon at least 12 to 18 weeks before the race. A carefully planned training schedule can help you avoid injury. Thirty percent to 50 percent of people who enter marathons drop out before the race, most often because of injury.

The most important element of marathon training is the long run. Many training schedules start with a long run of four to six miles in the first week, adding one mile each week to reach 20 to 22 miles, the longest run, a few weeks before the race. The training schedule alternates long runs with shorter, easier runs, rest days and cross-training (see the "Sample novice marathon training schedule" on page 317).

During a marathon, you may consider taking brief walking breaks (30 to 90 seconds) every mile or so. When you're training, include regular walking breaks in your long runs so that you can get a feel for how and when to walk in a race and how to start running again. Your long runs should also be at a slightly slower pace than your goal pace. You can do the shorter runs a little faster than your marathon pace.

Two ways to predict your marathon time — and thus determine your per-mile pace — are to multiply your best recent

Sample novice marathon training schedule

This chart presents a workout schedule for beginners who are training for their first marathon. Intermediate and advanced runners may want to seek out a more challenging schedule. On your rest days, you can cross-train with other activities, but make sure to take one day completely off each week.

Week	Mon	Tues	Weds	Thurs	Fri	Sat	Sun	Total
1	rest	3 miles	3 miles	3 miles	rest	6 miles	cross	15 miles
2	rest	3 miles	3 miles	3 miles	rest	7 miles	cross	16 miles
3	rest	3 miles	4 miles	3 miles	rest	5 miles	cross	15 miles
4	rest	3 miles	4 miles	3 miles	rest	9 miles	cross	19 miles
5	rest	3 miles	5 miles	3 miles	rest	10 miles	cross	21 miles
6	rest	3 miles	5 miles	3 miles	rest	7 miles	cross	18 miles
7	rest	3 miles	6 miles	3 miles	rest	12 miles	cross	24 miles
8	rest	3 miles	6 miles	3 miles	rest	13 miles	cross	25 miles
9	rest	3 miles	7 miles	4 miles	rest	10 miles	cross	24 miles
10	rest	3 miles	7 miles	4 miles	rest	15 miles	cross	29 miles
11	rest	4 miles	8 miles	4 miles	rest	16 miles	cross	32 miles
12	rest	4 miles	8 miles	5 miles	rest	12 miles	cross	29 miles
13	rest	4 miles	9 miles	5 miles	rest	18 miles	cross	36 miles
14	rest	5 miles	9 miles	5 miles	rest	14 miles	cross	33 miles
15	rest	5 miles	10 miles	5 miles	rest	20 miles	cross	40 miles
16	rest	5 miles	8 miles	4 miles	rest	12 miles	cross	29 miles
17	rest	4 miles	6 miles	3 miles	rest	8 miles	cross	21 miles
18	rest	3 miles	4 miles	2 miles	rest	rest	race	35 miles

Source: *Hal Higdon's Marathon: The Ultimate Training Guide, 2005.* Used with permission.

10K time by 4.65, or to multiply your half-marathon time by 2 and add 10 percent to that. In your first marathon, your goal should be to finish — don't worry about achieving a certain time.

Rest days are essential if you want to stay healthy. Take two or three days each week for rest. Don't work out at all on at least one day. On the other rest days, you can cross-train with cycling, swimming and strength training. Make stretching a part of your daily routine. Long runs tend to stiffen and shorten leg muscles, and as your mileage increases, so does your injury risk.

It's helpful to run a couple of other races, such as a 10K, during your training period. In the last two weeks of training, taper your mileage by 50 percent, with very little running the final two to three days before the marathon. This allows any damaged muscles to heal and promotes maximum glycogen storage in your muscles.

Triathlons. The first modern triathlon took place in 1974, and in 1978 the famous Ironman competition started in Hawaii. At the time, only a few highly trained athletes took part in the "hardest race of the world." The grueling Ironman races are still going strong, but shorter course races are far more popular, attracting millions of participants across the world to thousands of races each year. Triathlon events may range from 20 minutes to several days.

Training for a triathlon begins with establishing a solid foundation of overall fitness and a high level of aerobic and muscle endurance. For someone who's just starting out, endurance is the key to improvement and should be the primary focus of training.

Long swim, bike and run workouts are the primary ways to improve your endurance. These workouts train your muscles specifically for the activities of a triathlon. You can also cross-train with other aerobic activities, such as cross-country skiing, rowing and aerobics classes.

Most people who compete in triathlons spend the greatest portion of their training time in bike workouts. That's because the cycling leg of the race typically takes up about half the total race time. If you don't have a cycling background, make sure to learn proper techniques.

In addition to endurance training, strengthening and stretching exercises are important. Strength training can improve your speed and power, and flexibility is important for keeping your body balanced for optimal performance and may play a role in reducing the risk of injury. Overuse injuries are common among triathletes. The injuries are similar to those seen in swimmers, cyclists and runners and most often affect the lower extremities and back. The knees are the most common areas injured, and tendinitis is the most frequent problem.

Strength training should include all the major muscle groups, especially the core muscles. Use light weights.

How you organize your training each week will depend on several factors, such as your available time, work schedule and experience in the different sports. For most beginning triathletes, a schedule of doing one workout a day and alternating the sports every three days, with one day off a week, works well. For example, you can swim on Mondays, bike on Tuesdays, run on Wednesdays and rest on Thursdays. On Fridays, you begin the Monday through Wednesday cycle again.

Depending on how fit you are, you'll want to start training several weeks or months before your first triathlon. Begin with short, slow workouts and gradually progress to a combination of longer sessions at low intensity and shorter workouts at higher intensity. Aim for a balance of harder and lighter workouts, and don't increase your distance, duration or intensity by more than 10 percent at a time.

In the last two to three weeks before the race, include combined workouts such as swim-bike or bike-run. In the last week before the race, reduce your training and rest more.

KEEPING IT ALL IN BALANCE

Training for any sport can be a challenging and satisfying experience. From deciding that you want to regain some of the ability to perform that you've perhaps lost over the years, to carrying out a program that gets you to your goal, training may be one of the most satisfying things you do. Remember that keeping a balance is important. Backing off when your body tells you to and pushing when you feel

you have the extra energy are things you'll learn to do better as you progress. Most of all, try to enjoy the process toward your goal as much as you do achieving the end result.

Case studies

Learning from the experiences of others is a valuable way in which to gain insight into building an active lifestyle that leads to physical fitness. The case studies presented in this chapter incorporate many of the facts and concepts discussed in the first nine chapters of this book. The case studies show how different people can overcome common fitness barriers. Which person sounds most like you?

Before you read these case studies, here are some things to keep in mind:

- The exercise programs outlined are in their initial phases and are intended to be starting points.

- Each program represents just one of many possible options the individual could choose from. In almost all situations, alternative exercises are available.

- In general, the order of the types of exercises listed in each case study is warm-up (five to 10 minutes), balance, flexibility (as needed), aerobic, strength and cool-down (including flexibility). Balance exercises are best done early in the session, before you become fatigued

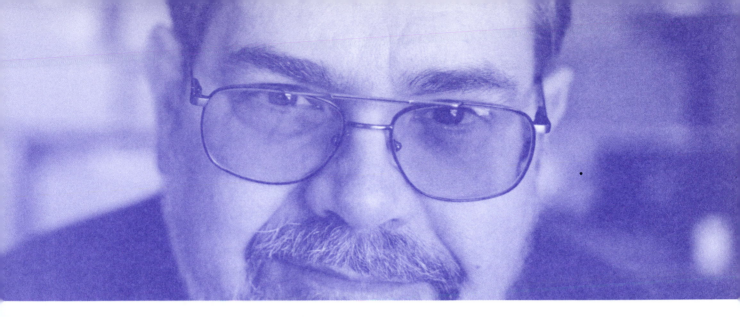

— when they're safer and more effective. Your individual priorities will determine the order of your exercises.

- Most strength exercises call for one set of eight to 12 repetitions, with just barely being able to complete the last repetition with good form. If you're specifically interested in toning your muscles, consider increasing the number of repetitions to 12 to 25. Before doing strength exercises, warm up with a low-intensity set of repetitions, using 50 percent to 60 percent of the weight you'll work with.
- In general, save stretching for after your workout. Exceptions might be to stretch beforehand any areas of your body that are recovering from injury, that are prone to injury or that feel tight. (See "Tight muscles," on page 83).
- Although you may identify with one of the case studies more than others, each has information that may be helpful in tailoring a program that's best for you.
- The "Exercise guide," beginning on page 134, has all of the exercises referred to in this chapter.

CASE 1: ROB

Rob is a 45-year-old businessman and father of three who wants to start an exercise program. He played football in high school, but for the past two decades he's been relatively inactive because of continual business and family obligations.

Rob's children are now in high school. His brother just died of a heart attack at age 47. Rob recently quit smoking, a habit he'd had since college. He has high blood pressure and high cholesterol. He is 5 feet 11 inches tall and weighs 215 pounds, giving him a body mass index (BMI) of 30.

Goals

In beginning an exercise program, Rob has five goals:

1. Improve general fitness
2. Reduce cardiac risk
3. Reduce high blood pressure
4. Reduce cholesterol
5. Reduce weight

Challenges

In meeting these goals, Rob faces three main challenges:

1. He needs a general physical and doctor's clearance before beginning an exercise program.
2. He often works 12-hour days, leaving little free time for exercise.
3. He travels 10 days out of each month. That means he needs an exercise plan that works on the road.

Resources and strategies

Rob is fortunate. He can afford exercise equipment and a membership at a local health club.

Rob's goals in beginning an exercise program are all geared toward improving his health, and they're all very reasonable. Regular exercise improves your body composition, endurance, strength and flexibility — all of which are components of general fitness. It also benefits your cardiovascular system in several ways, including strengthening your heart so that it can pump blood more efficiently. It helps to lower high blood pressure and improves the ratio of low-density lipoprotein (LDL) cholesterol (the "bad" cholesterol) to high-density lipoprotein (HDL) cholesterol (the "good" cholesterol) in your blood. This allows blood to flow through your arteries more smoothly.

Given all of these benefits, if Rob begins an exercise program and sticks with it, he'll likely reduce his blood pressure and cholesterol and his overall risk of dying of heart disease.

Rob's final goal of losing weight is also within his grasp. Exercise burns calories. By burning more calories than he takes in, Rob can reduce his body fat, leading to a healthier body composition. The longer he exercises, the more calories he'll burn.

Getting medical clearance

Rob should get his doctor's OK before beginning an exercise program. As a general rule, men over age 40, women over age 50 and people with chronic health conditions, such as heart disease or diabetes, need medical clearance before starting to exercise. Rob also has the risk factors of high blood pressure, high cholesterol, a family history of heart disease and a personal history of smoking. A checkup will allow Rob's doctor to assess whether he may have an underlying heart condition or other health problem that needs further investigation before starting his program. For example, his doctor may order an exercise stress test as part of this evaluation.

Home workout, health club or both?

Rob may want to consider the pros and cons of working out at home or at a health club, based on his needs, likes and dislikes. One benefit of having a home gym is convenience. The downside is that he'll need a place to put the equipment. If he joins a health club, he'll have easy access to equipment, the opportunity to work out with other people, and access to professional trainers. But he'll have to set aside the time to get to the club. Given his busy schedule, the required extra effort may squelch his motivation. To review the pros and cons of using a fitness facility versus home equipment, see Chapter 5.

Perhaps the best solution for Rob is to buy a treadmill or exercise cycle for home use and to join a health club close to his office. That way, he'll have the greatest chance of fitting exercise into his busy day. On days when he has an early meeting, perhaps he can go to the health club for a half-hour during lunch. This would also help him lose weight by necessitating that he eat a lighter lunch. On other days, he may work out at home on the treadmill first thing in the morning. For someone like Rob, having options is crucial to success. He should anticipate potential barriers to success, such as having limited time, and develop proactive solutions.

For more information on buying home exercise equipment and on choosing a health club, see Chapter 5.

Designing a program

At a minimum, Rob's exercise program should have three components: flexibility, aerobic training and strength (resistance) training. Becoming more flexible may reduce Rob's post-exercise soreness and lower his risk of injury — an important consideration for someone who hasn't exercised in a while.

Aerobic exercise will form the foundation of his program, given his goals of weight reduction and reduced cardiac risk. As discussed in Chapter 1, higher levels of aerobic capacity and increased aerobic capacity over time have been correlated with improved blood pressure and cholesterol and a reduced risk of death from all causes, including cardiac causes.

Strength training will be important because it can help Rob maintain muscle during his aerobic training. It will also help him maintain strong bones and tendons and increase his basal metabolic rate. Muscle is much more metabolically active than is fat. It burns calories even at rest. Because Rob is concerned about his weight, his strength training program should be tailored to build or maintain strength rather than to promote larger, heavier muscles.

Each workout should start with a general five-minute warm-up, consisting of walking, cycling or using other aerobic equipment at a slow pace. This will increase body temperature and muscle blood flow and prepare Rob's neurological system for exercise. At the end of each workout, Rob should perform a five- to 10-minute cool-down, similar to what he did to warm up. Following this, he should perform up to three 30-second stretches for each major body region, as discussed in Chapter 3, concentrating on those muscles that feel tight.

Rob should perform his aerobic exercises at least three days a week, starting at a moderate intensity for 20 to 30 minutes and increasing the duration toward 30 to 60 minutes, depending on the time he has available that day. Because weight loss is a primary goal, increasing duration is more important than increasing intensity.

As far as the choice of exercise, Rob may consider aerobic options such as taking a brisk walk, riding an exercise cycle or jogging. Swimming wouldn't be the best choice for Rob's particular goals because it tends to produce less weight loss than do other aerobic activities.

As time goes on, Rob can increase the frequency of his aerobic activities to four or five days a week, alternating between days of high and low intensity. This will increase his cardiovascular benefits and weight loss. (For more on aerobic activity, see Chapters 3 and 4.)

With strength training, the key for Rob is portability. Resistance bands and body-weight exercises are an ideal choice. Body-weight exercises, such as push-ups, squats, crunches and lunges, can be done anywhere. Resistance bands can be used at home, during lunch hours at the office or in a hotel room when on business trips. Most free-weight exercises can also be performed with a resistance band. Rob can choose several exercises that work major body regions, as detailed in the "Exercise guide" beginning on page 134.

Because Rob is interested in strength and not necessarily large muscle bulk, he should focus on one set of eight to 12 repetitions for each exercise, concentrating on using good form. He'll know he has found the proper resistance when he feels that he can just complete the 12th repetition. Rob should perform his strength training exercises initially twice a week, then increase to three times a week as his time allows. For details on developing a strengthening program, see Chapter 3.

Given his busy schedule, Rob must be flexible about when and where he exercises. Trying to adhere to a rigid routine may be counterproductive. When time permits, though, he should perhaps consider scheduling two of his workouts on weekend days. That will free up time during the workweek. He should also consider working out early in the morning, when he can. For someone as busy as Rob is, exercising at the end of the day may be very difficult. It's often better to start the day with your exercise program, giving yourself a sense of accomplishment.

Finding the time

Rob can slip some physical activity into his busy day in lots of ways. At work, he can take the stairs instead of the elevator or take a brisk walk during lunch. The cumulative amount of physical activity throughout the day is what counts, and all types of activities help. Walking briskly for 10 minutes three times a day may fit into his schedule better than one 30-minute session. This may not help as much with weight loss, but it will help him achieve his other health goals.

Multitasking is another good strategy for Rob. He can walk on a treadmill while watching the early morning news. Or he can buy a bookstand to place in front of his exercise cycle so that he can read the morning paper while he pedals. If he tries to multitask, though, he should be careful to use proper technique and maintain his exercise intensity.

Exercising on the road

Rob spends much of his working life traveling. Business travel can derail a fitness routine, but it doesn't have to. The keys to success are to plan ahead, create a portable workout and use the fitness resources available where you're staying.

To keep his fitness program on track while he travels, Rob should remember to pack his workout gear and swimming trunks so that he can go for a brisk walk around the hotel or swim laps in the hotel pool. He should also focus on creating a portable workout, that is, a routine made up of exercises he can do in his hotel room with little or no equipment. Good examples include push-ups, crunches, pull-ups and strengthening exercises using resistance bands. These bands, which are available at most fitness shops, come in varying degrees of resistance and can be used to do a variety of upper and lower body exercises. For information on buying resistance bands, see Chapter 5. For examples of resistance band exercises, see strength training, beginning on page 150.

Rob's initial exercise program

	Sunday	Monday*	Tuesday		Wednesday	Thursday	Friday	Saturday
Flexibility			✔			✔		✔
Aerobic training**			20-30 min. on treadmill or jogging outdoors			Same as Tue		Same as Tue
Strength training			•Squats: 1 set of 8-12 reps •Dumbbell rows: 1 set of 8-12 reps •Bench presses or push-ups: 1 set of 8-12 reps •Biceps curls: 1 set of 8-12 reps •Dumbbell shoulder presses: 1 set of 8-12 reps •Crunches: 1 set of 8-12 reps					Same as Tue

*Rob has Monday off because it tends to be a very busy day at work.

✔ Stretches as needed.

**After one to two months, Rob can add more days of aerobic training, depending on availability of time.

CASE 2: LAURIE

Laurie is a 40-year-old mother of two who gave birth to her second child two months ago. She gained 30 pounds with her first pregnancy, of which she lost only 20. She gained an additional 15 pounds with her last pregnancy. She now weighs 160 pounds, 25 pounds more than her pre-pregnancy weight of 135. She is 5 feet 4 inches tall, giving her a body mass index (BMI) of 27.5, which classifies her as overweight.

Laurie doesn't anticipate having any more children and wants to regain her pre-pregnancy weight and level of fitness. Laurie has a strong family history of osteoporosis but is otherwise healthy. She hasn't exercised regularly for about seven years, but now she's interested in a combination of aerobic exercise and toning exercises. One important goal is to firm up her abdomen and another is to increase overall strength. Laurie is currently a homemaker with a supportive husband. However, with the responsibilities of caring for her 6-year-old and new baby, she feels tired much of the time.

Goals

In starting an exercise program, Laurie has five goals:
1. Reduce weight
2. Improve abdominal (core) strength and endurance
3. Improve muscle tone
4. Prevent osteoporosis
5. Improve energy level

Challenges

In accomplishing these goals, Laurie faces five challenges:
1. She needs to find time in her busy day to exercise.
2. She's often fatigued from a poor night's sleep.
3. She usually must exercise at home.
4. She's concerned whether exercise is safe in the postpartum period.
5. She needs to exercise while her children are at home.

Resources and strategies

Laurie can afford to buy relatively low-cost exercise equipment. She can begin exercising to some degree soon after pregnancy, especially if the pregnancy was uncomplicated and delivery didn't involve a Caesarean section (C-section). It's a good idea for her to start out gradually, perhaps with some Kegel exercises (see page 269) and abdominal-hollowing exercises (see page 60) to strengthen the pelvic floor muscles and deep abdominal muscles. In addition, including brief walks will help to get her heart rate up. By about six weeks after the birth of a child, most women can get back into a full-fledged aerobic exercise routine. If you've had a C-section or a complicated pregnancy or delivery, ask your doctor when it's safe to begin exercising again. Even after a Caesarean delivery, most women can return to exercise by six to 12 weeks, but it's a good idea to ask your doctor before starting a high-intensity aerobic or strength training program.

It has been two months since the birth of her baby, and Laurie is ready to begin exercising. She wants to get fit again and lose those pregnancy pounds, and she's willing to do what it takes to make that happen. Her main concern is that exercising will make her more tired than she already is. Caring for an active 6-year-old and a new baby takes a lot of energy, to put it mildly.

When she begins exercising, Laurie should expect to feel tired in the short term, during and right after her exercise session. But these feelings will pass as she gains strength and endurance. Over the longer term, exercise will increase Laurie's stamina and energy, making her feel less fatigued. It will also help her meet another goal — preventing osteoporosis. Aerobic activity and strengthening exercises aimed at reducing her weight and increasing her strength and endurance will also help slow mineral loss in her bones that occurs with aging.

Designing a program

Laurie's exercise program should include a fairly rigorous weight-bearing aerobic component, a strengthening component and a flexibility component. Flexibility training may help reduce post-exercise soreness. Admittedly, flexibility may not be the highest priority for Laurie right now. Having just given birth, she has some of the most mobile joints around. Although she should end each workout with a short cool-down and some stretching, Laurie can probably be more selective in her stretching routine, targeting areas that she feels are tight or problematic. The lower back, hamstrings and chest muscles all tend to get tighter after pregnancy.

Because weight loss is one of her primary goals, she should aim for five aerobic workouts a week, at least 30 minutes each session. For weight loss, frequency and duration of aerobic activity are keys. Walking on a treadmill or working out with a low- to moderate-impact aerobics video are things she can do at home. When the weather is nice, she might put the baby in the stroller and go out for a brisk walk or go for a jog with a baby jogger, a special type of stroller that allows her to jog while pushing it. Laurie might start with adding brief periods of jogging to her walks, then increase to longer periods of jogging as her fitness improves. This may also help prevent injury by gradually increasing the impact and strain on her joints, particularly as she has been relatively inactive during her pregnancy. The intensity of her exercise should be moderate.

Laurie's strength training program should include exercises for her upper and lower body using resistance bands, light free weights, her own body weight or a combination of all three. In each case, she can do the exercises at home. Given her postpartum state and desire to firm up her abdomen, her program should also include a major component of core strengthening. In addition to losing weight, this is the best way to begin restoring muscle tone to her abdominal wall. Laurie's core strengthening program should initially include exercises intended to retrain her deep abdominal muscles (see core exercises on page 173) and later progress to static exercises, such as push-ups and bridging exercises. Subsequently, she can progress to abdominal crunches on the floor or on a stability ball, leg-lowering, cobras, tripods, bird-dogs and similar exercises. The great thing about deep abdominal training exercises, such as abdominal hollowing (see page 60), is that they can be done almost anytime and anywhere. For example, at home while she's making dinner, Laurie can lean forward over a counter for several seconds to work her abdominal muscles. Standing in line at the grocery store, she can do the same thing while leaning on the grocery cart. It's simply a matter of contracting and relaxing your abdominal wall in a very specific manner.

In addition, or alternatively, Laurie may want to get a Pilates video and start doing it at home. In most cases, Pilates would suffice for core training. However, Laurie should keep in mind that many of these exercises are challenging and can be difficult to perform properly without the assistance of an instructor, at least at first. She might consider taking a class on a weekend day, while her husband watches the kids, to get her started.

For more information on the specifics of a core strengthening program, see Chapter 3. For illustrated examples of at-home core strengthening exercises for the upper and lower body, see pages 173-180.

Finding the time

Laurie can usually fit in a workout on weekend days, when her husband is at home. It's the workweek that poses the problem. Her husband is supportive, so perhaps he and Laurie can work out a schedule so that he's home from work by 6 p.m. at least two days a week. That way, she can get on the treadmill for a half-hour while he's watching the kids and making dinner. This may also have another benefit. Often after a sustained, strenuous workout, you don't feel like eating. Exercising before the evening meal may help Laurie reduce her total daily calorie intake, helping her lose weight.

To get her third workout during the workweek, Laurie can probably walk on the treadmill or ride the exercise cycle while the baby is napping or strapped into the car seat next to her. The key is to be flexible. Babies don't always nap at the same time each day, so Laurie will have to go with the flow and grab time for exercise when the opportunity arises.

Overcoming fatigue

With a new baby in the house requiring round-the-clock feeding, Laurie is often simply exhausted. Exercising is often the last thing she feels like doing. After a night of poor sleep, it's OK to let up on her workout, perhaps just take a short walk or do a few abdominal crunches. Laurie doesn't want to wear herself out and get run down further. The key is to be flexible and make up the time later in the week.

That said, keep in mind that doing something is always better than doing nothing. On days when Laurie is especially tired, she might want to consider just taking a brisk walk for five or 10 minutes. Once she gets started, she may surprise herself and feel like doing more of her workout routine.

Laurie's initial exercise program

Note: Depending on how Laurie progresses, she may decide to challenge herself by using a stability ball to improve her balance and build core strength. Laurie can also achieve this by doing exercises while standing on one leg. For details on core strength building, see "Core stability training" on page 57.

	Sunday	Monday	Tuesday	Wednesday	Thursday	Friday	Saturday
Flexibility*	✔		✔	✔	✔		✔
Weight-bearing aerobic training**	30 min. walking or jogging		Same as Sun	Same as Sun	Same as Sun		Same as Sun
Strength training***	•Lunges: 1 set of 12-15 reps •Hip abductor walks with resistance band: 1 set of 8-12 steps •Modified push-ups: 1 set of 8-12 reps •Dumbbell rows: 1 set of 8-12 reps •Dumbbell shoulder presses: 1 set of 8-12 reps •Dumbbell or resistance band curls: 1 set of 8-12 reps •Resistance band trunk rotations: 1 set of 8-12 reps each side •Lying bridges: 1 set of 8-12 reps			Same as Sun			

Given the demands on Laurie's time and energy, flexibility is a relatively low priority. ✔ Stretches as needed.

**Laurie may substitute other weight-bearing activities, like working out to a moderate-impact aerobics video.*

***Laurie should also include abdominal hollowing exercises two to three times a day — three repetitions of 10 seconds each with 10-second rest periods in between — most days of the week.*

Exercising with kids around

Babies often rule the roost, dictating the activities of everybody else in the house. Even so, you can at times work caring for a baby into your workout. Many babies like the hum of a treadmill. When her baby is ready for a nap, Laurie might strap her into a car seat near the treadmill where the baby can see her mom. The humming of the treadmill motor may lull the baby to sleep.

When the baby is fussy, Laurie can hold her in her arms and gently bounce on a stability ball. Bouncing on the ball is a great way to get a baby to sleep, and it tones your abdominal and back muscles while you're at it. It also improves your balance. However, before bouncing with the baby, Laurie should try it alone to make sure she can do it safely. For more information on safety issues regarding the stability ball, see Chapter 5.

Laurie can also get the exercise she needs through recreation with her family. On weekend days, she may enjoy bike rides or nature hikes at the local park with her 6-year-old. Her husband can carry the baby in a backpack or front carrier or can push her in the stroller.

A final note. A key part of Laurie's success depends on something unrelated to exercise — that is, implementing and adhering to a reasonable diet. If weight loss is a primary goal of your exercise program, then it should be supported by an appropriate diet. There's no good evidence that "spot reducing" — taking off pounds from one particular part of the body — is possible with exercise alone. Like everything else, a healthy diet also requires planning. Although Chapter 7 contains relevant information, a full discussion of diet and nutrition is beyond the scope of this book. Just know that dietary indiscretions can sabotage your exercise success.

CASE 3: ELLEN

Ellen is a 70-year-old woman with osteoporosis who recently fell at home and broke her hip, requiring a hip replacement. After a short stay in a nursing home, she's now back home with her 71-year-old husband. Ellen has been told to start an exercise program to improve her balance and mobility, keep her muscles strong and maintain her bone density. She and her husband are both generally healthy. They live in a retirement community that has a fitness center and exercise classes.

Goals

In beginning an exercise program, Ellen has four goals:

1. Improve balance and prevent falls
2. Improve general strength and mobility
3. Maintain bone density
4. Protect the hip replacement

Challenges

In meeting these goals, Ellen faces four main challenges:

1. She needs to follow her doctor's orders about protecting her hip replacement.

2. She still lacks confidence on her feet, making her afraid to start walking for exercise.

3. She has never exercised before and is afraid she'll injure herself.

4. Her husband doesn't regularly exercise.

Resources and strategies

Ellen's retirement community has a fitness center and fitness classes. In addition, her husband is willing to help. Her children, who live in the area, check in with her regularly.

For Ellen, the whole concept of exercise is a bit odd. She's never done it before, so she lacks confidence. And she's just gotten over breaking her hip. Her doctor says she must protect the hip replacement, but at the same time tells her to begin exercising. How can she do both? Won't she just break another hip?

Ellen may not know it yet, but exercising is one of the best things she can do to avoid another hip fracture. Regular exercise will maintain, or even increase, the density of her bones, making them stronger and less prone to fracture. It will also strengthen her muscles and improve her overall fitness. Together, stronger bones and muscles will improve her posture and balance, reducing her risk of falling again.

Exercise will also help her new hip heal. Low-impact activity, such as walking, after joint replacement surgery increases bone density and may improve fixation of the prosthetic hip.

Overcoming fear

Because of Ellen's fears, inexperience with exercise and recent hip replacement, joining an exercise class in her retirement community is probably her best option. By exercising with people who have similar fears and challenges, she may be better able to overcome her own. Her retirement community may even have a class specifically designed for people recovering from hip replacement.

An exercise class also has the advantage of professional instruction. In Ellen's case, the instructor can help make sure she's not doing anything to jeopardize her new hip. In general, after a hip replacement, she should avoid the following:

- Bending her hip more than 90 degrees
- Letting her leg cross the midline of her body
- Twisting her hip inward
- Leaning over to pick things up off the floor or tie her shoes

Ellen may also have individual precautions that differ slightly from those just mentioned. She should discuss all precautions with her hip surgeon before starting her program. (See "Exercising after joint replacement surgery" on page 260.)

A group fitness program may also help Ellen stay motivated. She may feel obligated to show up for a class she has signed up for. Or she may want to socialize with new friends that she has made. Maybe her husband will decide he wants to join in, too.

Designing a program

Exercise programs for people with osteoporosis generally include flexibility exercises, weight-bearing activities, strength training (especially back and leg exercises), postural training (exercises that help draw back the shoulders) and balance exercises. Older adults tend to develop tightness of the hip flexors, abdominal wall and chest muscles, which can lead to

Ellen's initial exercise program

Note: The number of exercises in Ellen's program is low due to her inexperience with exercise.

	Sunday	Monday	Tuesday	Wednesday	Thursday	Friday	Saturday
Balance		Standing weight shifts*		Same as Mon		Same as Mon	
Flexibility	•Chest stretch in corner •Foam roller thoracic spine stretch •Prone push-ups •Supine hip flexor stretch •Deep-breathing exercises	Same as Sun	Same as Sun	Same as Sun	Same as Sun	Same as Sun	Same as Sun
Weight-bearing aerobic training**		Walk for 20-30 min.		Same as Mon		Same as Mon	
Strength training	•Chair squat: 1 set of 8-12 reps •Prone cobra: 1 set of 8-12 reps •Resistance band rows (sitting or standing): 1 set of 8-12 reps •Resistance band hip abduction: 1 set of 8-12 reps				Same as Sun		

*This exercise can be done in a doorway for added stability.

**Increase frequency to four to five days a week and duration up to 30 minutes as able.

a slouched posture. To help address this tightness, after her general warm-up Ellen should do one to three 30-second stretches for these regions.

Weight-bearing aerobic activities are those you do on your feet, with your bones supporting your weight, such as walking or doing low-impact water aerobics. Research has shown that weight-bearing exercise best facilitates the maintenance of bone density.

Strength training also maintains bone density because of the beneficial stress it places on bones through muscle tension. In particular, people with osteoporosis should focus on the entire lower body and upper back. Back-strengthening exercises can improve posture and help reduce the risk of developing the back hump that sometimes develops with osteoporosis.

Hip-strengthening exercises are a necessity after a hip replacement. Ellen's doctor may provide specific guidelines for hip strengthening following hip replacement surgery. In general, the exercises should not cause pain and should avoid extremes of motion. Many yoga positions, for example, aren't recommended without approval from your doctor.

Ellen is still a little unsteady on her feet, so she may not yet be ready to begin walking for exercise, or she may want to use a cane when she walks. And she needs to improve her balance. Her exercise class will probably provide a combination of strengthening and balance exercises, with a minor weight-bearing component. For additional exercise, Ellen can do low-impact water aerobics at the pool, use the exercise cycle, use the weight machines, or sit and lift light free weights. Individuals who have never lifted weights before should start with 1-pound weights or less or do the lifting motions without a weight. Over time, Ellen should slightly increase the weight amount or add a weight. These activities will help strengthen her bones and muscles, while posing minimal risk of falling. They'll also provide some aerobic benefits. Once Ellen's balance has improved, she should increase the weight-bearing component of her exercise routine. A daily walk or a low-impact aerobics class may be a good option.

Ellen should begin exercising gradually. She may be very deconditioned after her hip surgery. But it's imperative that she begin the process. If she wants to regain the use of her joint and muscles, activity and exercise must become part of her daily routine. Lower body exercises after hip surgery can help in regaining a more natural gait. In addition, calf exercises are important in helping to prevent blood clots. For more information on exercising with osteoporosis or after joint replacement surgery, see Chapter 8.

CASE 4: DON

Don is a 60-year-old man who tore some cartilage in his right knee while playing college football years ago. This required surgery, and he believes some of the cartilage was removed. For the past five years, Don's right knee has gotten more and more painful and it has started swelling. His doctor diagnosed it as arthritis but said that surgery wasn't needed. Because of his knee pain, Don has become progressively less active, having stopped jogging three years ago. He's gained about 20 pounds and now has high blood pressure and borderline high blood sugar. This concerns him because he has a family history of type 2 diabetes. Don currently takes ibuprofen, glucosamine and chondroitin for his arthritis. He wants to become more active, but he doesn't do any lower body strength training because he's concerned that it will aggravate his arthritic knee.

Goals

In beginning an exercise program, Don has five goals:

1. Reduce right-knee pain
2. Increase general activity level
3. Reduce weight
4. Reduce blood pressure
5. Reduce blood sugar and diabetes risk

Challenges

In meeting these goals, Don faces four primary challenges:

1. He can't tolerate impact activities because of the pain in his right knee.
2. His doctor said he should take it easy on his knee. However, during a recent physical, Don received a clean bill of health with respect to his heart.
3. He's concerned that weight training focused on his lower body will cause damage to his knee.
4. He doesn't have much experience with aerobic activities other than jogging and walking.

Resources and strategies

Don belongs to a well-equipped fitness center. And he's willing to work with a personal trainer to meet his goals.

Don considers exercise to be an all-or-nothing proposition. In his glory days of college football, aerobic exercise meant running laps. Strength training for your legs meant doing squats. Even later in his life, exercise meant jogging. Now that he has arthritis and can't perform at that level anymore, he's become a couch potato. He has taken his doctor's warning to take it easy on his knee as license to do nothing, which has led to weight gain, high blood pressure and increased risk of diabetes.

Don needs to readjust his ideas about aerobic exercise and strength training. Studies have clearly shown that regular aerobic exercise can reduce pain and improve function in people with knee arthritis. The key is choosing the correct aerobic and strength exercises.

Aerobic exercise doesn't necessarily mean doing high-impact, knee-stressing activities, such as running and jogging. In fact, these types of aerobic activities aren't generally recommended for people with arthritis of the knee. Instead, low-impact aerobic exercise is recommended, of which there are many types. The simplest is walking, but there are many others — several of which offer even less impact than does walking — such as swimming, water aerobics, pool walking, bicycling, or using a cross-country ski machine, elliptical trainer or rowing machine (see "Exercise for healthy joints" on page 40). If Don was to do any of these exercises on a regular basis, he would begin to experience some of the main health benefits of aerobic activity, including reduced knee pain, lower blood pressure and better blood sugar control, which comes with a reduced risk of developing diabetes.

Don's worry is that exercise — especially strength training — will further aggravate his knee injury, increasing his pain. In fact, the opposite may be true. Aerobic exercise can improve joint stability and strengthen your muscles. Building up your leg muscles with strength training offers further benefits. It strengthens your quadriceps muscles and hamstrings, helping to take pressure off the cartilage and bone of your knee joint. The strengthened muscles act as a natural brace for the arthritic knee, protecting it from injury. If Don was to enhance the structural support of his knee joint with stronger muscles, he would be able to take more force and load off his bones and cartilage, very likely resulting in reduced knee pain. As previously mentioned, studies have shown that aerobic activity and strength training can improve pain and function in people with arthritis of the knee, with slightly more benefit coming from doing

both than from doing either by itself.

The key is to perform the correct strength program. The old saying, "No pain, no gain," doesn't apply here. Exercise to strengthen the muscles around the knee shouldn't be painful. If an exercise does cause pain, modify the exercise by decreasing resistance or repetitions or replace it with an alternative exercise. After exercise, it's a good idea to apply ice to the arthritic knee. This helps to decrease the swelling and inflammation. If you use heat, reserve it for warming up the joint before exercise.

Designing a program

Don's exercise program should include a warm-up period, flexibility training, balance exercises, aerobic activity and strength training. Besides strengthening your muscles, balance training helps the muscles around your knees work together more effectively to brace and support your knees.

Given Don's past experience with team sports, exercising at the gym where he holds a membership is probably his best option. The interaction with other people and his competitive nature may help keep him motivated. Working with a certified personal trainer is also probably a good idea. By getting some instruction, Don will learn to use low-impact aerobic equipment that may be unfamiliar to him, such as a ski machine or elliptical trainer. He'll also learn to make modifications to standard leg-strengthening exercises that may be necessary to help protect his knee.

The support of a personal trainer may also help Don overcome some of the anxiety he feels about injuring his knee.

Because his knee is deconditioned due to previous injury and arthritis and probably tends to stiffen up, Don's first aim should perhaps be to improve his muscle flexibility and strength. He should make sure to perform stretches for his major lower body muscles (quadriceps, hamstrings, gluteals and calves) after each exercise session, holding each stretch for

Don's initial exercise program

	Sunday	Monday	Tuesday	Wednesday	Thursday	Friday	Saturday
Balance	Single leg stand: 3-5 reps each side		Same as Sun		Same as Sun		
Flexibility	✔		✔		✔		✔
Low-impact aerobic training*	Exercise cycle for 30 min.		Same as Sun		Same as Sun		Same as Sun
Strength training	• Squat: 1 set of 8-12 reps • Calf raise: 1 set of 8-12 reps • Bench press: 1 set of 8-12 reps • Dumbbell shoulder press: 1 set of 8-12 reps • Triceps extension: 1 set of 8-12 reps • Stability ball abdominal crunches: 1 set of 8-12 reps		• Hamstring curls: 1 set of 8-12 reps • Dumbbell rows: 1 set of 8-12 reps • Lat pull-downs: 1 set of 8-12 reps • Dumbbell biceps curls: 1 set of 8-12 reps • Hip abductor walks with resistance band: 1 set of 8-12 reps • Lying bridges		Same as Sun		Same as Tue

✔ Stretches as needed.

*May substitute other low-impact exercises. When Don is able to do so, he'll add a fifth day of aerobic exercise.

30 seconds. For strengthening, he should focus on improving the strength of his entire lower body using exercises such as hip abduction, hip extension, leg curls and either leg presses or body-weight squats.

Because many people with arthritis can't tolerate multiple sets, Don's strength program should consist of a single set of eight to 12 good-quality repetitions for each exercise. For more information on strength training progression, see Chapter 3.

To add a low-impact aerobic component to his routine, Don can use the gym's ski machine, elliptical trainer or exercise cycle. On days away from the gym, he may even want to take a bike ride with his grandchildren. Regardless of the type of activity, Don's goal should be some form of aerobic activity most days of the week.

Once Don has gotten into a good exercise routine, he may consider participating in recreational sports in his community. If he does, he'll want to avoid sports such as singles tennis, handball, racquetball, basketball, football and soccer because they make him twist and turn, start and stop — sudden movements that can injure his knees. Playing in a local golf league or playing doubles tennis with his wife could be good options for Don.

Don should ice his knee after exercise. By reducing swelling, he'll reduce stiffness and pain. During arthritic flares, when his pain is too much to do his usual aerobic activities, he may want to consider swimming or water aerobics. Although water-based activities aren't the ideal exercise for achieving weight loss, they are some of the least stressful exercises on the joints. Because water's buoyancy reduces stress on your joints, experts often recommend swimming and other water exercises for individuals who have arthritis.

For more information on exercising with arthritis, see Chapter 8. For illustrated examples of leg strengthening and balance exercises, see the section of the "Exercise guide" beginning on page 181.

CASE 5: KAY

Kay is a 50-year-old woman who has ongoing intermittent pain in her right shoulder. Her pain is possibly linked to her hobby of playing tennis.

Kay recently saw her doctor, who said she had rotator cuff tendinitis and prescribed physical therapy. Kay completed four therapy sessions, with reasonable reduction in her shoulder pain. She was about to return to tennis when she came down with influenza and was out of commission for two weeks.

Now she's feeling a little bit better and has returned to work. However, she didn't do any of her shoulder rehabilitation exercises during her recent illness. She is now concerned that she's lost all of her fitness gains during the past two weeks of inactivity, and she wonders what to do.

Goals

In starting up her exercise program again, Kay has four goals:

1. Reduce shoulder pain
2. Improve strength and endurance of her rotator cuff and shoulder girdle
3. Regain fitness after her recent bout with the flu
4. Return to doubles tennis

Challenges

In meeting these goals, Kay faces two particular challenges:

1. Her recent illness has led to deconditioning and a reduced capacity to exercise.
2. She's uncertain whether she should stop exercising if she becomes ill again.

Resources and strategies

Before her illness, Kay had established a home exercise program with resistance tubing and free weights. She also has a gym membership at the club where she plays tennis.

Kay had been faithfully following her rotator cuff rehabilitation program. Being ill changed all that, putting her in bed for several days. Kay made the right decision to stop exercising while she was ill. In general, if you have signs and symptoms of illness below the neck, such as vomiting or intestinal cramping, it's not recommended that you continue exercising. If your signs and symptoms are above the neck, such as nasal congestion, exercise is generally OK. For more information on exercising after an acute illness, see Chapter 8.

Getting back with the program

Now that she's feeling a little better, Kay should resume her rotator cuff rehabilitation program. Exercise therapy is the main treatment for rotator cuff injuries. The exercises are specifically designed to help heal the injury, improve the flexibility of the shoulder and strengthen the rotator cuff and other shoulder muscles so that they're better able to control the position of the arm. These include stretching exercises such as the inferior and posterior shoulder stretches (see "Exercise guide," page 140), and strengthening exercises, such as external and internal rotation, sidearm raises, rows and punches (see pages 150-156). By continuing her rehabilitation program, Kay is likely to meet her goals of reduced shoulder pain and improved shoulder strength and endurance.

That's not to say that Kay should just jump back into her old routine and expect to feel fine. After two weeks away from exercise, she's gotten a bit out of shape. Doctors call this deconditioning. She's also quite tired. Kay hasn't lost everything she worked so hard to achieve — her strength is probably about what it was before she got the flu — but she clearly doesn't have the endurance she had before the illness. To compensate for this, Kay should begin exercising again gradually, starting with shorter sessions. That way, she'll avoid becoming overly tired, which could cause a further setback. She should also consider exercising less frequently, maybe just three times a week at first, depending on her sense of recovery between exercise sessions.

Tennis, anyone? After a long time away, Kay is understandably eager to return to playing tennis. But she should probably wait just a bit longer. No matter what the setting, tennis is a competitive sport in which you keep score of who wins and who loses. In a competitive situation, Kay may push herself too hard without intending to. Her best strategy before she feels 100 percent well is to minimize the pressure on herself.

Once she feels completely back to normal, Kay can begin playing tennis again. But here, too, she should take it a little slow. During the early weeks back, she should merely hit against a backboard or practice with a partner. The return-to-tennis program outlined on the right side of this page is a guide to gradually increasing both intensity and volume of tennis activity. It can help Kay avoid re-injuring her shoulder. After that, she can progressively increase her participation by playing a few games, then one set, and so on. Once she feels ready for a full match, Kay should start by playing a doubles match and then, as her fitness improves, progress to a singles match. If at any time she feels overtired or her shoulder starts hurting, she should back off, rest for a day or two and then start again.

In addition to tennis, Kay may want to consider other forms of aerobic exercise that involve her lower body to help prevent overuse injuries.

Kay's return-to-tennis exercise program

Kay should progress to the next level only if she's pain-free.

Week 1
- Do three workouts a week.
- Hit 25-30 forehand shots and 15-20 backhand shots each workout, with a 10-minute break halfway through.
- Hit at 50 percent effort.

Week 2
- Do three workouts a week.
- Hit 50-60 forehand shots and 30-40 backhand shots each workout, with a 10-minute break halfway through.
- Hit at 75 percent effort.

Week 3
- Do three workouts a week.
- Hit 60-90 forehand shots, 50-60 backhand shots and 20-45 serves each workout, with a 10-minute break halfway through.
- Hit at 75 percent effort.
- Serve at 50 percent effort.

Week 4
- Do three workouts a week.
- Begin with 30 forehand shots, 30 backhand shots and 10 serves each workout, followed by a 10-minute break.
- Build up from playing three games during the first workout to a set in the second and 1½ sets in the third.
- Hit at 100 percent effort.
- Serve at 75 percent effort.

CASE 6: JACK

Jack is a 57-year-old recently retired executive who has ongoing intermittent low back pain. When he was in his 30s, he had low back disk surgery for sciatica. Since then he has had intermittent back pain. Jack retired hoping that he could spend more time playing golf — a great passion of his. However, he found that as he played more golf, his back pain increased. He saw his doctor, who diagnosed it as arthritis and recommended heat, anti-inflammatory medications and exercise. At 6 feet and 205 pounds, Jack's body mass index (BMI) is 27.8, which puts him solidly in the overweight category. Jack feels that he's in good shape. Other than borderline high cholesterol and being overweight, he's healthy. Jack jogs two to three miles three or four times a week, but otherwise is on no formal exercise program. His pre-golf warm-up routine is minimal. He stretches if he gets the chance.

Goals

In beginning an exercise program, Jack has four goals:

1. Reduce low back pain
2. Improve flexibility
3. Improve core strength and endurance
4. Improve golf game

Challenges

In meeting these goals, Jack faces two main challenges:

1. He needs rehabilitation for his low back pain.

2. He's skeptical that exercise can help ease his pain or improve his golf game.

Resources and strategies

Jack is fortunate. He will buy or do whatever it takes, as long as he's convinced it will keep him golfing.

Golfing seems so benign. You walk a little, take your shot and get back in the cart. But that's not the whole story. Golf is a casual sport for many, but it puts a tremendous amount of strain on your back. In fact, back pain is one of the most common complaints among golfers of all levels, even pros.

Jack is one of those golfers with back pain, but he's skeptical that exercise can help him. He runs three or four times a week, which certainly represents a good aerobic fitness program, but it doesn't help his back pain as much as he'd like.

Jack's problem is that he's missing two key components of fitness — strength and flexibility. By focusing only on aerobic exercise, Jack is doing little or nothing to strengthen his back and abdominal muscles. Why is that important? Conditioned back and abdominal muscles work together like a natural corset, keeping you upright, stabilizing your body and protecting your spine from injurious stress. For example, during a golf swing, enough compressive force is generated in the spine to crush a vertebra or herniate a disk. When you have good core stability, the muscles in your back, hips and abdomen work in harmony, providing support to your spine and

Jack's initial exercise program

	Sunday	Monday	Tuesday	Wednesday	Thursday	Friday	Saturday
Strength training*	• Squat: 1 set of 8-12 reps • Hip abductor walks with resistance band • Push-ups: 1 set to failure • Dumbbell shoulder press: 1 set of 8-12 reps • Abdominal hollowing in shortstop position: 5-10 reps, holding each rep 10 sec. • Lying bridge: 1 set of 8-12 reps • Abdominal crunches on stability ball: 1 set of 8-12 reps		• Bent-over dumbbell rows: 1 set of 8-12 reps • Prone cobra: 1 set of 8-12 reps • Dumbbell arm curls: 1 set of 8-12 reps • Trunk twists: 1 set of 8-12 reps each side or chop and lifts: 1 set of 8-12 reps on each side		Same as Sun		Same as Tues
Flexibility**	• Hamstring • Quads • Hip flexors • Prone press-up • Lats • Chest/pectorals • Shoulder • Neck • Trunk rotation • Knee to chest		Same as Sun		Same as Sun		Same as Sun
Aerobic training***		Running		Running		Running	

*As strength improves, incorporate more difficult balance exercises.

**Focus on stretches for the back and other areas that feel tight.

***See Chapter 4 for a number of sample aerobic training programs.

shielding your spinal structures from these potentially damaging forces. Conversely, the weaker your core muscles, the more likely you are to experience low back pain.

In addition, by only stretching occasionally, Jack isn't doing what it takes to maintain flexibility. If he began stretching more regularly, the increased flexibility in his hips and upper legs would allow for better alignment of his pelvic bones, improving how his lower back functions and feels. In golf, stretching is also important to make sure your body can move through the range of motion required in the golf swing without causing excessive stress on your muscles or joints.

Designing a program

A lower back stabilization program — an exercise program that incorporates core strengthening and flexibility — can help to reduce the frequency and severity of Jack's low back pain, making golfing more enjoyable. For golfers, doctors typically recommend strength training and flexibility in the lower back, abdomen and hips. The aim is to stabilize the back by creating balanced strength in the abdominal and lower back muscles and good flexibility in the legs.

Jack would also benefit from deep abdominal training. People with chronic back pain often have deficiencies in the use of these important, deep abdominal and spinal-stabilizing muscles. Abdominal hollowing (see page 60) and core exercises can help correct that. If Jack is having a difficult time with these exercises, a physical therapist or personal trainer can assist him. These exercises are the same as those suggested for Laurie on pages 327-328. In fact, Jack would benefit, at least initially, from the same core strength training program as is prescribed for Laurie (see page 329).

Jack's main complaint is his back. But his current lack of strength and flexibility training also puts him at risk of rotator cuff injury — common among golfers as they age. To help prevent this, Jack may also want to include shoulder-strengthening exercises, specifically for the rotator cuff and scapular stabilizers. Such exercises might include rows, lat pull-downs, push-ups (with a plus) and external and internal shoulder rotations with a resistance band or free weight. Balanced strength in the front and back shoulder muscles provides protective stability to the rotator cuff.

Balancing his aerobic exercise with strengthening and flexibility will make Jack's fitness regimen more rounded and complete. And it may even help him improve his golf game. The increased strength in his back and abdomen may increase his club-head speed, allowing him to hit a longer ball. In fact, studies have demonstrated improved club-head speed in golfers who improve flexibility or complete core training programs. For examples of shoulder stretches, see the "Exercise guide," pages 140-141. For examples of shoulder strengthening exercises, see pages 150-154.

NOW IT'S UP TO YOU

You may not fit exactly into one of the scenarios discussed in this chapter, but consider using these case studies for guidance as you design your own exercise program. Make sure to include the basic elements of fitness — strengthening exercises, flexibility stretches, aerobic training and balance exercises. Before you know it, you'll have a well-developed, personalized plan that makes exercise a regular part of your life. Then you'll be on your way to reaping the rewards from being physically fit. Remember, fitness is for everybody.

Additional resources

These Web sites offer information about the benefits of exercise and fitness. Some also have information about exercises that may be appropriate if you have a medical condition that limits physical activity.

American College of Sports Medicine ....*www.acsm.org*

American Council on Exercise ....*www.acefitness.org*

American Society for the Alexander Technique............*www.alexandertech.org*

Arthritis Foundation ....*www.arthritis.org*

American Heart Association ....*www.americanheart.org*

American Medical Association................................*www.ama-assn.org*

American Sports Medicine Institute..........................*www.asmi.org*

Centers for Disease Control and Prevention ....*www.cdc.gov*

Department of Health and Human Services ....*www.health.gov*

Feldenkrais Educational Foundation of North America *www.feldenkrais.com*

Hal Higdon's Training Programs ....*www.halhigdon.com*

MayoClinic.com..*www.MayoClinic.com*

**National Institutes of Health
Interactive Menu Planner** ....*http://hin.nhlbi.nih.gov/menuplanner/menu.cgi*

Glossary

A

adenosine triphosphate (ATP). A chemical in the body that carries energy to fuel all muscle contractions, ATP is the basic energy currency in the body. ATP reserves in a muscle are used up within 10 to 12 seconds of work, and must be replenished by energy systems (short-term and long-term systems) from outside the muscle.

aerobic activity. Activity that uses oxygen to generate adenosine triphosphate (ATP) for energy. Aerobic energy systems generate ATP slower than do anaerobic systems. Therefore, aerobic activity is typically of lower intensity but longer duration than is anaerobic activity.

aerobic fitness (aerobic capacity). The body's ability to take in and use oxygen to produce energy.

alignment. The position of your body. Optimal alignment in standing is when the ears are above the shoulders, the shoulders over the hips and the normal spine curves are maintained. In this book, alignment is used interchangeably with *form* and *posture*.

anaerobic activity. Activities that don't use oxygen to generate adenosine triphosphate (ATP) for energy. Anaerobic energy systems generate ATP faster than do aerobic systems, but are limited in capacity. Therefore, anaerobic activity is typically of higher intensity but shorter duration, compared with aerobic activity.

B

balance. The ability to control your center of gravity over your base of support.

basal metabolic rate (BMR). Your body's energy use at rest.

blood pressure. The force of blood pushing against the walls of the blood vessels.

body composition. The amount of body fat you have in comparison with muscle, bone and other tissue. Body composition is one component of fitness.

body mass index (BMI). The most commonly used tool to determine whether a person is normal weight, overweight or obese. Individuals with a BMI of 30 or greater are considered obese.

Borg ratings of perceived exertion scale. A scale from 6 to 20 used to gauge intensity of physical activity or exercise.

C

calcium. The mineral that makes bones hard and able to support weight.

calorie. A measurement of the amount of energy provided by a food. In reality, the unit of measure is kilocalorie (1,000 calories). However, when discussing calories for the purposes of diet, nutrition and exercise, most people just say "calories." In this book, the term *calorie* is used in this way.

cardiovascular disease. Deterioration of, or damage to, arteries, including those that supply blood and oxygen to the heart.

central nervous system. The brain and spinal cord, which coordinate and control all movements of the body.

chondroitin. A nutritional supplement taken to reduce the pain of osteoarthritis. *See* glucosamine.

chronic. A condition that's long lasting, typically six months or more in duration. Many diseases are considered chronic, such as osteoarthritis, osteoporosis and diabetes.

cool-down. Deliberate slowing of activity after exercise to allow your body to return to a level close to its resting state.

core muscles. The muscles located in your trunk, including the lower back, hips, abdomen and buttocks.

core stability training. A type of strength training that works the muscles at the core of the body.

creatine. An energy carrier in the cell. Creatine, in the form of creatine phosphate, rebuilds adenosine triphosphate (ATP) after it loses some of its energy to fuel muscle contractions. Although creatine occurs naturally in the cell, it's also taken as a nutritional supplement for ergogenic effects.

cross-training. Alternating between different activities or between a variety of exercises. Cross-training may prevent overuse injuries.

D

delayed-onset muscle soreness. Muscle soreness that follows a day or two after exercise.

detraining. The loss of the beneficial effects of fitness when you stop exercising.

diabetes. A disease in which the body doesn't produce or properly use the hormone insulin. Type 1 diabetes results from the inability to produce insulin. Type 2 diabetes, which is related to inactivity and obesity, primarily results from your body's inability to use the insulin it produces.

duration. The length of time you exercise or perform an activity during a single session.

E

endorphins. Brain chemicals (neurotransmitters) that produce feelings of well-being. Sometimes referred to as natural painkillers.

endurance. The ability to exert force (muscular endurance) or sustain an activity (aerobic endurance) over a period of time.

energy systems. The three systems that supply energy for muscle contraction during activity or exercise. These include the immediate (ATP-PC, or anaerobic), short-term (glycogen, anaerobic and aerobic) and long-term (oxygen, aerobic) systems. The capacity of the immediate system is 10 to 15 seconds, the short-term system is 30 seconds to two minutes. The long-term energy system can function from minutes to hours.

ergogenic aid. A substance taken to improve performance in sport or activity.

exercise. The planned, structured and repetitive movement done to improve physical fitness.

extensor. A muscle that contracts to extend or straighten a limb at a joint and move the limb away from the body.

F

Feldenkrais Method. Uses gentle movements designed to enhance flexibility and coordination. Goal is to increase awareness of movement through body feedback rather than prescribed positions.

fitness. The overall cardiovascular and musculoskeletal health of your body. Fitness consists of aerobic capacity, strength, core stability, flexibility and balance.

flexibility. The ability to bend joints and stretch muscles through a full range of motion.

flexor. A muscle that contracts to bend a limb at a joint and bring the limb closer to the body.

free weights. Barbells or dumbbells.

frequency. How many times you complete a particular exercise or exercise session.

G

glucosamine. A nutritional supplement sometimes taken to reduce the pain of osteoarthritis. Although the exact mechanism of its effect is unknown, it may help preserve cartilage and does have anti-inflammatory effects. Often taken with chondroitin sulfate, which has similar properties.

glycemic index. A system for classifying carbohydrates according to the effect they have on your blood sugar level. In general, foods with a higher glycemic index produce larger increases in blood sugar.

glycolysis. A series of chemical reactions that breaks down stored glycogen and glucose circulating in the blood to produce fresh supplies of adenosine triphosphate (ATP). Glycolysis is relatively fast acting but limited in capacity. It occurs with oxygen (aerobic glycolysis) and without oxygen (anaerobic glycolysis).

H

hypertension. Increased pressure in your blood vessels that continues on a persistent basis. Also called high blood pressure.

I

impingement. Pinching in the shoulder joint during repetitive activities, particularly during those in which the arm is overhead and outstretched. The condition is often associated with injury to, or inflammation of, the rotator cuff muscles.

insulin. A hormone that regulates the use of blood sugar by converting sugar, starches and other food into stored energy.

intensity. How hard you work as determined by intensity scales (Borg), by your heart rate or by how much oxygen you burn.

interval training. Training that consists of alternating short bursts of intense activity with less intense activity.

involuntary muscles. Typically classified as smooth muscles, involuntary muscles aren't consciously controlled. They include muscles of the stomach, blood vessels and intestines.

J

joint. The connection of bones in the body. Most joints are places in which movement, initiated by skeletal muscle, takes place.

L

lactic acid (lactate). A byproduct of the anaerobic metabolism of glycogen and glucose. Lactic acid contributes to the muscle burn associated with intense, fast-paced activity.

ligaments. The long, strap-like fibers that connect one bone to another.

M

metabolic equivalent (MET) level. A measurement of the amount of oxygen consumed during a physical activity to determine the intensity of that activity. One MET is equal to 3.5 milliliters (mL) of oxygen/kilogram (kg) of body weight/minute, and reflects the amount of oxygen typically consumed at rest.

metabolic syndrome. A cluster of signs and symptoms that increases the risk of developing diabetes, cardiovascular disease and stroke. Metabolic syndrome consists of high blood pressure, high insulin levels (insulin sensitivity), excess body weight and abnormal cholesterol levels.

metabolism. The complex process of digesting food to produce proteins, carbohydrates and fats to support bodily processes, such as the production of energy.

mode. The type of exercise or activity. For example, aerobic, flexibility, core, balance and strength training are modes of exercise.

multifidus muscles. The deep core back muscles important for spine stability. These muscles often become dysfunctional in people with low back pain.

muscle cramps. Sharp, stabbing, cramping or aching muscle pains that can range from mild to excruciating. The exact cause of muscle cramps is unknown, but they're thought to reflect a metabolic imbalance, such as dehydration or low sodium.

muscles. The contractile tissue that connects bones and joints, and which is responsible for movement. Muscles may be voluntarily controlled (skeletal muscles) or involuntarily controlled (cardiac and smooth muscle).

muscular fitness. The ability to generate force (strength) and maintain force (endurance).

musculoskeletal system. The system that allows the body to move. Formed by bones, muscles, tendons, ligaments and joints.

N

neurotransmitters. Chemicals used by your nerve cells to communicate with one another.

O

obese. An excess amount of body fat. Obesity is defined as a body mass index (BMI) of 30 or greater.

osteoarthritis. A type of arthritis characterized by degeneration of joint cartilage. Although it may have an inflammatory component, it's not a primary inflammatory arthritis like rheumatoid arthritis.

osteoporosis. A condition of decreased bone density and deterioration of bone, causing bone to become weak, porous and fragile.

overtraining. A situation in which you exercise so much that your body doesn't recover between workouts. Overtraining can produce fatigue, mood changes, and loss of weight, strength and endurance. It's a cause of plateaus in an exercise regimen.

P

peak bone mass. The highest amount of bone mass that you're able to attain as a result of normal growth. Peak bone mass typically occurs in the second or third decade of life.

perceived exertion. A reference for how hard you feel you're exerting yourself during an activity with regard to effort, physical stress and fatigue. Perceived exertion is typically measured using the Borg ratings of perceived exertion scale.

phosphocreatine (PC). A compound found in muscles that can rapidly regenerate adenosine triphosphate (ATP) for energy production. Phosphocreatine may be increased in some people through exercise, proper diet and supplementation with creatine phosphate.

physiatrist. A medical doctor specializing in physical medicine and rehabilitation. A physiatrist is trained to evaluate and treat a wide variety of musculoskeletal and neurological conditions and diseases.

physical activity. Any body movement that burns calories.

Pilates. A low-impact fitness technique designed specifically to strengthen the core muscles by developing pelvic stability and abdominal control. Helps improve flexibility, joint mobility and strength.

plantar fasciitis. An inflammation of the fibrous tissue that runs along the bottom of your foot.

plyometrics. A specialized form of strength training that capitalizes on the ability of muscles to generate more force after they've been stretched slightly. Plyometrics typically involves high-impact activities done at rapid speeds.

power. The ability to apply force during a short period of time. High-power activity involves rapid development of force. This is typically more stressful to joints, but is important for many sports in which speed is essential.

proprioceptive training. A specialized form of balance training that deliberately and incrementally challenges balance, similar to the way adding more weight challenges muscles in strength training. This training is used to improve overall balance, muscle coordination and sense of joint position. May involve one joint or a series of joints.

proprioceptors. Special receptors located in muscles, tendons, ligaments, bones and joints that send reports back to the brain about their movement, tension, pressure and position.

R

recovery time. The amount of time your body needs to rest and recuperate after exercise. Insufficient recovery time can lead to overtraining.

repetitions. The number of times a movement is repeated, such as lifting a weight or pushing against the resistance produced by a weight machine.

resistance bands and tubing. Elastic-like flat bands, tubes or cords that offer weight-like resistance when you pull on them. They come in different elasticities, offering differing levels of resistance. They simulate, but don't exactly replicate, the forces experienced when using free weights.

rheumatoid arthritis. A common form of arthritis primarily affecting the lining of the joints (synovium). The lining becomes chronically inflamed, causing stiffness, swelling and pain.

S

sedentary lifestyle. A lifestyle consisting of little or no exercise activity.

set. The number of times you perform a given number of repetitions of the same exercise.

side stitch. Muscle cramps that occur in the abdominal area.

skeletal muscles. Muscles under voluntary control. In general, exercises target skeletal muscles, which move your trunk, arms and legs to perform motion.

strength. A muscle's ability to generate force. *See also* muscular fitness.

strength endurance. The ability of muscles to maintain a force. *See also* muscular fitness.

strength training (resistance training). Training involving the use of free weights, body weight, resistance bands and tubing or weight machines to increase muscle strength and endurance. Strength training can also result in muscle growth.

synovial fluid. A joint lubricant produced by the body that allows joints to move freely and easily. In people with arthritis, synovial fluid is reduced in thickness.

synovium. Tissue that lines most joints in the musculoskeletal system. It generates synovial fluid and maintains an optimal chemical environment for joint functions.

T

tai chi. A form of ancient Chinese martial arts in which poses are performed slowly and gracefully, with smooth transitions.

tendons. Tough, cord-like tissues that connect muscles to bones.

transversus abdominis muscle. A corset-like muscle spanning across the deep abdomen. Its key function is to maintain spine stability and protect the spine during physical activity.

triathlon. A demanding athletic event that consists of swimming, cycling and running completed successively.

type I muscle fiber (slow twitch). Muscle fibers that produce energy and movement primarily through aerobic pathways. These fibers are supplied by energy that's generated at a relatively slow pace — thus the term *slow-twitch*. Type I fibers are used for endurance activities such as long-distance cycling and jogging.

type II muscle fiber (fast twitch). Muscle fibers that produce energy and movement primarily through anaerobic pathways. These fibers are supplied by rapidly available energy — thus the term *fast-twitch* — that's limited in quantity. Type II fibers contract more quickly and forcefully than do slow-twitch fibers, but can't maintain contractions for very long. These fibers are used for high-intensity, short-duration activities such as weightlifting, jumping and sprinting.

V

volume (of exercise). An indicator of the total amount of work done. May be expressed as the total number of miles run or pounds lifted, or the total number of repetitions (number of sets multiplied by number of repetitions per set) of a particular exercise.

voluntary muscles. These muscles are consciously controlled. Voluntary muscles are more sensitive to resistance-training techniques to improve strength, endurance and mass, than are involuntary muscles (smooth muscle and cardiac muscle), which can't be trained.

W

warm-up. Deliberate activity to prepare your body for exercise. Generally includes a short, low-intensity aerobic exercise, followed by any necessary stretching.

Y

yoga. A specialized fitness technique that combines deep breathing, movement and postures.

Index